Principles of Oral and Maxillofacial Surgery

Principles of Oral and Maxillofacial Surgery

Sixth Edition

Edited by

U J Moore

FDSRCS (Eng), PhD (Ncle)
Senior Lecturer in Oral and Maxillofacial Surgery
University of Newcastle-upon-Tyne

WILEY-BLACKWELL

A John Wiley & Sons, Ltd., Publication

This edition first published 2011
© 1965, 1981, 1984, 1991, 2001 by Blackwell Science Ltd
© 2011 by Blackwell Publishing Ltd

Blackwell Publishing was acquired by John Wiley & Sons in February 2007. Blackwell's publishing program has been merged with Wiley's global Scientific, Technical and Medical business to form Wiley-Blackwell.

Registered office: John Wiley & Sons Ltd, The Atrium, Southern Gate, Chichester, West Sussex, PO19 8SQ, UK

Editorial offices: 9600 Garsington Road, Oxford OX4 2DQ, UK
The Atrium, Southern Gate, Chichester, West Sussex PO19 8SQ, UK
2121 State Avenue, Ames, Iowa 50014-8300, USA

For details of our global editorial offices, for customer services and for information about how to apply for permission to reuse the copyright material in this book please see our website at www.wiley.com/wiley-blackwell.

Library of Congress Cataloging-in-Publication Data

Principles of oral and maxillofacial surgery / edited by U.J. Moore. – 6th ed.
        p. ; cm.
    Includes bibliographical references and index.
    ISBN 978-1-4051-9998-8 (pbk. : alk. paper) 1. Mouth–Surgery. 2. Maxilla–Surgery. 3. Face–Surgery. I. Moore, U. J. (Undrell J.)
    [DNLM: 1. Stomatognathic System–surgery. 2. Oral Surgical Procedures–methods.
3. Stomatognathic Diseases–surgery. WU 600]
    RK529.P752 2011
    617.5'22–dc22

                                                                    2010041320

A catalogue record for this book is available from the British Library.

This book is published in the following electronic formats: epdf 9781444393163; ePub 9781444393170

Set in 10/12.5 pt Times by Toppan Best-set Premedia Limited

1 2011

Contents

Preface to the Sixth Edition

Oral and maxillofacial surgery continues to develop, with new technologies being embraced. These developments have been incorporated into this new edition for the new generations of students; however, full attention is still paid to the fundamental basis of patient assessment and diagnosis, which form the cornerstone of any surgical specialty. Developing the decision-making process for the learner is one of the more difficult aspects of teaching and learning. We hope that this book still helps in this process.

Explanation of principles has remained the priority and this is still intended as an undergraduate and early postgraduate text.

Acknowledgements

This textbook had its inception in the early days of the specialty and much has changed within the discipline and the book since then. It is important to continue to acknowledge those who created the environment for these changes and influenced the contributions to this new edition.

I am grateful to Wiley-Blackwell, who have strongly supported the concept of developing a new edition. The process has been much facilitated by their steady yet insistent style of management and I can honestly say it has been a pleasure. It is invigorating to be part of something that feels very positive and my fellow contributors have been equally positive about the process. I would like to thank them for their prompt and relaxed style of authorship.

I am grateful also for any illustrations that have been permitted to be included, as they are essential to the understanding of the text.

Foreword to the First Edition

There is an increasing need for trained oral surgeons in the world today. An operative field that was a no-man's-land partly controlled by the general surgeon, partly controlled by the dental surgeon, has now come to be the field of a specialised branch of dentistry.

In the past we have had to use books written and published in America, and, fine though these books are, it is refreshing to find a book produced by a British oral surgeon, because in the world today, British oral surgery has undoubtedly the highest general level of training and achievement in the oral surgical field.

Mr J. R. Moore has had considerable practical experience as an oral surgeon in a consultative capacity before devoting his talents to teaching, and he has produced a book of great practical use both to the student or trainee learning oral surgery and also a book of great interest to the established specialist.

I deplore the fragmentation of the dental profession by dividing it into so many specialities, but in the field of oral surgery there are procedures which the dental surgeon would not wish to carry out. Therefore a knowledge of the difficulties and hazards of an oral surgical procedure is essential for the general dental surgeon, who should include this book in his library.

It is with great pleasure that I commend this work of Mr J. R. Moore of University College Hospital to the profession.

T G Ward

List of Contributors

Jonathan G Cowpe
BDS, FDSRCSEd, PhD, FDSRCSEng, FCDS (HK), FFGDP (UK), FDSRCPSGlas, FHEA
Director, Postgraduate Dental Education for Wales, School of Postgraduate Medical and Dental Education, Wales, Cardiff University and Professor/ Consultant in Oral Surgery, School of Dentistry, Cardiff University

Justin Durham
BDS, PhD, MFDS, RCS (Ed), FHEA
NIHR Academic Clinical Lecturer in Oral Surgery, School of Dental Sciences, Newcastle

Mark Greenwood
MDS, PhD, MB ChB, FDS, FRCS, FRCS (OMFS), FHEA
Consultant Oral and Maxillofacial Surgeon and Honorary Professor of Medical Education in Dentistry, Newcastle Hospitals NHS Foundation Trust and Newcastle University

John G Meechan
BSc, BDS, PhD, FDSRCS(Edin), FDSRCPS(Glas)
Senior Lecturer and Honorary Consultant in Oral Surgery, School of Dental Sciences, Newcastle

Francis Nohl
MB BS, BDS, MSc, MRD, FDS, RCS, DDS
Consultant and Honorary Senior Clinical Lecturer in Restorative Dentistry, Newcastle Dental Hospital and School

Keith R Postlethwaite
FRCS, FDSRCS, MB ChB, BDS
Consultant Oral and Maxillofacial Surgeon, Newcastle upon Tyne Hospitals NHS Trust

Peter J Thomson
BDS, MBBS, MSc, PhD, FDSRCS, FFDRCSI, FRCS(Ed)
Professor of Oral and Maxillofacial Surgery, Newcastle University

Chapter 1
The New Patient

- History
- Principles of examination
- Systematic procedure for examination of the oro-facial tissues
- Special investigation
- Diagnosis
- Treatment planning

It is difficult to overstress the importance of a good history and thorough clinical examination for every patient. It is on this that the diagnosis is made and the treatment plan based. A full, clearly written record of the original consultation is essential to assess progress following treatment. This is particularly true if a colleague should be called to see the patient in the practitioner's absence. The medico-legal importance of accurate records cannot be overemphasised.

In hospital and specialist practice this procedure can seldom be relaxed, but the student and the busy practitioner may find it irksome to maintain a high standard when faced with a series of apparently straightforward dental conditions. Nevertheless, sufficient time must be allowed for an unhurried consultation at the first visit. This will help to avoid errors of omission, and may contribute much to the success of treatment and to the interest of the practitioner. With experience, only important facts need be noted, the dental surgeon considering and setting aside the irrelevant points. This technique can be used with safety only after a long apprenticeship during which many histories and examinations have been methodically completed and all the information recorded. In this chapter a system for interviewing and examining patients, and recording findings, is briefly suggested.

History

At the first meeting it is important for the clinician to establish a rapport with the patient and to assess attitudes to the clinical situation. Behavioural issues

Principles of Oral and Maxillofacial Surgery, 6th Edition. Edited by U. J. Moore
© 2011 Blackwell Publishing Ltd

must be addressed, attempting to put the patient at ease in what is for many a confrontational situation. The interview must be planned to facilitate the process, seating the patient comfortably, adjusting the chair as required to show care, as well as addressing them by the correct name and title. Even at this stage it should be possible to determine whether the patient is anxious or relaxed. The general details of age, sex, marital status, occupation and contact details, together with the names of their general medical and dental practitioner, should be available in the notes but can be checked. The history is then recorded under the headings shown in italics.

The patient will seldom tell their story well. Some will be verbose, others reticent, while the sequence is usually in inverse chronological order with the most recent events first. The art of the good history lies in avoiding leading questions, in eliciting all the essentials, in censoring verbosity and in arranging the facts in their true order, so that the written record is short and logical. Allowing the patient initially to give the history and subsequently writing notes in chronological order while rechecking and summarising the facts verbally, helps the clinician obtain a concise and accurate account of the patient's symptoms.

Patient referred by

The name and professional status of the person referring is noted. This facilitates a reply to the referral in the form of a letter.

Complains of (CO)

The patient's chief complaint told *in their own words*. Opinions, professional and otherwise, repeated in an effort to help must be gently set aside and the patient encouraged to describe the symptoms they want cured, and not their views on the diagnosis.

History of present complaint (HPC)

This is an account *in chronological order* of the presenting complaint. When and how it first started, the suspected cause, any exacerbating factors and the character of the local lesion, such as pain, swelling and discharge. This includes remissions and the effects of any treatment received. General symptoms such as fever, malaise and nausea are also noted.

Previous dental history (PDH)

This records how regularly the patient attends for dental care and the importance they attach to their teeth. Any past experience of oral surgery is included, especially where difficulty occurred in the administration of anaesthetics, the extraction of teeth and the control of bleeding.

Medical history (MH)

A summary in chronological order of the patient's past illnesses. Details of prolonged illness or those requiring hospital admission are recorded. Current medication, which can give insight into the severity of any underlying conditions, and allergies of any kind, particularly drugs that might be prescribed and latex, must be noted. The more important medical conditions are discussed in Chapter 3.

The family history (FH)

Occasionally this is of importance in oral surgery. Hereditary diseases such as the haemophilias and hypodontia together with autoimmune disease may be relevant in management of the patient.

The social history (SH)

This includes a brief comment on the patient's occupation and social habits, such as exercise, smoking and drinking. The home circumstances are important when surgery is to be performed – that is, whether the patient has far to travel, lives alone or has someone to look after them. These factors may influence the decision to treat as an in- or outpatient.

Principles of examination

The basic principles of examination are the same in all fields of healthcare. It should be made according to a definite system, which in time becomes a ritual. In this way errors of omission are avoided.

From the moment the patient enters the surgery they should be carefully observed for signs of physical or of psychological disease which may show in the gait, the carriage, the general manner, or the relationship between parent and child. Too little time is often spent on visual inspection, both intra- and extraorally. Eyes first, then hands, should be the rule, not both together.

In palpation, all movements are purposeful and logical, and the touch firm but gentle. The tips of the fingers are used first to locate anatomical landmarks and then to determine the characteristics of the pathological condition. The patient's co-operation is sought so that areas of tenderness may be recognised and the minimum discomfort caused. Wherever possible the normal side is examined simultaneously. Only by such comparison can minor degrees of asymmetry be detected. Swellings situated in the floor of the mouth or in the cheek are felt bimanually with one hand placed inside, and one outside, the mouth. Both positive and negative findings are written down as later one may wish to check that at the first visit no abnormality was found in certain structures.

Systematic procedure for examination of the oro-facial tissues

Extraoral examination

This commences with a general inspection and palpation of the face, including the mandible, maxillary and malar bones, noting the presence of any abnormality, such as asymmetry or paralysis of the facial muscles. The eyes, their movements and pupil reactions are observed together with any difficulty in breathing.

The temporomandibular joints

(See also Chapter 17)

With the surgeon standing behind the patient, the site of the condyles are identified by palpation while the patient opens and closes their mouth. The joints are examined for tenderness and clicking or crepitus on opening and closing. The range of opening and left and right lateral excursion are checked and abnormalities noted.

The muscles of mastication

The muscles of mastication are palpated for tenderness. From extraoral, principally this means masseter and temporalis muscles, although medial pterygoid insertion can be palpated at the lower border.

The maxillary sinuses

In disease these may give rise to swellings, redness and tenderness over the cheek and canine fossa, nasal discharge and fistulae into the mouth, often through a tooth socket.

The lymph nodes

The operator stands behind the patient, who flexes their head forward to relax the neck muscles. Enlarged submental and submandibular nodes can be felt with the fingertips by placing these below the lower border of the mandible and rolling the nodes outwards. The upper deep cervical group can be found by identifying the anterior border of the sternocleidomastoid muscles at the mastoid process and rolling the skin and subcutaneous tissues between fingers and thumb. Working down this muscle to the clavicle and then ascending the neck to palpate the trachea and hyoid regions, the nodes may be felt against other structures such as muscles and underlying bones. With practice, tenderness, consistency and degrees of mobility will be recognised.

The lips

These are inspected for lesions such as fissuring at the angles of the mouth, or ulceration.

The cranial nerves

In some circumstances examination of all the cranial nerves is undertaken as part of the general examination. In particular this will be when neurological defects are noted and the possibility of intracranial lesions is suspected. The orofacial region encompasses the activity of the majority of the cranial nerves. and a degree of familiarity with their action and testing is to be encouraged (Table 1.1). Facial trauma is often implicated in damage of the cranial nerves

Table 1.1 Cranial nerves. The cranial nerves are listed with their area of activity in which testing must take place. The principal actions are indicated; S = sensory, M = motor (bold indicates main action of nerve, lower case indicates lesser action of nerve)

Number	Name	Action	Function
1	Olfactory	**S**	Smell
2	Optic	**S**	Sight
3	Oculomotor	**M**	Extrinsic muscles of eye
4	Trochlear	**M**	Superior oblique muscle
5	Trigeminal	**S** + m	Sensory to face, mouth, teeth; motor to muscles of mastication
6	Abducent	**M**	Lateral rectus muscle
7	Facial	**M** + s	Motor to face; taste
8	Vestibular-cochlear	**S**	Hearing
9	Glossopharyngeal	S + **M**	Sensation to posterior tongue; motor for swallowing
10	Vagus	**M** + **S**	Motor to pharynx, larynx; sensory to viscera; autonomic to gastrointestinal tract
11	Accessory	**M**	Trapezius, sternocleidomastoid
12	Hypoglossal	**M**	Muscles of tongue

either intracranially or more peripherally, and even the most superficial dental examination will test branches of the 5th, 7th and 12th cranial nerve.

Intraoral examination

Mirror examination

An initial mirror examination of all the structures visible in the mouth, both soft tissues and hard, should be undertaken first to give a clear survey of the general state of the mouth.

The mucous membranes

The cheeks, lips, palate and floor of the mouth are examined for colour, texture and presence of swelling or ulceration. Comparison of both sides by palpation is essential to discover any abnormality.

The tongue

Movements, both intrinsic and extrinsic, are tested, as limitation is an important clinical sign in inflammation and early neoplasia. The dorsum is best seen by protruding the tongue over dental gauze with which it can be grasped, drawn forward and, with the aid of a mouth mirror, examined over its length for fissures, ulcers, etc.

The tonsils

These are seen by depressing the tongue with a spatula and asking the patient to say 'Ah'.

The pharynx

Again the tongue is depressed, the patient asked to say 'Ah'. In good light, a small, warm mirror is passed over the dorsum of the tongue, past the uvula, and rotated to show the naso- and oropharynx. This can be demanding both for the surgeon and the patient, particularly those with a pronounced gag reflex.

The salivary glands

The examination of these is described in Chapter 16.

The periodontal tissues

The colour and texture of the gingivae are noted, and the standard of oral hygiene classified, including charting the presence of plaque and calculus. Recession, pocketing and hyperplasia of the gums are measured, and the mobility of the teeth assessed.

The teeth

These are charted for caries and fillings with a mirror and probe. Loose teeth, crowns or fillings are noted.

Edentulous ridges

These are examined for the form of the ridge, retained roots and soft tissue or bony abnormalities. Dentures worn should be inspected *in situ* before being removed to examine the underlying tissues

The occlusion

This is best analysed by taking study models and mounting them on an anatomical articulator and is usual only for assessment of orthognathic cases. However, the occlusal function of natural teeth, bridges and dentures should be assessed at the same time as the teeth are charted.

Presenting lesion

This is the examination of the lesion for which the patient has sought treatment. It may have been included in the general examination mentioned above, but frequently there is a swelling, ulcer, fistula or other disease that requires special attention, the details of which are best recorded under one heading easily referred to throughout treatment.

It is important in examining such pathological entities to determine their site, size, shape, colour, the character of their margins and whether they are single

or multiple. Tenderness, discharge and lymphatic involvement are also important. Swellings should be palpated to determine whether they are mobile or
fixed to the skin or to the underlying tissues. They may be either fluctuant or
solid. Solid swellings may be very hard (like bone) or firm (like contracted
muscle), soft (like relaxed muscle) or very soft (like fat). Induration is a firmness
particularly associated with neoplastic lesions. Where a collection of fluid is
suspected, fluctuation is elicited by placing two fingers of one hand on each side
of the swelling and pressing centrally with a finger of the other hand. Where
the lesion is fluid a thrill will be felt. This must be elicited in two directions at
right angles, as muscle fluctuates in the longitudinal but not the transverse plane.
All pulsatile swellings must be checked to establish whether the pulsation is
true or transmitted from an underlying artery.

Special investigation

The history taken and the examination of the patient having been completed,
a differential or provisional diagnosis should be made. This should attempt to
establish the disease process and relate it to the tissue involved. It is always
useful to consider the main pathological categories (Table 1.2), rejecting those
that do not fit the presenting situation. Similarly, the tissues in the area from
which the lesion could arise should be identified. In this way a sensible argument
may be sustained to support a definitive or differential diagnosis. Special investigations may be necessary to differentiate between these or to confirm a clinical
finding. These are not indicated for every patient; indeed, their cost and the
delay involved in completing them make it necessary to limit their use. Such
investigations are an aid to diagnosis and may also be required for treatment
planning. It is convenient to divide the more usual procedures into the four
main categories shown in Box 1.1.

   The oral surgeon must be quite clear about how the necessary specimens are
collected and, even more important, understand the clinical significance of the
results. These have been dealt with extensively in other works and the methods
of collection of certain specimens are described later in this text in the appropriate chapters.

Diagnosis

When the special investigations have been completed the surgeon should be
able to make a final diagnosis and it is important that this be clearly stated in
the notes. Diagnosis is not a matter of intuition but is a 'computer' exercise in
which all the information is sorted and analysed. Sometimes it is impossible to
reach a decision because of lack of information or knowledge, in which case the

Table 1.2 The surgical sieve. The consideration of possible pathological processes and the tissues involved may be considered as a 'surgical sieve' into one of the holes of which the diagnosis may fit

Pathological categories	Tissue involved									
	Epithelium	Connective tissue	Fat	Muscle	Bone	Blood vessels	Lymphatics	Nerves	Dental tissues	Salivary gland
Hereditary										
Developmental										
Traumatic										
Inflammatory (acute)										
(chronic)										
Cystic										
Neoplastic (benign)										
Neoplastic (malignant)										
Degenerative										
Medical										
Endocrine										

surgeon will need to consult textbooks or papers and may need to seek the opinion of a colleague.

Treatment planning

Only when the diagnosis is established can a satisfactory treatment plan be made. This should be divided into preoperative, operative and postoperative care, each of which should be planned in a logical sequence, constantly bearing in mind that the ultimate aim is to cure the patient with the least risk and minimal inconvenience.

Box 1.1   Special investigations commonly used in oral surgery

Local dental investigations

A Performed in the surgery
   (1) Percussion of teeth for apical tenderness
   (2) Vitality tests on teeth
        (a) Thermal
        (b) Electrical
   (3) Radiography
   (4) Diagnostic injections of local anaesthetic solutions in facial pain
   (5) Study models for studying the occlusion
   (6) Photography as a comparative record

B Requiring special facilities
   (1) Bacteriological investigations, including sensitivity tests
   (2) Aspiration of cystic cavities
   (3) Biopsy of tissue

General investigations

A Performed in the surgery
   (1) Temperature of body
   (2) Pulse rate
   (3) Blood pressure
   (4) Respiration rate
   (5) Cranial nerve testing (see Table 1.1)

B Requiring special facilities
   (1) Urinalysis
        Physical examination for colour, specific gravity
        Chemical tests for sugar, acetone, albumen, chlorides, blood
        Microscopic examination for cells, bacteria, blood
        Bacteriological culture
   (2) Blood investigations
        Haemoglobin estimation
        Red cell, white cell and platelet count
        C-reactive protein (CRP)
        Bleeding and clotting mechanisms
        Grouping and cross-matching for transfusion
        Blood chemistry and electrolytes – calcium, inorganic phosphorus, alkaline phosphatase,
          serum potassium, chloride, albumen, globulin, urea, glucose (see appendix)
        Serology
   (3) Radiographs, CT, MRI scans
   (4) Electrocardiograph
   (5) Tests for allergy

Further reading

Douglas G, Nicol F, Robertson C (eds) (2009) *Macleod's Clinical Examination*, 12th edn. Churchill Livingstone, Elsevier.

Meechan JG (2006) *Minor Oral Surgery in Dental Practice*. Quintessence, London.

Thomas J, Monaghan T (2007) *Oxford Handbook of Clinical Examination and Practical Skills*. Oxford University Press, Oxford.

Chapter 2
General Patient Management

- Surgical patients
- Inpatient care
- Intensive care
- Outpatient care
- Follow-up

Surgical patients

The management of surgical patients can be considered under three headings: preoperative, operative and postoperative. These should form a programme planned to meet the patient's therapeutic need. This chapter is concerned with the pre- and postoperative care, excluding the medically compromised patients, who are the subject of Chapter 3.

Once the treatment has been planned it must be decided whether the patient requires admission to hospital or can be treated on a day-case basis or as an outpatient. Admission as an inpatient ensures more comprehensive care, which can be extended both pre- and postoperatively until the patient is both fit for the procedure and able to be discharged home. Much of the responsibility for the provision of care is entrusted to the nursing staff. Optimal conditions can be maintained with administration of intravenous drugs and appropriate nutrition catering for the particular patient needs. This provides an environment that can seldom be achieved at home, although early discharge is to be encouraged to increase efficient bed use. With this in mind, day-stay facilities where the patient is admitted in the morning to return home postoperatively, some hours after recovery, are increasingly popular. The advantage of this is postoperative supervision by nursing staff during the period when complications related to surgery or anaesthesia may occur, while allowing the patient to return home as soon as possible. However, the home circumstances must allow the patient to be adequately looked after and the patient must be within reasonable distance of help postoperatively should unexpected complications occur. In oral surgery, the majority of outpatients are treated using local anaesthesia, sometimes in conjunction with sedation techniques. Inpatients usually have endotracheal

Principles of Oral and Maxillofacial Surgery, 6th Edition. Edited by U. J. Moore
© 2011 Blackwell Publishing Ltd

general anaesthesia of a longer duration than should be administered on a day-stay basis.

The indications for admitting patients to hospital are surgical, medical and social.

Surgical

The length of surgery – a day case should ideally be around 30 minutes in duration, anything longer than this may require overnight admission, although improvements in general anaesthetic agents have allowed more rapid recovery. If there is a risk of complications such as haemorrhage or fracture of the jaw, or if major surgery is being undertaken with consequent increased morbidity, the need for admission increases.

Medical

The patient requires collateral management by a physician (e.g. management of diabetes), needs special therapy or skilled nursing care.

Social

The patient's home conditions are poor, they are living alone, live far away or are anxious to be treated as an inpatient.

Inpatient care demands a wider application of the general principles that underlie the management of surgical patients. It is therefore considered first, though no important difference is implied between the needs of in- and outpatients.

Inpatient care

The date of admission to hospital can be arranged at the time of consultation and waiting lists thereby avoided. Where a waiting list is used it is important to give adequate warning that a bed is available and also to recognise certain surgical priorities, such as the following.

Emergency

Conditions requiring instant admission, such as acute infections or traumatic injuries.

Urgent

Conditions that can progress to emergencies if treatment is long delayed, for example subacute infections and neoplasms.

Routine

Those of no urgency who may take their turn in chronological order.

A patient who is fit and only requires routine surgery is normally admitted the day before the operation, although pre-admission clinics (PAC) can usefully highlight management issues that can be addressed prior to the actual admission date. Problems related to the administration of a general anaesthetic should be anticipated and an anaesthetic opinion sought (see below). Where special preparation is needed, such as blood investigation, or consultation with other specialists, the time of admission must be calculated to allow for these procedures to take place first.

The patient should be visited by the surgical team within a few hours of admission and findings made at the outpatient examination reviewed and revised if necessary. The pulse, temperature and blood pressure are recorded. Blood tests may be required and should be sent off in time to allow analysis before surgery. The mouth must be carefully examined and the area of surgery reassessed. If teeth are to be removed, any change to the dentition should be noted to enable those beyond conservation to be extracted under the same anaesthetic. Insecure dressings should be replaced to prevent their being dislodged into a socket or wound. Before a general anaesthetic, loose or crowned teeth are noted and the anaesthetist warned. Where extensive haemorrhage is anticipated blood is taken for grouping and cross-matching, and the necessary amount for replacement is ordered. Where grouping is done only as a precautionary measure the serum may be kept for cross-matching if required, but no blood ordered. The nature of the operation and likely complications should be explained to the patient and informed consent obtained in writing for both the anaesthetic and the operation.

It is the role of the surgeon not only to carry out the local treatment but also to supervise the day-to-day care.

Relations with the nursing staff

The surgeon must understand the routine of the wards and the way the patients are nursed. Though it is essential to make daily visits to assess progress and give treatment, these must be arranged to avoid awkward times when the wards are normally closed. The nursing staff spend much time with the patient and have opportunities to hear complaints and observe minor changes that the surgeon may overlook. Their role in motivating the patient during the postoperative period should not be underestimated and their comments can therefore be of great help. They are an essential member of the ward round and should be consulted about progress daily.

Informed consent

Before any procedure is undertaken the patient's informed consent must be obtained. The proposed operation or investigation should be explained in simple language which can be understood by the lay person. The more common complications must be mentioned without causing undue distress. Where a general anaesthetic or sedation is proposed the consent should be in writing. For those under 16 years of age, it must be given by their parent or guardian.

Major points on informed consent:

- It is required for any surgical procedure on children under 16.
- It is required for all patients undergoing general anaesthesia or sedation.
- It requires careful explanation by staff who fully understand the procedure.
- Full warnings of recognised complications must be noted.
- Nervous patients may have little recall of information given.

Diet

A knowledge of the principles of nutrition is essential to understand the dietetic problems of the patient, and the following summary is presented with this in mind. The diet can be broadly divided into its fluid and solid content.

Fluid intake and output

The water intake is approximately the sum of the weight, expressed in grammes, of fluid and of solid food ingested, because solid food when digested and metabolised yields three-fifths its own weight as water. The water intake should be about 2500 ml daily, half of which is taken as drinks.

Water is excreted as exhaled air (400 ml), evaporation including sweat (500–1000 ml), urine (1200 ml) and faeces (200 ml). Water lost by exhalation and evaporation is used for heat regulation and the quantity lost varies widely according to the circumstances. Insufficient fluid intake shows as a decrease in urine output. The absolute daily minimum of urine is the 600 ml required to carry the 50 g of urinary solids excreted daily; below this volume toxic metabolites are returned to the blood. At this concentration the specific gravity is raised from 1.015 to 1.030. All patients who have difficulty in feeding because of acute trismus or mouth injuries should have a fluid balance chart. This shows on the credit side all fluid taken in 24 hours, including metabolic water, and on the debit side the urine passed plus an estimate for water lost by evaporation, which may be very high in febrile states. For all practical purposes the urine output is a measure of the water balance.

In the adult, the daily output should be at least 1000–1500 ml. This simple but accurate criterion is satisfactory unless cardiovascular or renal disease is present, when overenthusiastic pressing of fluids beyond the power of the kidney to excrete may result in fluid overloading and excessive stress on the heart. Fluids may be administered by several routes, of which only the oral and intravenous are much used. The safest, most convenient and effective way of giving fluids is by mouth if not contraindicated, and should be preferred to all others. Up to three litres of water, flavoured attractively, can be taken each day. Where the intraoral route cannot be used, fluids may be given intravenously.

Solid food

A balanced diet includes carbohydrates, fats, proteins, vitamins and mineral salts.

Fats, the highest calorie provider, are not easily digested by the sick and their intake may have to be markedly reduced. They are, however, important as a vehicle for the fat-soluble vitamins A, D, E and K. In starvation, the body's fat reserves may be mobilised, but a certain minimum daily quantity of carbohydrate is needed for their physiological use and to prevent ketosis. Only 100 g of glycogen is stored in the liver, which is less than a one-day requirement. Protein is essential for the repair of tissues and for maintaining the circulation. A deficiency may occur after extensive haemorrhage or burns and may increase the susceptibility to shock, impede the healing of wounds, impair circulatory efficiency and lower resistance to infection. Patients in bed undergo protein wastage, which is best prevented by a high carbohydrate and protein diet. Vitamins and mineral salts are essential and are supplied therapeutically, if deficient.

Food must be attractively prepared, and even if sieved or in fluid form it should not lose its identity. Each meal should bear some resemblance to its usual form; most foods can easily be liquidised and baby foods, though expensive, are useful in this respect.

Special dietary requirements must be discussed with the dietitian and the ward sister. The total calories, the amount of water, protein and vitamins, together with proprietary preparations and the number and the kind of supplementary feeds, must be specified. The rule 'a little and often' will help to avoid indigestion and ensure an adequate intake, particularly when the jaws are wired together. Supplementary feeds should be considered so that the daily routine includes early morning tea, breakfast, 'elevenses', lunch, tea, dinner, supper and nightcap.

Certain patients may have to be fed through a nasogastric (Ryle's) tube. This is a small-bore plastic tube passed through the nose so that about 5 cm lies in the stomach. The normal length of tube from the nose is 50 cm; any excess interferes with gastric peristalsis and may cause anorexia and nausea. Its presence in the stomach is confirmed by radiographs and by aspirating gastric contents up the tube before feeding is started. Feeding may be continued in this way indefinitely if the tube is brought out, cleaned and replaced through the other nostril every two or three days. Feed is pumped from a calibrated dispenser at a controlled rate to ensure that it is tolerated. This is initiated at 5 ml/hour and gradually increased to full strength over 24 to 48 hours. Before disconnecting the syringe the nasogastric tube must be clamped off. All patients on special diets should be weighed weekly as a check on their progress. For those patients unable to swallow, particularly those undergoing surgery for neoplasia, percutaneous endoscopic gastrostomy (PEG) feeding may be established to allow nutritional input to be controlled over the longer term.

Preoperative diet

Patients for operation under local anaesthesia may take their normal meals. If the patient has missed a meal they should be given a glucose drink before the local anaesthetic is administered. Where a general anaesthetic is to be administered, a light meal, chiefly of protein and carbohydrate, is advised the night before. On the day of operation those on the morning list are starved, but those for the afternoon list may be given a small breakfast of tea and toast. No food must be taken for 4 hours nor clear fluids for 2 hours before operation. The patient's normal medication should be maintained after consultation with the anaesthetist.

Postoperative diet

Each patient must be considered individually, but feeding should be started as soon as possible to avoid nausea. Many can manage the ordinary food provided, but others, because of tenderness or trismus, require specially prepared food. Where necessary, the patient should receive dietary advice before discharge home.

Excretion

Micturition

This reflex act occurs when the pressure in the bladder rises sufficiently to cause the sphincter to relax and the detrusor muscle to contract. The ability to delay micturition is the inhibition of the normal reflex response to distension. In patients with head injuries, the apparently insane desire to get out of bed is often for the purpose of emptying the bladder or bowel, as the wish to go to the right place is strongly imbued and may persist despite gross craniocerebral disturbance. Retention can be organic, as in men suffering from prostatic enlargement, or a functional disorder. It may occur after general anaesthesia but should cause no undue anxiety up to 24 hours, unless the bladder becomes distended or symptoms of overflow occur. Micturition can be encouraged by getting the patient up, but if this fails catheterisation may be necessary. Any urinary catheter, placed perioperatively for patients undergoing procedures of more than 4 hours' duration, should be removed as soon as the patient is mobilised in order to avoid an ascending urinary infection.

Sweat

Sweat contains 0.5% of solids, chiefly sodium chloride. In fever or in hot weather sweating may be greatly increased and as much as 10 g of sodium chloride can be lost in an hour, and must be replaced in the diet.

Defecation

The bowels should be opened regularly and the fact noted, but too much attention can be paid to irregularity. In constipation one must first decide whether the cause is organic or functional. Organic irregularity is due to partial obstruction of the lumen, often by a tumour. Functional irregularity may be due to defective movements of the colonic musculature or a deficiency in the bulk of faeces due to feeding with fluid diets. It may arise in hospital as a result of a sudden change in routine and of diet.

It is treated either by feeding fruit, vegetables and wholemeal cereals or by giving laxatives. It is stressed that wherever there is doubt as to the cause a general surgeon's opinion should be sought.

Sleep

Sleep is distinguished from other unconscious states by the ease with which the sleeper may be roused. Disturbed sleep may be due to pain, external stimuli, worry or change of habit. It is important to recognise the cause before considering treatment. Where the cause is pain, hypnotics must not be given until its source has been investigated, removed if possible, or analgesics prescribed. If these are effective the patient should sleep naturally. External stimuli should be reduced by keeping the wards dark at night, and by providing side wards for night admissions and for noisy or restless patients. Worry or change of habit, particularly dozing by day, can lead to insomnia in the convalescent or fit adult. Hypnotic drugs may be prescribed, but only if really necessary, because they are habit forming.

Hygiene

General and oral hygiene is the responsibility of the ward sister, but mouth hygiene is supervised by the surgical team. On admission the patient should have their oral hygiene assessed and appropriate instructions given. This might include rinsing the mouth preoperatively with 0.2% aqueous chlorhexidine.

In the badly injured, the elderly and those recently operated on, a modified technique is necessary either to avoid causing pain or because they need assistance. No cleansing of the mouth is advised for the first 24 hours after operation and may indeed do harm by starting haemorrhage. Thereafter, mucous membranes and teeth may be cleansed with a soft toothbrush or foam pads attached to orange sticks, and the mouth irrigated with 0.2% aqueous chlorhexidine after every meal. Intraoral sutures also require care as they tend to trap food over the wound. Clinging debris should be removed by swabbing with cotton wool each day. A hypertonic saline mouth bath, as hot as the individual can bear without scalding, may be used and allowed to lie over the wound until cool, but unlike the mouthwashes used preoperatively, no violent flushing is advised. Mouth brushing is started on normal teeth and gingivae as soon as possible and the patient encouraged at an early stage to carry out their own oral hygiene. This not only occupies their time usefully, but the techniques may be supervised before discharge, ensuring satisfactory home care.

Arch bars

Arch bars may be cleaned with a toothbrush and paste, and chlorhexidine mouthwash can be employed with obturators.

Where gutta-percha moulds are used to hold skin grafts in position, the mouth is cleansed using only the blandest mouthwashes. After the first 10 days (by which time the graft should have taken) a syringe may be introduced between the graft and the mould to clean the dead space gently but thoroughly.

Premedication and sedation

See Chapter 5.

Postoperative care

On arriving in the recovery room after an operation the patient is immediately put into bed and laid on their side with a pillow behind the shoulders in the position of sleep in such a way that drainage may take place from the mouth. The arms are kept folded over the chest. Under no circumstances should the arms be elevated above the head for fear of damage to the brachial plexus.

During the uneasy period before complete consciousness is regained, and especially where the jaws are wired together, a trained recovery nurse must sit with the patient to watch the airway, suck out the mouth and oropharynx, and to ensure that no injury is suffered by pulling at sutures or splints. Cot sides should be raised to avoid falling out of bed. A careful watch for vomiting and haemorrhage is a priority, and the pulse, blood pressure, respirations and level of consciousness is recorded.

Postoperative medication

Analgesics should be given to reduce postoperative pain. Hypnotics should not be prescribed for semi-conscious patients where the jaws are wired together (see Chapter 5).

Postoperative complications

These can include fever, vomiting, conjunctivitis, sore throat, pharyngitis and pulmonary complications.

Fever

Raised temperature is a natural reaction to infection, but a slight fever is common for two to three days after an operation where a haematoma or necrotic material is present. A large haematoma may keep the temperature up for a week. After a general anaesthetic a chest complaint must be considered as a cause of fever and any sputum sent for culture. More rarely, a temporary upset of heat regulation does occur after an anaesthetic or a head injury.

The primary treatment must be that of the underlying cause, whether local or general. The symptomatic treatment includes confinement to bed, liberal administration of fluids and a high carbohydrate diet, which has been found to prevent the breakdown of body proteins. At temperatures of 39.4°C and above, the body may be sponged down with tepid water at 27°C, which cools the patient. The use of paracetamol is indicated and attention to adequate fluid intake is also important.

Vomiting

This does occur following operation, usually due to the anaesthetic or swallowed blood, though the nervous disposition of the patient is a factor. Persistent vomiting for more than 8 hours is part of a vicious circle characterised by an upset of the acid–base equilibrium, in which the alkali reserve is reduced with increased urinary acidity and ketonuria. The anaesthetist should be consulted about the treatment for this. However, it can often be avoided by energetic treatment earlier. This consists of giving milk or alkaline drinks with glucose, which should be sipped very slowly but frequently. An antiemetic may be prescribed (see Chapter 5).

Conjunctivitis

Conjunctivitis can be caused by anaesthetic vapours, blood, antiseptics or towels entering the eye, or by the eye being open and drying up during the operation. This can be prevented by keeping the eyes closed with eyepads, but should contamination occur the eye can be gently irrigated with normal saline. Chloramphenicol eye drops will afford relief.

Sore throat or pharyngitis

This is usually caused by trauma from the endotracheal tube, excoriation from a dry pack or desiccation. It may be treated with gargles (see Chapter 5).

Pulmonary complications

Routine postoperative breathing exercises will reduce the incidence of pulmonary complications, but it must be borne in mind that these may occur. They may range from a minor inflammation of the trachea or bronchi to pulmonary collapse or postoperative pneumonia. Where they are suspected, a chest radiograph should be taken and the anaesthetist immediately informed. General management will include the use of antibiotics, physiotherapy, humidified oxygen, sedatives and mucolytic drugs. Frequent hot drinks help to relieve spasm and loosen secretions.

Progress

Routine monitoring of inpatients should include:

● vital signs:
  – temperature, pulse, blood pressure

- fluid balance chart
- bloods:
  - full blood count, haemoglobin, electrolytes
- bowel habit
- dietary intake
- drug requirements:
  - analgesics, antibiotics, normal medications.

The patient should be visited daily by the surgeon, who should first ask how the patient feels and about the day-to-day care, diet and oral hygiene. This is followed by a careful examination of the operation site, a check of the temperature chart, drug sheet, etc., and questions to the nursing staff where necessary. The response to treatment is assessed and should be recorded in the notes, together with any changes to be made to the treatment. Before discharge the patient's final condition should be summarised. The importance of these records cannot be overstressed, as it is difficult to compare progress over a long period without them.

Discharge

When the patient is fit for discharge home the patient or the relatives must be informed of the regimen and treatment to be followed and when to attend for review. Sick notes, where appropriate, must be completed and adequate transport, if necessary, arranged both to the patient's home and for their return for review.

The patient's doctor and dentist should receive notification that the patient is being discharged, including an outline of the operative procedures and condition on discharge. In this way, if called in an emergency, they are informed of all that has gone before and are able to prescribe for any drugs or dressings required at home.

Intensive care

Not all patients will follow the above routine; some will be admitted shocked, unconscious or both. Some will require special management after operation and the condition of others may deteriorate while they are on the ward. The management of respiration may require intubation or tracheostomy and a ventilator. These critically ill patients are treated in an intensive care unit (ICU) with one-to-one nursing and moment-by-moment management of their condition until they are fit to be moved either to a general ward or, if they still require intensive nursing care, to a high dependency unit (HDU). Within oral and maxillofacial surgery this most often applies to the polytraumatised patient and those suffering overwhelming infection that continues to threaten the airway.

Such care is entirely within the realm of specialist anaesthetists (intensivists). Fluids and feeding for these patients is given intravenously. All prolonged intravenous infusion requires the most careful continual monitoring as it is all too easy to upset the delicately balanced homeostasis.

Intravenous fluids

The solution must be sterile and is contained in a bottle or bag into which a polythene tube is inserted. All air should be removed from the tube by running the fluid through it with the stop clamp open. A suitable vein, not too superficial or near a joint, is chosen and a tourniquet is placed above the selected point. An indwelling plastic cannula is inserted over a needle, which is then withdrawn and the giving set attached. The cannula is secured in place and the flow adjusted according to the patient's needs. Usually this is about 1 litre over 8 hours.

The fluids that may be given in this way are whole blood, plasma and saline, dextrose or fat solutions. The decision as to which fluid to use will depend on the clinical needs of the patient. Blood may be given as a replacement following loss from trauma or surgery, and saline or dextrose solutions during long operations and in the immediate recovery period. Where the use of intravenous fluids goes beyond the short term, monitoring is performed using a central venous pressure line and by taking blood samples and estimating blood sugar and electrolytes. Where feeding using fat solutions is necessary, urinary urea estimation and body weight will indicate the nitrogen to be replaced and the calories required.

Outpatient care

All the principles of management of inpatient care, particularly those relating to diet, hygiene and progress, are applicable, with modification, to outpatients. The salient points with regard to outpatients are summarised here.

Day cases

Where outpatients are having minor operations under endotracheal anaesthesia, they may be operated on during the morning but kept in a suitably equipped recovery room or ward under adequate professional and nursing supervision. As it is usual for these patients to stay on the premises all day and be discharged home in the evening, they are known as 'day cases', although otherwise their general care is the same as that of other outpatients. However, they must be adequately assessed and height/weight criteria may be applicable before they are accepted for outpatient anaesthesia. Suitable transport must be available and they will require rest and care on their return home. Careful enquiry should be made as to the patient's home circumstances to ensure that adequate support can be provided.

Finally, both the anaesthetist and the surgeon should be able and experienced in their fields so that the patient is not exposed to risk due to lack of skill or judgement.

Pre-admission clinics

Nurse-run pre-admission clinics (PAC) are often used to improve day-case services. The patient attends some weeks before surgery and the details of the patient's fitness to undergo surgery are confirmed. The consent is checked and the patient encouraged to ask questions about the procedure to allay fears. The date of the surgery is confirmed to minimise the chance of non-attendance.

Preoperative instructions for outpatients

The nature of the operation must be explained and the patient's permission obtained in writing for both general anaesthetic and surgery. Outpatients should be instructed to come accompanied and told whether or not it will be safe to take alcohol, drive a car or bicycle, or operate machinery (including cooking) after the operation. Instructions should be given about diet before a local anaesthetic – something light and easily digested. Where a general anaesthetic is to be administered, they are instructed to come accompanied, not to wear restrictive clothing and to fast from food or drink for at least 6 hours before the operation; in this respect children require particular supervision. Patients having sedation should be given similar instructions to those having a general anaesthetic. Of particular importance is the advice that the patient must not drive a motor vehicle or operate machinery until the following day. Before commencing surgery they are asked to remove their dentures, contact lenses and earrings, and to empty bowel and bladder.

Preoperative dental treatment

Preoperative prophylaxis and instruction in oral hygiene is given to those about to undergo a dental operation. Many patients fail to appreciate the importance of this measure. All doubtful teeth should be assessed and insecure dressings replaced so that those beyond conservation can be extracted under the same anaesthetic. Before a general anaesthetic very loose teeth should be noted and the anaesthetist warned.

Pre- and post-medication

This is discussed in Chapter 5.

Postoperative care

Before discharging the patient a reasonable time should be allowed for recovery. This applies equally to those treated under local or general anaesthesia, and particularly to day-case patients.

Adequate instructions should be given for home treatment. If possible these should be stated in the presence of a relative or written down, as the patient

---

Box 2.1   Specimen of postoperative instructions to patient

Your mouth will be numb for up to 3 hours after the operation – be careful not to damage your mouth by biting areas that you cannot feel.

To prevent bleeding:
AVOID mouthwashing for 24 hours
            hot drinks, hot food and alcohol
            exercise or effort

If bleeding occurs:
Apply pressure by biting on to a clean, rolled handkerchief
Rest sitting in an upright position
If bleeding is not controlled by these measures contact us by telephone by day on _____, by night on _____

If in pain:
Take two 500 mg paracetamol tablets or 400 mg ibuprofen as required **(DO NOT EXCEED SAFE DOSAGE)**
If pain is persistent or severe contact the dental surgery

After 24 hours:
Mix one teaspoonful of salt in a tumbler of hot water
Take a mouthful and tilt head so that the water lies over the extraction site
Hold water over area, spit it out and repeat until the tumbler is empty
Repeat this 3 to 4 times daily, especially after food

If for any reason you are worried about the healing of the operation site contact the surgery at the number above

Operation ....
Anaesthetic ....
Operator ....

---

may not be sufficiently alert after the surgical ordeal to remember details. They should include diet, oral hygiene, analgesics and the rest period required before return to work. The date and time of the next appointment must also be clearly stated, together with the action to be taken should a postoperative emergency, such as haemorrhage, arise (Box 2.1).

The operator *must be easily available* to the patient to deal with any surgical complications that may arise. Where a general anaesthetic has been given, the general medical practitioner should be informed.

Follow-up

It is the duty of the surgeon to assume responsibility for the patient's after-care until all possibility of postoperative complications is passed. The patient should be encouraged to return if their postoperative symptoms do not settle satisfactorily, and the surgeon should be prepared to see them at short notice. Long-term follow-up should be carried out personally in cases where the postoperative course is unpredictable, as through it much may be learned, which will benefit both the surgeon and their patients. Before final discharge, the surgeon should refer back through the notes and establish that not only have the operations been successful, but that the patient has been relieved of their original complaint and that any subsequent complications incurred during treatment have been cured.

Further reading

Barrett K (2010) *Ganong's Review of Medical Physiology*, 23rd edn. Lange Basic Science, McGraw Hill Medical.
Gwinnutt C (2008) *Lecture Notes in Clinical Anaesthesia*, 3rd edn. Wiley-Blackwell, Oxford.
Shaw IH, Kumar C, Dodds C (2010) *Oxford Textbook of Anaesthesia for Oral and Maxillofacial Surgery*. Oxford University Press, Oxford.

Consent

www.nhs.uk/conditions/Consent-to-treatment/Pages/Introduction.aspx
www.dh.gov.uk/prod_consum_dh/groups/dh_digitalassets/@dh/@en/documents/digitalasset/dh_075159.pdf
www.dh.gov.uk/prod_consum_dh/groups/dh_digitalassets/documents/digitalasset/dh_103653.pdf

Chapter 3
Problems Related to Certain
Systemic Conditions

- Physiological conditions
- Endocrine disorders
- Allergy
- Cardiovascular disorders
- Respiratory disorders
- Disorders of the blood
- Musculoskeletal disorders
- Systemic diseases of bone
- Epilepsy
- Psychiatric illness
- Liver disorders
- Renal disorders
- Conclusion

Patients referred for oral and maxillofacial surgical procedures may be suffering from systemic disorders or undergoing treatment with drugs. Either of these situations may complicate the operation, including the choice and administration of an anaesthetic, sedation or local anaesthesia. A full medical history is therefore essential and should be rechecked periodically if the patient attends for a prolonged period. With certain systemic disorders, liaison with the surgeon or physician treating these disorders is important. Advances in drug therapy occur rapidly and where a patient is taking medication with which the oral surgeon is not familiar, reference should be made to the current *British National Formulary* or a similar publication.

A medical history must cover certain areas to be complete. The overall scheme may vary between clinicians, but most follow a pattern similar to that described in Chapter 1. After taking the medical history a patient may be assigned to a category derived from the American Society of Anesthesiologists (ASA) Physical Status Classification System. The purpose of this system is to assess the degree of a patient's 'sickness' prior to sedation, an anaesthetic or before performing surgery. Describing a patient's preoperative physical status

Principles of Oral and Maxillofacial Surgery, 6th Edition. Edited by U. J. Moore
© 2011 Blackwell Publishing Ltd

Table 3.1   ASA Physical Status (PS) Classification System

ASA PS category	Preoperative health status	Comments, examples
ASA PS1	Normal healthy patient	No organic, physiologic or psychiatric disturbance; excludes the very young and very old; healthy with good exercise tolerance
ASA PS2	Patients with mild systemic disease	No functional limitations; has a well-controlled disease of one body system; controlled hypertension or diabetes without systemic effects, cigarette smoking without chronic obstructive pulmonary disease (COPD); mild obesity, pregnancy
ASA PS3	Patients with severe systemic disease	Some functional limitation; has a controlled disease of more than one body system or one major system; no immediate danger of death; controlled congestive heart failure (CHF), stable angina, old heart attack, poorly controlled hypertension, morbid obesity, chronic kidney disease, bronchospastic disease with intermittent symptoms
ASA PS4	Patients with severe systemic disease that is a constant threat to life	Has at least one severe disease that is poorly controlled or at end stage; possible risk of death; unstable angina, symptomatic COPD, symptomatic CHF, hepatorenal failure
ASA PS5	Moribund patients who are not expected to survive without the operation	Not expected to survive >24 hours without surgery; imminent risk of death; multiorgan failure, sepsis syndrome with haemodynamic instability, hypothermia, poorly controlled coagulopathy
ASA PS6	A declared brain-dead patient whose organs are being removed for donor purposes	

in this way is used for record keeping, for communicating between colleagues and to create a system that facilitates statistical analysis. It is not intended as a measure to predict operative risk. The classification system consists of six categories as shown in Table 3.1.

Physiological conditions

Pregnancy

It is best to try to avoid prescribing drugs during pregnancy. This is not always practical but in certain groups, particularly those with a history of spontaneous abortion, treatment should be delayed until after parturition, if possible.

Use of local anaesthetic with adrenaline is acceptable in pregnant patients. With general anaesthesia, one danger to the foetus is hypoxia, which must be prevented by adequate oxygenation. Patients should be treated in the left lateral position to avoid pressure from the gravid uterus on the inferior vena cava, which if not done could lead to the supine hypotension syndrome. Ideally general anaesthesia during pregnancy should be avoided, but if this is not possible, specialist anaesthetic services must be available.

The optimum time for operation is the second trimester, i.e. fourth, fifth and sixth months of pregnancy, as danger to the foetus is least at this time. In the second and third trimesters the foetus is growing but is still susceptible to the effects of infections and drugs.

A hypersensitive gag reflex may be present in some pregnant patients. Apart from the avoidance of drug prescriptions wherever possible during pregnancy, this is another reason why extensive oral surgery under local anaesthesia may best be postponed until after parturition.

Intravenous sedation must be avoided in the first trimester and the last month of the third trimester; ideally it is best avoided altogether during pregnancy. Nitrous oxide can interfere with vitamin B_{12} and folate metabolism and should not be used in the first trimester, although it does not appear to be teratogenic. The duration of exposure if used should be less than 30 minutes and 50% oxygen should be administered with avoidance of repeated exposures.

In general anaesthesia, there is an increased likelihood of vomiting during induction of anaesthesia in the third trimester. Another concern is the risk late in pregnancy of general anaesthesia inducing respiratory depression in the foetus. There is little evidence of teratogenic effects in humans of general anaesthetic agents.

All drugs should be considered as potentially being teratogenic and should therefore be avoided wherever possible, but particularly in the first trimester. It is important to check in the *British National Formulary* before any prescriptions are written in this group of patients.

Breast-feeding

Drugs taken by the mother while breast-feeding can be transferred to the breast milk in some cases and therefore the infant could be affected. The *British National Formulary* includes an appendix highlighting which drugs are implicated.

Endocrine disorders

Diabetes mellitus

Diabetes mellitus is a disease characterised by a rise in blood glucose levels and urinary excretion of glucose. Osmotically, increased amounts of water are also excreted (polyuria). Such patients have an increased susceptibility to infection.

It is the most common endocrine disorder likely to be encountered by the oral surgeon. The main subdivisions of diabetes mellitus are into type I and type II. Type I diabetes mellitus has an autoimmune origin whereas type II has a genetic background and these patients are usually overweight. Due to the so-called 'obesity epidemic', type II diabetes is becoming more common in younger people. Emotional stress or infection may increase the severity of the disease.

Type I diabetes mellitus is usually treated with insulin, type II diabetes mellitus is usually treated with dietary control with or without oral hypoglycaemic agents. In uncontrolled diabetes mellitus hyperglycaemia may occur, but this is of slow onset and the patient is so obviously ill that it is unlikely to present as an emergency in the dental surgery.

Hypoglycaemia

Hypoglycaemia on the other hand, can occur with alarming suddenness. Weakness, hunger, pallor, a rapid pulse, confusion/aggression and loss of consciousness are all signs. Treatment is to give sugar by mouth if conscious or 1 mg glucagon intramuscularly if not. Preparations such as GlucoGel® (formerly Hypostop Gel) have been developed for use as an oral preparation. It is important to observe the patient after treatment for hypoglycaemia to ensure that no relapse occurs.

Local anaesthesia

Where a diabetic patient is to have an operation under local anaesthesia, normal diet and insulin should be taken at the usual time and the patient treated first on the list. It is not necessary to use adrenaline-free local anaesthetic solutions, but the operation should not be unduly prolonged, nor must the patient miss meals or snacks.

General anaesthesia

Patients taking insulin who have a severe acute infection or need a general anaesthetic should be admitted to hospital. It is wise to obtain the advice of a diabetologist in such cases. When a general anaesthetic is to be given, the physician will advise according to the following broad principles. Patients taking long-acting insulin are changed to the soluble form and rebalanced. All but the most severe diabetic patients will then receive their normal insulin and carbohydrate till midnight on the day before operation. Next morning they should be first on the operating list. Blood glucose estimations are carried out and an infusion of glucose, potassium and insulin (GKI) is usually administered to keep blood glucose at optimal levels.

Postoperative care

The surgeon must take measures to minimise/control infection at the operative site by careful oral prophylaxis, and antibiotics may be prescribed. Blood glucose estimates are continued until the patient resumes normal diet and controlling medication.

Adrenal corticosteroids

The adrenal cortex produces hormones that are of importance to the surgeon since among their functions they affect the balance of electrolytes, depress the immune response and play a significant part in the body's reaction to stress. Their secretion is stimulated by the adrenocorticotrophic hormone (ACTH) produced by the anterior lobe of the pituitary gland via a feedback loop (the hypothalamo-pituitary-adrenal (HPA) axis). When the amount of ACTH in the circulation reaches the necessary level, its production is inhibited.

Corticosteroids, or their synthetic equivalents, are used in medicine for replacement therapy of insufficiency, which may be chronic and primary as in Addison's disease, or chronic and secondary as in hypopituitarism. They are also used in the treatment of a wide variety of medical conditions such as asthma and the collagen disorders.

Adrenal crisis and supplemental steroids

Adrenal crisis may result from adrenocortical hypofunction, leading to hypotension, shock and death. The use of supplemental steroids prior to dental surgery in patients at risk of adrenal crisis is a contentious issue. The rationale for steroid supplementation is as follows: a normal physiological response to the stress of trauma is to increase corticosteroid production. If, due to hypoadrenalism, this response is absent, hypotension, collapse and death will occur if no treatment is provided (see Chapter 4). The HPA axis will fail to function if either the pituitary or the adrenal cortex ceases to function. This happens in secondary hypoadrenocorticism since administration of corticosteroids leads to negative feedback to the hypothalamus causing decreased ACTH production and adrenocortical atrophy. The atrophy means that an adequate endogenous steroid boost cannot be produced in response to stress.

Recent studies suggest that dental surgery may not require supplementation. Certain procedures, however, such as third molar surgery or the treatment of very apprehensive patients, may still require 'steroid cover' (see Chapter 4). If supplementary steroids are not used in patients at possible risk from an adrenal crisis, it is wise to monitor the blood pressure. If the diastolic pressure falls by more than 25%, an intravenous steroid injection (100 mg of hydrocortisone) is indicated.

Patients with Addison's disease should receive steroid cover. If a patient is under the care of an endocrinologist and taking steroids, it is wise to consult with them prior to carrying out surgery.

Thyroid disorders

Disorders of the thyroid gland should be considered by the surgeon if a history of thyroid problems is elicited. Improved pharmacological control of thyroid disorders has considerably reduced risk in this group of patients undergoing surgery/anaesthesia but the considerations below are still potentially important.

Hyperthyroidism

If hyperthyroidism is poorly controlled, this group of patients may have sympathetic overactivity which makes them more prone to fainting. There is no particular risk associated from adrenaline in local anaesthetics exacerbating sympathetic overactivity when normal doses are used. Use of intravenous sedation may heighten the effects of antithyroid drugs, and this should be remembered.

Hypothyroidism

Intravenous sedatives should be avoided or low doses used as "myxoedema coma" may be induced in these patients if the replacement therapy (usually thyroxine) is inadequate. Local anaesthesia is safe in this group. Similar comments apply to general anaesthesia and the possibility of associated ischaemic heart disease should be borne in mind in these patients.

Allergy

Anaphylaxis

See Chapter 4.

Angioedema

Angioedema is a disorder in which there is widespread oedema due to increased vascular permeability as a result of an allergic reaction. Two forms exist; one is hereditary and is an apparently exaggerated response to minor trauma. It is characteristically shared by other genetically related members of the family. The disorder is due to a lack of C1 esterase inhibitor and a consequent initiation of the complement cascade. Administration of fresh frozen plasma (FFP) prior to surgery provides sufficient inhibitor to prevent the problem. In the event of a spontaneous oedematous episode, the patient should be treated with systemic steroids.

The non-hereditary type is a kind of urticaria in which there is an allergic response to food and certain drugs. Trauma seldom produces serious complications but the use of allergenic substances may do so. Should an acute reaction occur it should be treated as for anaphylactic shock as described in Chapter 4.

Cardiovascular disorders

There are many cardiovascular conditions but the oral surgeon is concerned principally with those that affect the efficiency of the heart as a pump. The damaged valvular endocardium and infective endocarditis, while still of interest to an oral surgeon, is nowadays considered to be of lesser significance in the context of oral surgery and other bacteraemia-producing dental procedures than in the past and is discussed later.

Hypertension

Patients with hypertension should have their blood pressure controlled before elective surgery is carried out. The surgeon should remember that hypertensive patients may have associated cardiac and renal problems. Postural hypotension is more likely if the patient is using antihypertensive drugs and such patients are more susceptible to the hypotensive effects of general anaesthetics. The raised blood pressure can contribute to postoperative bleeding.

Coronary artery disease

Partial occlusion of coronary vessels, usually due to atheromatous disease, may lead to angina pectoris with the characteristic chest pain, which may radiate into the left arm. This occurs during physical or emotional stress because the demand for blood by the myocardium outstrips the possible supply. Treatment includes the use of vasodilators (usually glyceryl trinitrate, GTN) when pain is experienced. Details of the frequency of need for such medication will give an indication of the severity of the disease. Where use of a drug is frequent, increasing in frequency or needed at rest, advice should be sought from the patient's physician. Complete occlusion of a coronary artery leads to myocardial infarction (MI). Chest pain not responding to GTN after around 3 minutes should be considered to be an MI until proved otherwise and treated accordingly (see Chapter 4).

Patients taking anticoagulants require special considerations (see later). Those patients with angina treated under local anaesthesia may require premedication to allay anxiety. In unstable angina, the treatment is best deferred. Adequate analgesia must always be given to these patients.

Should an attack of angina occur, the patient should use their GTN spray and oxygen is administered at a high flow rate (10 l/min). Where the severity of the attack does not respond to GTN and is marked by cyanosis, nausea and dyspnoea, this further suggests an MI. The patient should then be given aspirin 300 mg to be chewed, providing they are not allergic to this, and urgent help must be obtained.

Cardiac failure

Symptoms of heart failure include reduced exercise tolerance, dyspnoea and oedema of the lower extremities. Left ventricular failure produces pulmonary oedema, whereas right-sided heart failure produces peripheral oedema. Patients in the early stages of cardiac failure may be relatively asymptomatic, but the loss of cardiac reserve may become apparent only when the extra demands of physical exercise or hypoxia cannot be met.

Cardiac failure, along with all other cardiac conditions, should be optimised before surgical treatment is carried out.

Infective endocarditis

The endocardium of the heart may be damaged congenitally or after certain illnesses such as rheumatic fever. Colonisation of these damaged areas by micro-organisms can lead to infective endocarditis. In the UK, prophylactic antibiotics are no longer prescribed prior to dental procedures in patients at risk of infective endocarditis as they are thought to be ineffective in the face of the transient bacteraemias produced by mastication, particularly on mobile, periodontally involved teeth, and oral hygiene procedures, which occur on a daily basis. It is now felt that the risk of anaphylaxis to the antibiotics is higher than the risk of infective endocarditis arising from this cause.

Ventricular shunts and prosthetic joints

Patients with congenital hydrocephalus may have artificial drainage pathways inserted to relieve increased intracranial pressure. There is no evidence to suggest that these patients are at risk of infection when a bacteraemia occurs.

There is an increase in the number of patients who have prosthetic joint replacements, e.g. of hip and knee. In the past, these patients have received prophylactic antibiotics prior to dental extraction. There is no evidence to suggest that these prostheses are susceptible to infection from bacteraemias produced during dental treatment.

In none of the above situations is prophylactic antibiotic cover prescribed prior to dental surgery.

Respiratory disorders

Chronic obstructive pulmonary disease (COPD)

COPD comprises emphysema and chronic bronchitis and is a condition that has seasonal exacerbations. It is often associated with other conditions, particularly upper respiratory tract infections and bronchiectasis.

All patients with respiratory conditions should be examined thoroughly. Although routine chest radiography is not required, spirometry will assess the condition of the patient in a more objective way. In patients with respiratory impairment, optimisation of their condition should be carried out prior to any sedation or general anaesthesia, and they may benefit from preoperative physiotherapy or nebulisers.

Asthma

Asthma is a paroxysmal disorder in which there are attacks of bronchospasm leading to dyspnoea. Some patients are under treatment with bronchodilators in the form of an inhaler, while others may use corticosteroid aerosol inhalers. General anaesthesia is not generally contraindicated, but it is important to assess the severity of a patient's asthma before surgical treatment using any anaesthetic modality. Frequency of attacks, efficacy of treatment and the need for hospital admissions should all be taken into account.

In an acute asthma attack it is important that the patient is allowed to sit up as they will find it easier to breathe. To relieve spasm, inhalation of the bronchodilator should help, but if this fails further emergency measures outlined in Chapter 4 will be required.

Disorders of the blood

Anaemia

The oral surgeon must be satisfied that the patient is not clinically anaemic before operation. Where doubt exists, a haemoglobin estimation and blood film examination should be arranged. It should be remembered that there are several different forms of anaemia and that it can be a manifestation of serious disease such as leukaemia or other malignancy, which requires further investigation by an appropriate specialist. In severe anaemia, operation is delayed until it has responded to treatment. It is important that a cause for any anaemia is found.

Sickle cell anaemia

Sickle cell anaemia is a haemoglobinopathy that is inherited. It is found in individuals of African, Asian and Mediterranean origin. The abnormal haemoglobin (HbS) in lowered oxygen tension (such as may occur during a general anaesthetic) results in red blood cells becoming sickle shaped, leading to an increased blood viscosity and capillary thrombosis. It can present as either true sickle cell anaemia or a sickle cell trait, in which there is a variable proportion of affected haemoglobin, the remainder being normal.

All patients who may have inherited the disease and require a general anaesthetic should be tested for sickle cell trait or disease. These patients may require further investigation by a haematologist to differentiate those with the trait from those with sickle cell anaemia. This is usually done by haemoglobin electrophoresis. Both groups are more safely treated under local anaesthesia, but when a general anaesthetic is necessary the patient should be referred for hospital specialist anaesthetic opinion.

Thalassaemias

Thalassaemias are inherited disorders (autosomal dominant) in which either alpha or beta globin chains have a decreased rate of synthesis and as a result allow less haemoglobin A to be produced. Patients with thalassaemia suffer from haemolytic anaemia and are seen in Mediterranean races. Local anaesthesia is safe, but general anaesthesia should only be carried out after full assessment by a specialist anaesthetist.

Leukaemias

All forms of leukaemia are a contraindication to any form of oral surgery without full investigation and liaison with a haematologist because of the potential difficulty in controlling postoperative bleeding and infection. In such cases a conservative approach to dental care should be adopted until the leukaemia is in remission or the patient is free of the disease following treatment. If oral or maxillofacial treatment is unavoidable, full liaison with the patient's oncologist must be carried out.

Haemorrhagic diseases

Arrest of haemorrhage is brought about in three ways, first by the contraction of vessel walls, second by plugging of small deficiencies by platelets and third by the clotting of the blood. Clinically, patients with haemorrhagic disease can be divided into those where bleeding is profuse at operation and continues – these have a prolonged bleeding time but clotting may be normal; and those where bleeding is stopped for a short period after operation but persistent haemorrhage occurs later owing to failure of the blood to clot – these may have a normal bleeding time but an abnormality of coagulation.

Prolonged bleeding time

Prolonged bleeding time is found where vascular damage prevents arrest of haemorrhage by the contraction of the walls of cut vessels, or in platelet abnormalities in which there is ineffective plugging of small deficiencies.

Disorders of blood vessels

Disorders of blood vessels occur in conditions such as Henoch-Schonlein purpura. Symptomatic purpura can occur in severe infections such as scarlet fever, following the use of certain drugs and in hereditary haemorrhagic telangiectasia.

Platelet abnormalities

There are two main types of platelet abnormality. First, thrombocytopaenia, where there is a low platelet count. This may be primary, idiopathic or secondary to drugs or other blood diseases such as leukaemia. Essential thrombocythaemia is a disorder characterised by a high platelet count (thrombocytosis). The platelet morphology and function is abnormal and presentation could be by thrombosis or bleeding.

Abnormal coagulation

Haemostasis is the process whereby blood coagulation and clot breakdown are initiated and ended in a regulated way. The traditional model of the coagulation cascade has been superseded by the concept of a 'coagulation network'. This is summarised in Figure 3.1.

The coagulant and anticoagulant components are normally balanced. If this balance is disturbed, bleeding or thrombosis may occur, depending on which components are affected.

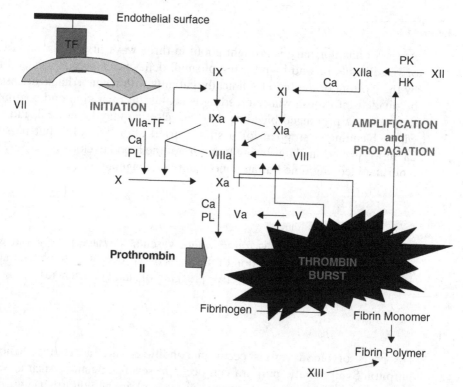

Figure 3.1 The coagulation network. The Roman numerals refer to the various clotting factors. Reproduced with permission from Greenwood *et al.* (2009) © John Wiley & Sons, Inc.

Coagulation defects are relatively rare and they arise from a deficiency of any of the factors concerned with the mechanism. The most common disease is haemophilia A, a sex-linked disease mainly of males, caused by an insufficiency of factor VIII. Females, if affected, are usually carriers and have lowered levels of factor VIII, which may require correction before surgery. Deficiency of factor IX causes haemophilia B (Christmas disease), seen in males.

Clotting failure may also occur due to a deficiency of prothrombin, which is formed in the liver and requires vitamin K for its synthesis.

Fibrinolysis

Normal circulating blood contains plasminogen, which is the precursor of plasmin, a proteolytic enzyme that breaks down fibrin and fibrinogen and thereby causes the destruction of clots. Though playing a physiological role in the organisation of clots, excessive fibrinolysis can occur in a wide variety of conditions such of sepsis, acute haemorrhage or after major surgery, thus delaying haemostasis.

von Willebrand's disease

von Willebrand's factor prolongs the life of factor VIII in the circulation and stabilises platelet plugs. Deficiency affects the level of factor VIII and platelet function. The disease is seen in males and females.

Anticoagulant therapy

There will be certain patients who are being treated with anticoagulant drugs following thrombosis or cardiac surgery. Two main types of anticoagulants are in use. First, the rapid and short-acting heparin group, which are antithrombins and thereby prevent the conversion of fibrinogen to fibrin. Second, the longer-acting oral group (such as warfarin), which reduce the amount of circulating prothrombin by preventing its formation in the liver.

The therapeutic range for warfarin is usually between 2.0 to 4.0. For most surgical dental treatment it is not necessary to discontinue warfarin but the International Normalised Ratio (INR) must be checked either on the day of surgery or within 24 hours of surgery if the general level of INR is well controlled. The degree of control can be ascertained from the patient's warfarin record booklet. If the INR level is 4 or less it is considered safe for surgical dental treatment. It is important after treatment that local haemostatic measures are carried out involving suturing the surgical site with a resorbable suture and in the case of tooth sockets placing oxidised cellulose (Surgicel®).

Liver disease

Many of the factors involved in the clotting mechanism are synthesised in the liver and thus any possibility of impaired liver function should be investigated. A history of liver disease should always prompt the surgeon to think about implications for haemostasis. Cirrhosis of the liver, usually secondary to alcohol abuse, may only manifest itself as an increased tendency to bleed after injury.

Careful enquiry should be made about the patient's alcohol intake. Recommended units per week of alcohol in males and females are 21 and 14 respectively. Impaired hepatic function also has implications for the use of the benzodiazepine sedative drugs, which are metabolised by the liver. Further factors to be considered in patients with liver disorders are discussed later in the chapter.

Investigation of post-extraction haemorrhage

The history of excessive bleeding is most commonly due to local factors, but particular attention should be paid to those who on several occasions have undergone repeated attempts to arrest post-extraction or other haemorrhage. These patients need careful investigation to eliminate a possible systemic cause. Petechial haemorrhage (purpura) and bruising are typical of generalised vascular damage and platelet inadequacy, but not of clotting disorders. Recurrent haemarthrosis is suggestive of haemophilia A and B, but not of platelet or vascular disorders. The family history is important, as many of the conditions are hereditary.

Wherever the surgeon's suspicions are aroused the patient must be referred to a haematologist for full investigation before operation, as the diagnosis can only be made in the laboratory.

Management of bleeding disorders

Patients with systemic haemorrhagic disease should be admitted to hospital for surgery and treated in conjunction with a haematologist. In vascular disorders, management depends on local measures.

In platelet disorders secondary to other diseases, the cause must be dealt with first. Patients with idiopathic thrombocytopaenia may be given steroid therapy to raise the platelet count. Other thrombocytopaenic patients may be given preoperative platelet infusions.

In clotting disorders, the essential treatment is usually to replace the missing factor. For haemophilia A and von Willebrand's disease, factor VIII is available and given by intravenous injection. For patients with mild diseases, DDAVP (desmopressin) will raise the patient's endogenous factor VIII. Tranexamic acid is an antifibrinolytic agent used to prevent the destruction of clots and should be given for 10 days, commencing 1 day preoperatively, and can also be used as a mouthwash postoperatively at 5% concentration.

Choice of anaesthetic

In general, all local anaesthesia may be used but due care should be taken. It is permissible, so long as the INR is within accepted range, for inferior dental blocks to be carried out on patients taking warfarin, but these are still best avoided if possible.

In patients with clotting disorders undergoing general anaesthesia, most anaesthetists would prefer whenever possible to use an oral endotracheal tube as opposed to a nasal tube.

Musculoskeletal disorders

The surgeon should consider general issues such as patient mobility and impairment of manual dexterity, which may significantly affect compliance with oral healthcare. Other general issues include the degree of mouth opening that is possible and likewise the ability to extend the neck. The latter is clearly important in the provision of general anaesthesia and opening of the airway, for example in cardiopulmonary resuscitation. The best method of opening the airway when there are cervical spine problems, either acutely as a result of injury or chronically as a result of disease, is to use a jaw thrust.

Patients with disorders such as rheumatoid arthritis will often have an anaemia that is normocytic and normochromic – the so-called anaemia of chronic disease. Such anaemia is also seen in patients with chronic kidney disease. This may have significant implications for oxygenation, particularly during sedation or anaesthesia.

Muscular disorders may be of relevance from the point of view of provision of treatment under local anaesthesia, but also enhanced effects of drugs used in intravenous sedation. Myasthenia gravis is an autoimmune disease of the neuromuscular junction involving the post-junctional acetylcholine receptors and is characterised by muscle weakness. Patients with myasthenia gravis should not be given benzodiazepine sedation due to the muscle relaxant properties of this group of drugs. In muscular dystrophy patients, cardiomyopathy and respiratory disease should be considered. These patients are also sensitive to the muscle relaxant suxamethonium and are predisposed to developing malignant hyperthermia if general anaesthesia is used.

Patients who have undergone radiation to the head and neck region are at risk of a condition known as osteoradionecrosis due to a diminution of the blood supply to the bone secondary to a condition known as endarteritis obliterans, where the size of the lumen of the vessel is decreased. Procedures such as dental extractions can result in necrotic bone, which is problematic. The best management of osteoradionecrosis is prevention. It is important to complete any oral surgical or restorative treatment prior to radiotherapy. Osteoradionecrosis is more common in the first six months after radiotherapy and it is particularly important to avoid extraction in the first six months to one year.

When pre-radiotherapy extractions are needed, particular care should be taken to ensure that bone is covered by mucosa. Post-radiotherapy extractions should be avoided if possible, but if unavoidable, trauma should be kept to a minimum. Local anaesthetic without vasoconstrictor should be used and raising of periosteum should be minimised. Any sharp bone edges should be gently

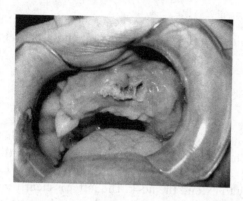

Figure 3.2   Osteonecrosis following a dental extraction on a patient who has been prescribed bisphosphonates.

trimmed. Soft tissue should be closed accurately and prophylactic antibiotics should be prescribed until the sockets have healed.

Osteonecrosis is a condition that is recognised in patients taking bisphosphonates to alter bone metabolism in conditions such as osteoporosis or in the management of metastatic disease in bone. The bisphosphonates may be administered orally or intravenously and both have been associated with osteonecrosis, particularly after dental extractions (Figure 3.2). The intravenous type produces an increased risk. Dental extractions are best avoided in this group whenever possible, but where unavoidable, management is similar to that of patients who have undergone radiotherapy.

Systemic diseases of bone

Bone disorders may affect the oral and maxillofacial surgeon in several ways. Difficulties in extraction of teeth may be encountered due to hypercementosis (osteitis deformans, or Paget's disease of bone) or sclerosis of bone (osteopetrosis, acromegaly). The bone may be fragile and prone to fracture even though minimal force is used during operations (osteogenesis imperfecta). The incidence of postoperative infection is increased (osteitis deformans) and there may be a risk of causing an exacerbation of the disease (fibrous dysplasia).

Epilepsy

Intermittent abnormal electric activity in a part of the brain may manifest as seizures. Such seizures can take many different forms. There may be a prodromal period that can last for hours or days preceding a seizure. This is not part of the seizure itself, however. An *aura* is part of the seizure and is a warning to the patient that a seizure is about to happen.

There are several different types of seizure, which can be classified into partial seizures, generalised seizures (incorporating petit mal and grand mal) and unilateral seizures. Petit mal is of a relatively minor character in which, without warning, the patient loses consciousness or awareness for a few seconds but seldom falls or has convulsions. Grand mal is characterised by generalised convulsions and possible loss of consciousness.

It is important to find out in the history the degree of control of epilepsy and the effectiveness of medication. The patient must always have taken their epilepsy medication on the day of an appointment. The management of a patient having an epileptic seizure is discussed in Chapter 4.

Epileptic patients who are scheduled for general anaesthesia should not be given methohexitone or enflurane since both are epileptogenic. Intravenous sedation is useful in managing epileptic patients. The benzodiazepines have anticonvulsant properties and anxiolysis should decrease the chances of a fit. When treating epileptic patients with sedation, supplemental oxygen should be provided via a nasal cannula. The use of the benzodiazepine reversal agent flumazenil should be avoided in patients with epilepsy as this drug can precipitate convulsions.

Psychiatric illness

Psychiatric illness is common and affects up to 1 in 4 people in the UK to some degree at some time in their lives. It is thus probable that a surgeon will encounter psychiatric problems at some point. It is beyond the scope of this book to discuss the whole field of psychiatric illness but some important points are summarised.

The Mental Capacity Act of 2005 (introduced into practice in 2007) is an important piece of legislation that is designed to protect the rights of individuals to make their own decisions and provide guidelines to address this. It is important to remember that many patients with psychiatric illness still have the capacity to make their own informed decisions. The Act referred to above sets out guidance for decision making on behalf of people who lack decision-making capacity and applies to all people aged 16 and over in England and Wales.

Decision-making capacity is considered to be task specific, relevant only to specific decisions at a given time, and should not be applied to other situations and decisions.

Some of the drugs that may be used in the treatment of psychiatric illness have effects that are of interest to the surgeon. Some of the more important examples are given in Box 3.1.

Liver disorders

Patients with liver disorders are of interest to the surgeon in terms of their ability to metabolise drugs, possible effects on haemostasis and the risk of infection in cases of infectious hepatitis.

Sedatives and general anaesthetics are potentially dangerous in liver disorders due to impairment of detoxification. With halothane, a hepatitis may follow its use, especially in obese patients, smokers, middle-aged females and if an

---

Box 3.1 Side effects of drugs used to treat psychiatric illness

Antidepressants

- *Tricyclics* (amitriptyline, clomipramine)
  Local anaesthetic (LA), sympathomimetics (e.g. adrenaline) → hypertension and arrhythmias
  General anaesthetic (GA) → ↑ risk cardiac arrhythmias and hypotension
- *MAOIs* (monoamine oxidase inhibitors, e.g. phenelzine)
  GA and sympathomimetics used in LA (e.g. adrenaline) → hypertension and arrhythmias
  Risk of hypertensive crisis – MAOI should be stopped 2 weeks before anaesthetic

Mood stabilisers

- *Lithium*
  Antibiotics, particularly metronidazole, may cause lithium toxicity
  NSAIDs, e.g. ibuprofen, diclofenac, may cause lithium toxicity

Antipsychotics

GA → enhanced hypotensive effect
Antibiotic
Erythromycin → ↑ risk convulsions with **clozapine**

Dementia drugs

Ketamine → toxic combination with **memantine**

ADHD drugs

GA → hypertension with **methylphenidate**

---

anaesthetic using halothane has been given in the last 3 months. The precise mechanism for this is unknown. Newer agents such as enflurane and sevoflurane are less hepatotoxic.

Patients who give a history of physical signs suggestive of a liver disorder or a high alcohol intake should have blood taken for clotting studies and liver function tests (LFTs).

In some liver disorders brain metabolism is altered, leading to its sensitivity to certain drugs. Encephalopathy can be triggered by sedatives or opiates.

Any patient with jaundice has increased risk of bleeding excessively following a surgical procedure. A perioperative infusion of fresh frozen plasma will often be required if surgery is unavoidable, and full liaison with the relevant physician should always be carried out. If the patient is severely jaundiced a general anaesthetic may precipitate renal failure, the hepatorenal syndrome.

Most of the amide local anaesthetics undergo biotransformation in the liver. Articaine is metabolised partly in the plasma and some of the metabolism of prilocaine is in the lungs; the liver, however, is the main site of metabolic break-down. All of a local anaesthetic injection dose will eventually reach the circulation and if liver metabolism is affected, the plasma concentration will slowly increase as approximately only 2% of the drug will be excreted unchanged. Signs of central nervous system (CNS) toxicity may therefore occur with as little as two cartridges in an adult patient in cases of severe liver disease.

Viral hepatitis is important in terms of the potential for hepatic impairment, but also due to the risk of transmission of infection. Efficient cross-infection control minimises the risk.

Renal disorders

Renal disease should be taken into account when prescribing drugs, as many that are prescribed by oral and maxillofacial surgeons are excreted by the kidney. If the drug or its metabolites are not excreted, toxicity may result. Clearly any drug that is nephrotoxic should be avoided and other drugs may require dose reduction. Erythromycin is contraindicated in patients who have had a kidney transplant and are taking ciclosporin. The metabolism of the latter is reduced, leading to an increase in toxicity.

Antimicrobials such as aciclovir, amoxicillin, ampicillin, cefalexin and erythromycin should all be used with dose reduction in patients with renal impairment. Tetracyclines other than doxycycline should be avoided. Non-steroidal anti-inflammatory drugs (NSAIDs) should not be prescribed in those with more than mild renal impairment. Drugs used in intravenous sedation should be used with caution, as a greater effect than normal may be produced.

The *British National Formulary* contains useful information with regard to prescribing in patients with renal disorders.

Conclusion

It is important for the surgeon to have a sound knowledge of applied medicine and surgery. Safe practice is dependent on it.

Further reading

British National Formulary (published biannually) BMJ Group and RPS Publishing, London (available online at http://bnf.org/bnf/).

Greenwood M, Seymour RA, Meechan JG (eds) (2009) *Textbook of Human Disease in Dentistry*. Wiley-Blackwell, Oxford.

Longmore M, Wilkinson I, Davidson E, Foulkes A (2010) *Oxford Handbook of Clinical Medicine* (Oxford Handbooks Series). Oxford University Press, Oxford.

Chapter 4
Medical Emergencies

- Contents of an emergency drug box
- Staff training
- The 'ABCDE' approach to an emergency patient
- Use of defibrillation
- Fainting
- Hyperventilation
- Asthma
- Chest pain of cardiac origin
- Epileptic seizures
- Diabetic emergencies
- Allergies/Hypersensitivity reactions (including anaphylaxis)
- Choking and aspiration
- Adrenal insufficiency
- Stroke
- Local anaesthetic emergencies

It is important that medical emergencies are recognised and the practitioner becomes competent to carry out initial management if they occur. The commonest emergencies seen are faints, hypoglycaemia, asthma, anaphylaxis, angina and seizures.

All members of the clinical team need to be aware of what their role would be in the event of a medical emergency and should be trained appropriately with regular practice sessions. Successful patient management starts with anticipation of the more likely potential medical emergencies that could arise by taking a thorough history.

Contents of an emergency drug box

Medical emergencies may require equipment, drugs or both in order to manage them effectively. If these are not readily available, patients should not be treated.

Principles of Oral and Maxillofacial Surgery, 6th Edition. Edited by U. J. Moore
© 2011 Blackwell Publishing Ltd

Box 4.1 Contents of an emergency drug box, with routes of administration	
Drug	Route of administration
Oxygen	Inhalation
Glyceryl trinitrate (GTN) spray (400 µg per actuation)	Sublingual
Dispersible aspirin (300 mg)	Oral (chewed)
Salbutamol aerosol inhaler (100 µg per actuation)	Inhalation
Adrenaline injection (1:1000, 1 mg/ml)	Intramuscular
Glucagon injection (1 mg)	Intramuscular/subcutaneous
Oral glucose solution/gel (GlucoGel®)*	Oral
Midazolam 10 mg or 5 mg/ml (buccal or intranasal)	Buccal sulcus/inhalation

* Alternatives:
  – 2 teaspoons of sugar/3 sugar lumps
  – 200 ml milk
  – Lucozade (non-diet) 50 ml
  – Coca-Cola (non-diet) 90 ml
If necessary this can be repeated after 10–15 minutes

It is also important to check that the drugs are within their expiry date. Remember that different drugs have different 'shelf lives'.

Drugs to be included as a minimum in the emergency drug box are summarised in Box 4.1. The list is based on that given in the Resuscitation Council (UK) document on Medical Emergencies and Resuscitation in Dentistry, revised in 2008. Clearly, in a hospital environment the availability of emergency drugs is significantly increased. A practitioner registered with the General Dental Council (GDC) should administer only those drugs that they feel competent to handle.

All drugs should be stored together, ideally in a purpose-designed container.

The optimum route for delivery of emergency drugs is usually the intravenous route, but dentists are often inexperienced in this route of delivery. Formulations have now been developed that allow for other much quicker and more user-friendly routes to be used, and the intravenous route for emergency drugs is no longer recommended as routine for dental practitioners. Oxygen should always be available, deliverable at adequate flow rates (10 l/min).

Staff training

Staff should be trained in the management of medical emergencies to a degree that is appropriate to their level of clinical responsibility. Skills should be updated on an annual basis.

Box 4.2 The ABCDE approach to an emergency patient

A Airway
B Breathing
C Circulation
D Disability (or neurological status)
E Exposure (in dental practice, to facilitate placement of AED paddles) or appropriately exposing parts to be examined

The 'ABCDE' approach to an emergency patient

Medical emergencies can sometimes be prevented by early recognition. An abnormal patient colour, pulse rate or breathing can signal some impending emergencies.

It is important to have a systematic approach to an acutely ill patient and to remain calm. The principles are summarised in the 'ABCDE' approach (Box 4.2), but it is useful to start with a brief discussion of some general points. First, ensure that the environment is safe, and note that it is important to call for help at a very early stage. Continuous reappraisal of the patient's condition should be carried out and their airway (A) must always be the starting point for this. Without appropriate oxygen delivery, all other management steps will be ultimately futile. It is important to assess the success or otherwise of manoeuvres or treatments given, bearing in mind that treatments may take time to work.

If the patient is conscious, ask them how they are. This may give important information about the problem (for example, the patient who cannot speak or tells you that they have chest pain). If the patient is unresponsive, they should be shaken and asked 'Are you all right?' If they do not respond at all, have no pulse and show 'no signs of life' (breathing (B) and circulation (C)), they have had a cardiac arrest and should be managed as described later. They may respond in a breathless manner and should be asked 'Are you choking?'

Airway (A)

Airway obstruction is a medical emergency and must be managed quickly. Usually, a simple method of clearing the airway is all that is needed. A head tilt, chin lift or jaw thrust (the latter avoids cervical spine extension) will open the airway. Patients who are unable to speak are to be feared and establishing a patent airway is vital. It is important to remove any visible foreign bodies, blood or debris. The careful use of suction may be beneficial. Clearing the mouth should be done with great care (a 'finger sweep' in adults) to avoid pushing material further into the upper airway. Simple airway adjuncts, such as an oropharyngeal airway (Figure 4.1) may be used if the patient is unconscious. An impaired airway may be recognised by some of the signs and symptoms summarised in Box 4.3.

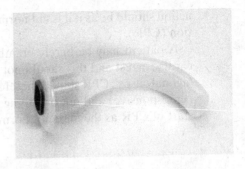

Figure 4.1   An oro-pharyngeal airway.

Box 4.3   Signs of airway obstruction

- Inability to complete sentences or speak
- 'Paradoxical' movement of chest and abdomen ('see-saw' respiration)
- Use of accessory muscles of respiration
- Blue lips and tongue (central cyanosis)
- No breathing sounds (complete airway obstruction)
- Stridor (inspiratory) – obstruction of larynx or above
- Wheeze (expiratory) – obstruction of lower airways, e.g. asthma or chronic obstructive pulmonary disease
- Gurgling – suggests liquid or semi-solid material in the upper airway
- Snoring – the pharynx is partly occluded by the soft palate or tongue

It is important to administer oxygen at high concentration (10 l/min) via a well-fitting face mask with a port for oxygen. Even patients with chronic obstructive pulmonary disease who retain carbon dioxide should be given a high concentration of oxygen. Such patients may depend on hypoxic drive to stimulate respiration, but in the short term a high concentration of oxygen will do no harm, so its avoidance in the acute situation is unnecessary.

Breathing (B) and Circulation (C)

The clinician should look, listen and feel for signs of respiratory distress. This should be done while keeping the airway open. The clinician should:

- look for chest movement
- listen for breath sounds at the patient's mouth
- feel for air on the rescuer's cheek with the rescuer's head turned against the patient's mouth.

This should be done for no more than 10 seconds to determine whether there is normal breathing. If there is any doubt as to whether breathing is normal, action should be as if it is not normal, i.e. commence cardiopulmonary resuscitation (CPR).

A patient may be barely breathing or gasping in the first few minutes after cardiac arrest and this should not be mistaken as normal breathing – so-called 'agonal gasps'. CPR should therefore be carried out if the patient is unconscious (unresponsive) and not breathing normally. Agonal gasps should not delay the start of CPR as they are not normal breathing.

If the patient is breathing normally

- The patient should be turned into the recovery position (essentially on their side – best learnt as a practical exercise).
- Send for help.
- Ensure that breathing continues.

If the patient is not breathing normally

- Ensure help is obtained.
- Start chest compressions:
  - kneel at the side of the victim
  - place the heel of one hand in the centre of the patient's chest and the other hand on top of the first hand – it will usually be possible to do this without removing the patient's clothes. If there is any doubt, outer clothing should be undone/removed
  - interlock the fingers of both hands – do not apply pressure over the ribs, upper abdomen or the lower end of the sternum
  - the rescuer should be positioned vertically above the patient's chest. With straight arms, the sternum should be depressed 4–5 cm
  - after each compression all the pressure should be released so that the rib cage recoils to its rest position, but the hands should be maintained in contact with the sternum
  - the rate should be approximately 100 times per minute (a little less than two compressions per second).
- After 30 compressions, the airway should be opened using head tilt and chin lift and two rescue breaths should be given. This may be carried out using a bag and mask or mouth-to-mouth (with the nostrils closed between thumb and index finger) or mouth-to-mask.
- Practical skills are best learnt on a resuscitation course.

If rescue breaths do not make the chest rise

- Check for visible obstruction in the mouth and remove if possible.
- Make sure that the head tilt and chin lift are adequate.
- Do not waste time attempting more than two breaths each time before continuing chest compressions.

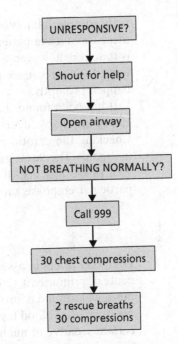

Figure 4.2 The Basic Life Support Algorithm (reproduced with permission from Resuscitation Council (UK)).

Box 4.4 Simple methods of circulatory assessment

Signs
- Are the patient's hands blue or pink, cool or warm?
- What is the capillary refill time?*
- Pulse rate (carotid or radial artery), rhythm and strength

Symptoms
- Is there a history of chest pain/does the patient report chest pain?

* If pressure is applied to the fingernail to produce blanching, the colour should return in less than 2 seconds in a normal patient. Remember that local causes such as a cold environment could also delay the response.

Carrying out these manoeuvres is tiring and if there is more than one rescuer CPR should be alternated between them every 2 minutes. The algorithm for adult basic life support is given in Figure 4.2.

Factors to consider in assessing circulation (C)

Assessment of the circulation should never delay the start of CPR. Simple observations to make a gross assessment of circulatory efficiency are given in Box 4.4. By far the most common cause of a collapse that is circulatory in origin is the simple faint (vasovagal syncope). A rapid recovery can be expected in these cases if the patient is laid flat and their legs raised. Prompt management is required, however, as cerebral hypoxia has devastating consequences if prolonged. Other causes than a faint must be considered if recovery does not happen promptly.

It has been found that checking the carotid pulse to diagnose cardiac arrest can be unreliable, even sometimes when attempted by healthcare professionals. Checking the carotid pulse should only be carried out by those proficient in doing this. The latest guidelines highlight the need to identify agonal gasps (as well as the absence of breathing) as a sign to commence CPR and place no particular emphasis on checking the carotid pulse.

Disability (D)

Disability refers to assessment of the neurological status of the patient. In this context, primarily it refers to the level of consciousness (in trauma patients a more widespread neurological examination is required). Hypoxia or hypercapnia (increased blood level of carbon dioxide) are possible causes, together with certain sedative or analgesic drugs.

It is important to exclude hypoxia or hypotension, and attention to the airway, giving supplemental oxygen and supporting the patient's circulation (by lying them supine and raising their legs) will in many cases solve the problem. Unconscious patients who are breathing and have a pulse should be placed in the recovery position if they are unable to maintain their own airway.

A rapid gross assessment can be made of a patient's level of consciousness using the AVPU method:

* are they **A**lert?
* do they respond to **V**ocal stimuli?
* do they respond to **P**ainful stimuli?
* or are they **U**nresponsive?

A lapse into unconsciousness may be due to hypoglycaemia – if the blood glucose level is less than 3 mmol/l as checked by a glucose-measuring device, 1 mg glucagon should be given intramuscularly.

Exposure (E)

Exposure refers to loosening or removal of some of the patient's clothes, for example for the application of defibrillator paddles or for examination purposes if the patient has been involved in a traumatic incident. It is important to bear in mind the patient's dignity as well as the potential for clinically significant heat loss.

Cardiac arrest can occur for a variety of reasons, summarised in Box 4.5.

> **Box 4.5**   Potential causes of cardiac arrest
>
> - Arrhythmia (most common type ventricular fibrillation or VF)
> - Myocardial infarction (may lead to an arrhythmia)
> - Choking
> - Bleeding
> - Drug overdose
> - Hypoxia

Use of defibrillation

Defibrillation is the term used to describe a controlled electrical shock administered to the fibrillating heart, which may restore an organised rhythm enabling the heart to contract effectively. It is now well recognised that early defibrillation in cardiac arrest is important. Ventricular fibrillation (VF) is the most common cause of cardiac arrest. It is a rapid and chaotic rhythm and as a result the heart is unable to contract effectively and unable to sustain its function as a pump. The only effective treatment for VF is defibrillation and the sooner the shock is given, the greater the chance of survival.

The provision of defibrillation has been made easier by the development of automated external defibrillators (AEDs). AEDs are sophisticated, reliable, safe, computerised devices which use voice and visual prompts to guide rescuers. The device analyses the victim's heart rhythm, determines the need for a shock and then delivers it if advised. The AED algorithm is given in Figure 4.3. CPR should not be interrupted or delayed to set up an AED. A typical AED is shown in Figure 4.4.

Placement of AED pads

Use of the AED is a skill that requires practical training and experience. One pad should be placed to the right of the sternum below the clavicle. The other pad should be placed in the left side mid-axillary line, centred on the fifth intercostal space. This electrode works best if orientated vertically. This position should be clear of any breast tissue. Although most AED pads are labelled or carry a picture of their position, it does not matter if they are reversed.

Signs, symptoms and management of specific medical emergencies will be discussed.

Fainting

Vasovagal syncope or a simple faint is a loss of consciousness due to inadequate cerebral perfusion. It is a reflex mediated by autonomic nerves leading to widespread vasodilatation in the splanchnic and skeletal vessels, and bradycardia,

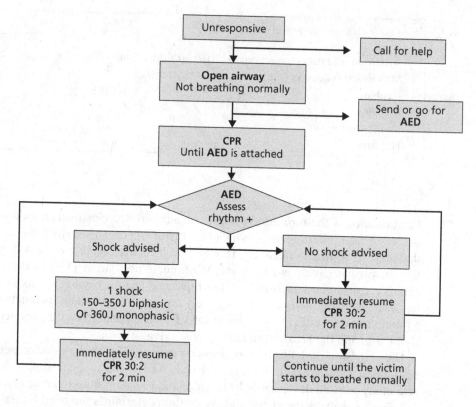

Figure 4.3   AED algorithm (reproduced with permission from Resuscitation Council (UK)).

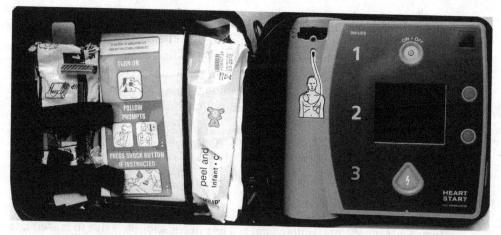

Figure 4.4   An automated external defibrillator (AED).

resulting in diminished cerebral perfusion. Fainting can be precipitated by pain or emotional stress, changes in posture or hypoxia. Some patients are more prone to fainting than others and it is wise to treat fainting-prone patients in the supine position.

A similar clinical picture may be seen in 'carotid sinus syndrome'. Mild pressure on the neck in such patients (usually elderly) leads to a vagal reaction producing syncope. This situation may progress to bradycardia or even cardiac arrest.

Signs and symptoms

- Patient feels faint/light headed/dizzy
- Pallor, sweating
- Pulse rate slows
- Low blood pressure
- Nausea and/or vomiting
- Loss of consciousness.

Treatment

- Lie the patient flat and raise their legs – recovery will normally be rapid.
- A patent airway must be maintained.
- If recovery is delayed, oxygen (10 l/min) should be administered and other causes of loss of consciousness be considered.

Hyperventilation

When hyperventilation persists it can become extremely distressing to the patient. Anxiety is the principal precipitating factor.

Signs and symptoms

- Anxiety
- Light headedness
- Dizziness
- Weakness
- Paraesthesia
- Tetany (see below)
- Chest pain and/or palpitations
- Breathlessness.

Treatment

A calm and sympathetic approach from the practitioner is important. The diagnosis, particularly in the early stages, is not always obvious.

- Exclude other causes for the symptoms before diagnosing hyperventilation.
- Encourage the patient to rebreathe their own exhaled air to increase the amount of inhaled carbon dioxide – a paper bag placed over nose and mouth allows this.
- If no paper bag is handy, the patient's cupped hands would be an alternative, but less satisfactory.

Hyperventilation leads to carbon dioxide being 'washed out' of the body, producing an alkalosis. If hyperventilation persists, carpal (hand) and pedal (foot) spasm (tetany) may be seen. Rebreathing exhaled air helps to return the situation to normal.

Asthma

Severe asthma is a potentially life-threatening condition and should always be taken seriously. An attack may be precipitated by exertion, anxiety, infection or exposure to an allergen. It is important to gain some idea of the severity of attacks from the history. Clues include precipitating factors, effectiveness of medication, hospital admissions due to asthma and the use of systemic steroids.

It is important that asthmatic patients bring their usual inhaler(s) with them – if they have not brought their inhaler, then unless there is one in the emergency kit, treatment should be deferred. If the asthma is in a particularly severe phase, elective treatment may be best postponed. Non-steroidal anti-inflammatory drugs (NSAIDs), may worsen asthma and are therefore best avoided.

Signs and symptoms

- Breathlessness (rapid respiration – more than 25 breaths per minute)
- Expiratory wheezing
- Use of accessory muscles of respiration
- Tachycardia.

Signs and symptoms of life-threatening asthma

- Cyanosis or slow respiratory rate (fewer than 8 breaths per minute)
- Bradycardia
- Decreased level of consciousness/confusion.

Treatment

- Most attacks will respond to the patient's own inhaler, e.g. salbutamol (may need to repeat after 2–3 minutes).
- If no rapid response, or features of severe asthma, call an ambulance.

- A medical assessment should be arranged for patients who require additional doses of bronchodilator to end an attack.
- A spacer device may be used if patient has difficulty using an inhaler.
- If the patient is distressed or shows any of the signs of life-threatening asthma, urgent medical assessment should be arranged.
- Ten litres of oxygen per minute should be given while awaiting transfer. Four to six actuations from the salbutamol inhaler via a spacer device should be used and repeated every 10 minutes.
- If asthma is part of a more generalised anaphylactic reaction, an intramuscular injection of adrenaline should be given (see section on anaphylaxis).

Chest pain of cardiac origin

Most patients who suffer chest pain from a cardiac origin in the dental surgery are likely to have a previous history of cardiac disease. If a patient uses medication to control known angina they should have brought this with them or it should be readily to hand in the emergency kit. Similarly, it is important that the patient has taken their normal medication on the day of their appointment.

Classically, the pain of angina is described as a crushing or band-like tightness of the chest, which may radiate to the left arm or mandible. There are many variations, however. The pain of myocardial infarction (MI) will often be similar to that of angina, but more severe, and, unlike angina, will not be relieved by glyceryl trinitrate (GTN). In cases of angina, the patient should use their GTN spray, which will usually relieve the symptoms. Surgical treatment may be best left until another day if there is an attack, according to the practitioner's discretion and patient's wishes. More severe chest pain always warrants postponement of treatment.

A list of possible causes of chest pain is given in Box 4.6. It is clearly important to exclude angina and myocardial infarction in the patient complaining of chest pain. If in doubt, treat as cardiac pain until proven otherwise.

Box 4.6   Possible causes of chest pain

- Angina
- Myocardial infarction (MI)
- Pleuritic, e.g. pulmonary embolism
- Musculoskeletal
- Oesophageal reflux
- Hyperventilation
- Gall bladder and pancreatic disease

Signs and symptoms of MI

- Severe, crushing chest pain, which may radiate to the shoulders and down the arms (particularly the left arm) and into the mandible
- The skin becomes pale and clammy
- Shortness of breath
- Pulse becomes weak and patient may become hypotensive
- Often there will be nausea and vomiting
- Not all patients fit this 'classic' picture and may exhibit only some of the signs and symptoms above.

Treatment of MI

- The practitioner should remain calm and be a reassuring presence
- Call for help immediately
- Most patients are best managed in the sitting position
- Patients who feel faint should be laid flat
- Give high flow oxygen (10 l/min)
- Give sublingual GTN spray
- Give 300 mg aspirin orally to be chewed (if no allergy) – ensure that when handing over to the receiving team they are made aware of this
- A patient who has had surgical dental treatment should be highlighted to the receiving team, as any significant risk of haemorrhage may affect the decision to use thrombolytic therapy
- If the patient becomes unresponsive, the clinician should check for 'signs of life' (breathing and circulation) and start CPR if necessary.

Epileptic seizures

The medical history will usually reveal the fact that a patient has epilepsy and should obtain information with regard to the nature of any seizures, their frequency and degree of control. The type and efficacy of medication should be determined. Signs and symptoms vary considerably.

Signs and symptoms

- The patient may have an 'aura' that a seizure is going to happen
- Tonic phase – loss of consciousness, patient becomes rigid, falls and becomes cyanosed
- Clonic phase – jerking movements of the limbs, tongue may be bitten
- Frothing at the mouth, urinary incontinence
- The seizure often gradually abates after a few minutes but the patient may remain unconscious and may remain confused after consciousness has been regained

- Hypoglycaemia may present as a fit and should be borne in mind (including in epileptic patients) – blood glucose measurement at an early stage is therefore wise.

In patients with a marked bradycardia (fewer than 40 beats per minute) the blood pressure may drop to such an extent that it causes transient cerebral hypoxia leading to a brief fit. This is not a true fit and represents a vasovagal episode.

Treatment of a fit

The decision to give medication should be made if seizures are prolonged (active convulsions for 5 minutes or more (status epilepticus) or seizures occur in quick succession). If possible, high-flow oxygen should be administered. The possibility of the patient's airway becoming occluded should be constantly remembered and the airway must therefore be protected.

- As far as possible, ensure safety of the patient and practitioner (but do not attempt to restrain).
- Midazolam given via the buccal or intranasal route (10 mg for adults). The buccal preparation is marketed as 'Epistatus' (10 mg/ml).
- For children:
  - child 1–5 years 5 mg
  - child 5–10 years 7.5 mg
  - child over 10 years 10 mg.
- The parents of some children with poorly controlled epilepsy will carry rectal diazepam. As part of pre-treatment preparation, it is wise to arrange with the parent for them to be on hand to administer this should a fit arise.
- In the absence of rapid response to treatment, call an ambulance.

Diabetic emergencies

The medical history should be used to assess the diabetic control achieved by the patient. A history of recurrent hypoglycaemic episodes and markedly varying blood glucose levels (from the patient's measurements) suggest that a patient attending for treatment is more likely to develop hypoglycaemia. It is wise to treat diabetic patients first on any list and ensure that they have had their normal medication and something to eat prior to attending.

Signs and symptoms of hypoglycaemia

- Trembling
- Hunger
- Sweating
- Headache
- Slurring of speech

- 'Pins and needles' in lips and tongue
- Aggression and/or confusion
- Seizures
- Unconsciousness.

Treatment of hypoglycaemia

- Lay the patient flat (remember A, B, C).
- If the patient is conscious, give oral glucose (3 lumps of sugar or 2–4 teaspoons of sugar) or GlucoGel®.
- If the patient is unconscious give 1 mg glucagon intramuscularly (or subcutaneously).
- Get medical help.

Patients who do not respond to glucagon (a rarity) or those who have exhausted their supplies of liver glycogen will require 20 ml of intravenous glucose solution (20–50%) and should be managed under medical supervision. It can take glucagon 5–10 minutes to be effective and the patient's airway must be protected at all times. Once the patient regains consciousness and has an intact gag reflex, they should be given glucose orally and, if possible, a high carbohydrate food.

The principle of treatment of hyperglycaemia is through intravenous rehydration. This should be carried out under medical supervision.

Allergies/Hypersensitivity reactions

Anaphylaxis

Anaphylaxis is a type I hypersensitivity reaction involving IgE. Free antigen binds to IgE, leading to the release of vasoactive peptides and histamine. Penicillin and latex are the most likely causes in oral surgery. Local anaesthetics are rarely responsible.

Signs and symptoms

- Itchy rash/erythema
- Facial flushing or pallor
- Upper airway (laryngeal) oedema and bronchospasm leading to stridor, wheezing and possibly hoarseness
- A respiratory arrest may occur, leading to cardiac arrest
- Vasodilatation leading to low blood pressure and collapse, which may progress to cardiac arrest.

Initial treatment

- The ABCDE approach should be used while the diagnosis is being made.
- Manage airway and breathing by administering 10 l/min of oxygen.
- Restore blood pressure by lying the patient flat and raising their legs.

In life-threatening anaphylaxis (hoarseness, stridor, cyanosis, dyspnoea, drowsiness, confusion or coma), adrenaline should be administered.

- Administer 0.5 ml of 1 in 1000 adrenaline intramuscularly and repeat at 5-minute intervals if no improvement.
- The optimum site for injection is the anterolateral mid-third of the thigh but the deltoid muscle may be used.

Chlorphenamine (antihistamine) and hydrocortisone (steroid) need not be given by non-medical 'first responders'. As a result, the only drug required to be administered by dental practitioners is adrenaline. The other drugs may be administered if the practitioner is competent to do so.

Many patients with a history of anaphylactic reactions carry an EpiPen, which contains 300 µg of epinephrine. This may be used if such a patient has an anaphylactic reaction in the outpatient department (Figure 4.5). Variation in the doses of adrenaline that may be given to different age groups are summarised in Box 4.7.

Angioedema

Angioedema is triggered when mast cells release histamine and other chemicals into the blood, producing rapid swelling, which may be life-threatening if the airway is involved. It may be precipitated by substances such as latex and penicillin. There is a hereditary component.

Hereditary angioneurotic edema (HANE) is caused by complement activation resulting from a deficiency of the inhibitor of the enzyme C1 esterase. It is

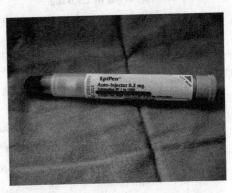

Figure 4.5   An EpiPen for use in anaphylactic reactions. It contains 300 µg of adrenaline.

Box 4.7   Variation in the dose of intramuscular adrenaline with age

- Adult (or child over 12 years) – 500 µg
- Child (6–12 years) – 250 µg
- Child (less than 6 years) – 150 µg
- Less than 6 months – 50 µg

usually inherited as autosomal dominant and may not present until adulthood. C1 esterase inhibitor concentrates are available to supplement the deficiency. Such supplements should be administered prior to surgical treatment.

Choking and aspiration

If a patient is suspected of having aspirated a foreign body, they should be allowed to cough vigorously in attempt to clear the airway and 'cough up' the object. An inhaled foreign body may lead to either mild or severe airway obstruction. Signs and symptoms that aid in differentiation of the degree of airway obstruction are shown in Box 4.8. In a conscious victim it is useful to ask the question 'Are you choking?' An algorithm for the management of a choking patient has been published by the Resuscitation Council (UK) and is given in Figure 4.6.

Back blows should be delivered by standing to the side of the patient and slightly behind. The chest should be supported with one hand and the victim leant well forwards so that when the obstruction is dislodged it is expelled from the mouth rather than passing further down the airway. Up to five sharp blows should be given between the shoulder blades with the heel of the other hand.

Box 4.8   Signs and symptoms that can be used to assess the severity of choking

General signs of choking
- Attack occurs while eating/misplaced dental instrument/restoration
- Victim may clutch their neck

Signs of mild airway obstruction
Response to question 'Are you choking?'

- Victim speaks and answers 'Yes'

Other signs
- Victim is able to speak, cough and breathe

Signs of severe airway obstruction

Response to question 'Are you choking?'
- Victim unable to speak
- Victim may respond by nodding

Other signs
- Victim unable to breathe
- Breathing sounds wheezy
- Attempts at coughing are silent
- Victim may be unconscious

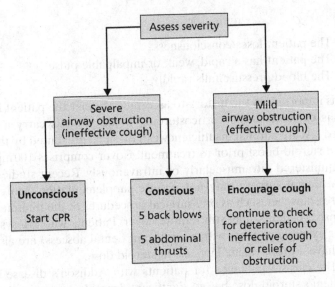

Figure 4.6   Algorithm for the management of a choking patient. The abdominal thrusts should not be used in children due to the risk of damaging organs.

After each back blow a check should be made to see if the obstruction has been relieved.

If back blows fail, up to five abdominal thrusts should be given.

- Stand behind the victim and put both arms around the upper part of the abdomen and lean them forwards.
- The rescuer's fist should be clenched and placed between the umbilicus and lower end of the sternum.
- The clenched fist should be grasped with the other hand and pulled sharply inwards and upwards.
- This should be repeated up to five times.
- The back blows and abdominal thrusts should be continued in a cyclical fashion.

If it is suspected that a foreign body has been inhaled the patient must be referred for chest radiography. Radiographs will be taken in two planes (postero-anterior and lateral). The foreign body is most likely to be seen in the right lung or right main bronchus, as the latter is more vertical than the left. Bronchoscopy or even thoracotomy may be needed to retrieve it.

Adrenal insufficiency

Adrenal crisis is discussed in Chapter 3. It is rare that this would happen as a result of dental treatment and if a patient collapses other causes are much more likely and should be considered first.

Signs and symptoms of adrenal crisis

- The patient loses consciousness.
- The patient has a rapid, weak or impalpable pulse.
- The blood pressure falls rapidly.

It is important in the history to ascertain whether the patient has recently used or is currently using corticosteroids. Some patients carry a 'steroid warning card'. Acute adrenal insufficiency can often be prevented by the administration of a steroid boost prior to treatment. Cover comprises 100 mg hydrocortisone administered intramuscularly or intravenously. Recent studies have suggested that dental surgery may not require supplementation. More invasive procedures, however, such as oral surgical procedures or the treatment of very apprehensive patients, may still require cover. Patients who are systemically unwell (for example patients with a significant dental abscess) are also recommended to have a prophylactic increase in steroid dose.

The current guidance for patients with Addison's disease is to double the patient's steroid dose before significant dental treatment under local anaesthesia and continue this for 24 hours.

Treatment of adrenal crisis

- Lay the patient flat and raise their legs.
- Ensure a clear airway and administer oxygen.
- Get help.
- If competent, give 200 mg hydrocortisone intravenously.

Stroke

Stroke may be either haemorrhagic or embolic in aetiology but clinically the effects are essentially the same. Signs and symptoms vary according to the site of brain damage. There may be loss of consciousness and weakness of limbs on one side of the body. One side of the face may become weak. As stroke causes an upper motor neurone lesion the forehead muscles of facial expression will be unaffected. Speech may become slurred.

Initial management

- The airway should be maintained and medical review arranged.
- High flow oxygen (10 l/min) should be given.
- The patient should be carefully monitored for any further deterioration.

Local anaesthetic emergencies

Allergy to local anaesthetic is rare but should be managed as any other case of anaphylaxis. When taken in the context of the number of local anaesthetics administered, complication rates are low. The signs and symptoms in allergy are those of anaphylaxis.

Fainting in association with the injection of local anaesthetic is more common and can usually be avoided by administering the local anaesthetic while the patient is supine.

Conclusions

Medical emergencies can occur at any time and the surgeon must be proficient at diagnosing them and instigating initial management. A sound knowledge of the potential signs and symptoms of medical emergencies and regular updates facilitate safe practice.

References

Medical Emergencies and Resuscitation Standards for Clinical Practice and Training for Dental Practitioners and Dental Care Professionals in General Dental Practice – a statement from the Resuscitation Council (UK) July 2006. Revised May 2008. Resuscitation Council (UK) (www.Resus.org.uk).

Chapter 5
Pharmacology and Oral Surgery

- Preoperative medication
- Perioperative medication
- Postoperative medication
- Traumatic injuries
- Infections
- Medication of packs for socket
- Adverse drug reactions
- Impact of prescribed medication on the practice of oral surgery

The successful practice of oral surgery depends on the use of certain drugs. Principally these are medications involved in the management of pain and anxiety, and in control of infection. These drugs may be:

- administered by the dentist or oral surgeon
- recommended for purchase over the counter by the dentist
- prescribed by the dentist.

Many drugs that the dentist can prescribe (such as ibuprofen and paracetamol) are cheaper when bought over the counter. When prescribing any drug it is important to consider the following points.

The pharmacological action of the drug

At no time should any drug be prescribed if its action is not clearly understood. In this respect side effects should be carefully considered. The *British National Formulary*, published twice-yearly and available online at http://bnf.org/bnf/index.htm, gives a good outline of action and side effects. It should be consulted if there is any doubt about the suitability of a particular drug or any possible interactions. There is a specific formulary for children. It is a good principle to have a repertoire of a few well-tried drugs, which meet the needs of day-to-day practice, and to understand them well, rather than to experiment with a wide range.

Principles of Oral and Maxillofacial Surgery, 6th Edition. Edited by U. J. Moore
© 2011 Blackwell Publishing Ltd

Contraindications and incompatibility of drugs

In certain medical conditions some drugs are contraindicated, for example aspirin in severe renal disease. Incompatibility of drugs only arises occasionally, though it should be borne in mind, but a more common and dangerous complication is an anaphylactic reaction in those patients sensitive to a drug (e.g. penicillin). It is therefore important to question the patient carefully about previous treatment and reactions, and any history of urticaria or asthma, as sufferers from these conditions seem more likely to be sensitive. Wherever there is doubt about the proposed drug an alternative should be used.

Dosage

Today the formularies make it unnecessary to give details of the constituent parts of medicines, but the correct title and strength of the drug, together with the four 'Hows' must be clearly stated.

- *How much* of the drug is to be taken in each individual dose.
- *How often* it is to be taken, expressed as the number of doses in each 24 hours.
- *How long* the course is to run, expressed in days, so that it is not continued overlong or stopped before the clinician thinks fit.
- *How* it is to be administered, by mouth, intramuscularly, etc.

The *British National Formularies* give suggested doses of accepted remedies for adults and children, to which reference should be made before prescribing. Excretion of drugs in the elderly may be slow and particular care is needed when prescribing drugs for them.

The importance of giving adequate doses for a specific purpose cannot be overstressed. Low doses must be avoided if drug therapy is to be effective.

An example of wording on a prescription is shown in Figure 5.1.

Methods of administration

The routes of administration of a drug are divided into enteral and parenteral. Enteral routes are gastrointestinal and include:

- oral
- sublingual
- rectal.

Parenteral modes of administration are:

- topical
- inhalational
- by injection: subcutaneous or intramuscular
- by intravenous infusion.

Dentists may use some of these routes to administer drugs. The timing of the administration of drugs can be divided into:

- preoperative
- perioperative
- postoperative.

Preoperative medication

Preoperative drugs may be used for the following reasons:

- anxiolysis
- pre-emptive analgesia
- prophylaxis to prevent infection.

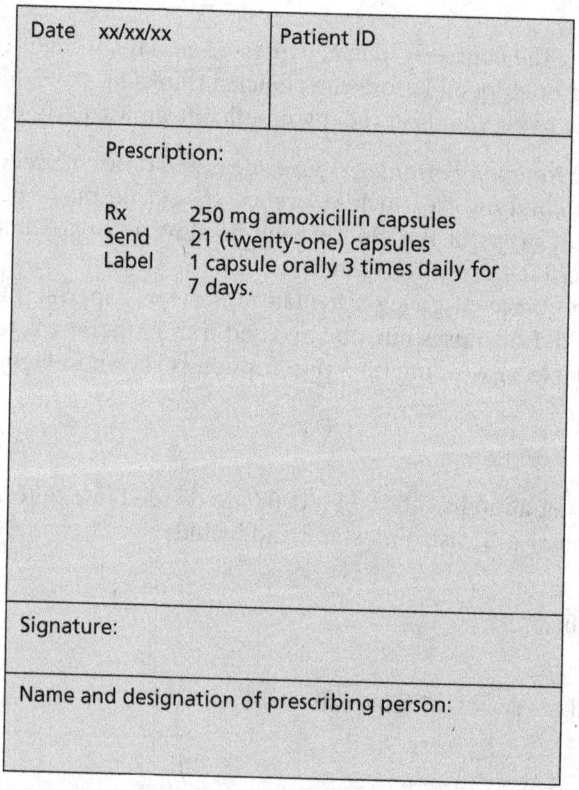

Date xx/xx/xx	Patient ID
Prescription: Rx 250 mg amoxicillin capsules Send 21 (twenty-one) capsules Label 1 capsule orally 3 times daily for 7 days.	
Signature:	
Name and designation of prescribing person:	

Figure 5.1   Prescription for 250 mg amoxicillin capsules. Note the simple explicit language used.

Anxiolysis

The most commonly used drugs at present for reduction of anxiety prior to surgical treatments are the benzodiazepines. When used for this purpose these drugs are taken orally. In addition to producing anxiolysis these agents are also hypnotics and thus can ensure a good night's sleep prior to surgery. Commonly used preparations for anxiolysis are diazepam and temazepam. Nitrazepam is a good hypnotic. In children, chloral hydrate may be useful.

Pre-emptive analgesia

Postoperative pain is a consequence of most surgical procedures, and operations performed in the mouth and jaws are no exception. The initiators of the pain process are produced by tissue damage. Therefore it is sensible to obtain adequate plasma levels of analgesic drugs at the time of tissue damage. Thus analgesics should begin prior to surgery. Non-steroidal analgesics such as ibuprofen taken orally 40 minutes before surgery or diclofenac administered per rectum in those having general anaesthesia should be considered.

Some operators prescribe corticosteroids preoperatively in an attempt to reduce postoperative swelling. In some instances this is legitimate; however, for routine surgical procedures such as the removal of impacted third molar teeth it is probably unwarranted.

Infection prophylaxis

The use of antibiotics prior to oral surgical procedures may be used to prevent infection of the surgical wound. Wound infection is not common after oral surgical procedures and thus antibiotics are not routinely prescribed. The indications for the use of prophylactic antibiotics to prevent wound infection are:

- in a patient with reduced host resistance
- when inserting foreign material (implants)
- transplantation of teeth
- for procedures lasting longer than 2 hours.

When prescribing antibiotics for the prevention of wound infection it is important to administer a bactericidal antibiotic at the correct dose at the correct time. Maximal plasma levels of the drug should be present at the time the blood clot is forming. This is achieved by administering at least twice the normal therapeutic dose orally 1 hour before clot formation is anticipated, or intravenously during the procedure. A single dose is sufficient. The use of antibiotics to *prevent* wound infection after clot formation has occurred does not make sense. A suitable drug for use in wound prophylaxis is amoxicillin; in those allergic to penicillin a single dose of clindamycin is an alternative.

The use of antibiotics to prevent infection at a distant site (such as damaged heart valves) from a bacteraemia resulting from an oral surgery procedure has been abandoned in the UK following recommendations from the National Institute for Health and Clinical Excellence (NICE), but this stance is not necessarily adopted in other parts of the world.

Perioperative medication

Sedative and anaesthetic drugs are used to allow the successful practice of oral surgery. The use of general anaesthesia for minor oral surgical procedures in adults should be discouraged. Nevertheless, this form of anaesthesia is still required for major procedures and for some minor operations in young children. However, even in children, the use of sedation enables operations that previously were performed under general anaesthesia to be carried out.

Intravenous sedation

The drug of choice in adults at present is the benzodiazepine midazolam, although other drugs such as propofol are used in some centres.

Midazolam is administered intravenously in 1.0 mg increments every minute until a state of sedation is reached. The average dose for sedation is in the range 0.07–0.1 mg/kg. Local anaesthetic may then be administered. Propofol is delivered by slow intravenous diffusion. This can be regulated by the operator, the patient, or effect-site controlled.

When performing intravenous sedation a second appropriately trained person must be present throughout the procedure, and adequate chaperoning of the patient must be arranged. Monitoring the patient's responses both visually and mechanically is essential when performing intravenous sedation; the use of a pulse oximeter is considered essential. Oxygen, adequate suction equipment and the benzodiazepine reversal agent flumazenil must be at hand. Intravenous sedation with midazolam provides between 30 minutes and 1 hour of sedation and this is ideal for many oral surgery procedures. In addition to the sedative properties of midazolam it is an excellent amnesic drug. Patients must be advised prior to the sedation appointment that on the day of surgery they should not drive, operate machinery or sign important legal documents. In addition an appropriate adult must accompany them home after they are sedated.

Inhalation sedation (relative analgesia)

Although inhalation sedation is used in adults for oral surgery it is more commonly used in children. In addition to producing sedation, the mixture of nitrous oxide and oxygen produces a degree of pain control in its own right (hence the name relative analgesia). In this technique the gaseous mixture is inhaled via a nasal mask. The concentration of nitrous oxide in the mixture is slowly increased until an appropriate level of sedation is achieved. Usually the concentration of nitrous oxide in the inhaled gas is in the range 30–50%. The use of inhalation sedation in combination with local anaesthesia allows the performance of some procedures in children that might otherwise require general anaesthesia.

Local anaesthesia

Local anaesthetic drugs may be used to reduce operative pain either alone or in combination with sedation or general anaesthesia. The use of local anaesthesia during general anaesthesia offers a number of advantages. These include:

- reduced dose of general anaesthetic
- operative haemostasis
- reduced postoperative pain
- reduced postoperative analgesic intake.

When used alone for operative procedures local anaesthetics can be used:

- topically
- as infiltration anaesthesia
- as regional block anaesthesia
- as intraosseous (including intraligamentary) anaesthesia.

Since its introduction in the late 1940s the gold standard local anaesthetic for most intraoral techniques in many countries including the UK is 2% lidocaine with adrenaline (epinephrine). This provides reliable anaesthesia following injection and good haemostasis. The introduction of 4% articaine with adrenaline into the UK in the late 1990s has led to a re-evaluation of the role of 2% lidocaine with adrenaline. Indeed, the former is the most commonly used dental local anaesthetic in some countries such as France and Germany. In most studies, 2% lidocaine and 4% articaine have similar efficacy. The only technique in which the latter has been shown consistently to be superior is in obtaining pulpal anaesthesia in the mandibular permanent dentition after buccal infiltration in the lower jaw. The concentration of adrenaline varies in different parts of the world (in the UK 1:80000 is the standard when used with 2% lidocaine; in other countries 1:50000 to 1:200000 are used). The maximum dose of lidocaine is 4.4 mg/kg. When adrenaline has to be avoided, an alternative vasoconstrictor is felypressin, which is supplied in combination with the local anaesthetic agent prilocaine (3% prilocaine with 0.03 IU/ml felypressin). The maximum dose of prilocaine is 6.0 mg/kg. If a vasoconstrictor-free solution must be used (for example if local vascularity is severely compromised after therapeutic irradiation) then 4% prilocaine plain or 3% mepivacaine plain are the solutions of choice. The maximum dose of mepivacaine is 4.4 mg/kg.

When performing surgical procedures that produce significant postoperative pain, the use of a long-acting local anaesthetic should be considered. Drugs such as bupivacaine and levobupivacaine can produce long-lasting anaesthesia (6–8 hours) when administered as a regional block. Bupivacaine is available as 0.25% and 0.5% solutions plain and with adrenaline at a dose of 1:200000. The maximum dose of bupivacaine is 1.3 mg/kg. It should be noted that conventional preparations such as lidocaine and articaine produce better operative anaesthesia than the long-acting solutions, so drug combinations may need to be used.

Control of haemorrhage

Appropriate prophylactic measures to reduce postoperative haemorrhage must be taken in the at-risk patient, for example the provision of platelets to those who are thrombocytopaenic. Physical measures such as suturing, packing with haemostatic gauze and diathermy are also important in arresting bleeding in the oral surgery patient. Tranexamic acid is a useful outpatient pharmacological adjunct. A 5% solution can be used postoperatively as a mouthwash four times a day for two days to reduce fibrinolysis that can cause early postoperative bleeding. The effect of prescribed medication on haemostasis is discussed below.

Postoperative medication

Postoperative problems following oral surgery include pain, swelling, trismus and (if a general anaesthetic has been used) nausea. Some of these problems can be prevented by pre-emptive medication and a careful surgical technique. Postoperative analgesic medication is usual after some procedures.

Postoperative analgesia

Most of the pain caused by oral surgery is inflammatory in nature. Therefore analgesic drugs with an anti-inflammatory action are recommended. The mainstays of postoperative analgesia therapy are non-steroidal anti-inflammatory drugs (NSAIDs) such as aspirin, ibuprofen and diclofenac. In patients who cannot take this type of medication paracetamol is the second choice. Patients should be advised to take analgesics following surgery as a routine if that particular procedure is known to produce pain. Third molar surgery, for example, can produce significant pain for three days after surgery, therefore patients having this procedure should be prepared to take analgesics for this time and not wait for the discomfort to occur. The use of opioid analgesics for post-oral surgery pain is not as effective as the anti-inflammatory type; indeed, some opioids have been shown to be less effective than placebo following the removal of lower third molar teeth.

Postoperative vomiting

Nausea may occur after a general anaesthetic and this can be controlled by the use of an intravenous antiemetic medication such as ondansetron or the intramuscular agent prochlorperazine. Although oral antiemetic preparations are available, their use in the control of postoperative vomiting is unlikely to be successful.

Traumatic injuries

See also Chapter 14.

Analgesics and hypnotics

In traumatic injuries these may be prescribed as necessary, provided the patient's reflexes are not so depressed that the airway may obstruct from bleeding or other causes. Similarly, in a suspected head injury, opiate analgesics or sedative drugs could mask the signs of progressive intracranial pressure and thus are to be avoided. All drugs given to patients must be carefully recorded and if the patient is transferred elsewhere the record must be sent with them.

Antibiotics

Antibacterial drugs are used prophylactically for a few days where there is a large haematoma that may become infected, and for a longer period where the deeper tissues, and particularly bone, have been contaminated.

In maxillary fractures that involve the cranial fossae with loss of cerebrospinal fluid (CSF) through the nose, ears or pharynx, the use of prophylactic antibiotics to prevent intracranial infection is controversial.

In all penetrating wounds contaminated with road dirt or soil, the need for tetanus prophylaxis must be considered. In patients who have not been immunised or where 10 years have elapsed since the last reinforcing dose, 0.5 ml of absorbed tetanus vaccine should be given by intramuscular injection

The common prescriptions of analgesics and antibiotics are summarised in Tables 5.1 and 5.2.

Infections

See also Chapter 12.

Antibacterial drugs play an important part in the treatment of acute infections but they should not be considered a substitute for any necessary surgery. They

Table 5.1   Some analgesic drug regimens

Drug	Oral dose	Oral dosing schedule	Intravenous dose	Intravenous dosing schedule
Aspirin	300–900 mg	6 hourly		
Codeine phosphate	30–60 mg	4 hourly	30–60 mg	4 hourly
Diclofenac	25–50 mg	8 hourly	75 mg	Maximum 150 mg/day
Ibuprofen	200–400 mg	6–8 hourly		
Paracetamol	500 mg–1 g	6 hourly	1 g	6 hourly
Pethidine	50–150 mg	4 hourly	25–50 mg	4 hourly
Tramadol	50–100 mg	4 hourly	50–100 mg	4 hourly

are useful as a preparation or adjunct to such treatment. The only cure for an infection is removal of the cause and this normally indicates a surgical procedure. The object of chemotherapy is to select the agent that gives the best therapeutic result with minimal side effects. In an ideal world this would be decided by determining the causative bacteria and assessing the drug sensitivity of those organisms. This is currently performed by culturing the bacteria and so an early result is not possible. Therefore most acute infections are treated empirically. Advances in the speed of bacterial typing will allow a more scientific approach in the future.

Once an antibacterial drug is chosen a regimen of sufficient concentration and duration that prevents formation of resistant strains is provided. A satisfactory concentration in the blood is obtained by administering the drug parenterally wherever possible, and a high initial 'loading' dose is to be recommended. The drug should be changed if there is no response after 48 hours. Generally the agents of choice are a penicillin such as amoxicillin, clindamicin or metronidazole. Combinations of antibacterial drugs must be used with caution. Some combinations are effective, for example amoxicillin and metronidazole. Drug therapy ceases when clinical resolution has occurred.

Medication of packs for sockets

It is often necessary to dress bone cavities after oral surgery. Medicaments may be used on ribbon gauze as a pack. Some agents that were popular in the past such as Whitehead's varnish (an iodoform) are no longer readily available; however, bismuth, iodoform and paraffin paste (BIPP) can still be obtained. BIPP may give rise to toxic symptoms from absorption of the bismuth, but this is most unusual on small packs in sockets, though it may occur if used on large packs in big cavities. Custom-designed medications such as Alvogyl, which contains a topical anaesthetic, and iodoform and eugenol may also be used to treat 'dry socket'.

In addition to local treatments the use of NSAIDs should be recommended to alleviate the discomfort of this painful condition.

Table 5.2 Some antibacterial regimens

Drug	Oral dose	Oral dosing schedule	Intravenous dose	Intravenous dosing schedule	Spectrum of activity
Amoxicillin	250–500 mg (3 g as loading dose)	8 hourly (2 doses 8 hours apart)	500 mg–1 g	6–8 hourly	Broad spectrum
Cefuroxime	250 mg	12 hourly	750 mg–1.5 g	6–8 hourly	Broad spectrum
Clindamycin	150–300 mg	6 hourly	600 mg	6 hourly	Gram positive cocci/ anaerobes
Doxycycline	100–200 mg	200 mg first day then 100 mg daily			Broad spectrum
Flucloxacillin	250–500 mg	6 hourly	250 mg–2 g	6 hourly	Beta-lactamase-producing staphylococci
Metronidazole	200–500 mg	8 hourly	500 mg	8 hourly	Anaerobes and protozoa

71

Adverse drug reactions

Occasionally a patient will report an unexpected adverse reaction to a drug or medicament. In an attempt to identify such problems at an early stage, a system of individual reporting of occurrences has been developed. The Committee on Safety of Medicines (CSM) collates the information and suitable forms for reporting will be found in the British National Formulary. When prescribing a medication to a patient it is essential to confirm that there is no allergy to that drug. Any concurrent medication must be recorded and potential drug interactions considered by reference to an authoritative source such as Appendix 1 of the British National Formulary. It is important to remember that even topical application of a drug can produce a drug interaction, for example the topical antifungal agent miconazole can increase the anticoagulant effect of warfarin to such an extent that spontaneous haemorrhage can occur.

Impact of prescribed medication on practice of oral surgery

See also Chapter 3.

Medications taken by patients can affect the mouth and perioral structures; for example, xerostomia is an unwanted effect of many drugs and others may produce lichenoid reactions. The practice of oral surgery can be affected by concurrent drug therapy. The two major areas of impact are in haemorrhage control and postoperative healing.

Drugs interfering with haemostasis

Anti-platelet medication

Oral surgery patients may be receiving therapy that interferes with haemostasis. Aspirin and other anti-platelet drugs such as clopidogrel and dipyridamole are not a concern and therapy does not need to be adjusted before surgery. A number of prescribed medications can produce a thrombocytopaenia as an unwanted effect and a full blood count is indicated if this is a concern. A platelet count of less than $50 \times 10^9/l$ precludes elective surgery and requires a platelet transfusion. When the platelet numbers are less than $100 \times 10^9/l$ it is wise to pack and suture extraction sockets to aid haemostasis. A suitable pack in such circumstances is Surgicel, which is oxidised regenerated cellulose and is absorbed during healing.

Oral anticoagulants

Outpatient anticoagulant therapy is provided by low molecular weight heparins or the coumarin warfarin. The low molecular weight heparins do not require alteration prior to treatment; however, warfarin therapy may need to be altered in conjunction with the patient's supervising physician. The efficacy of warfarin treatment is assessed by measuring the International Normalised Ratio (INR), which is a measure of the prothrombin time. A normal INR is 1.0. As long as the INR is below 4.0, straightforward treatments such as extractions can be performed provided suitable local measures such as packing and suturing are performed. An INR above 4.0 is outside the therapeutic range and the patient should be referred to their physician for amendment of therapy prior to surgery.

Drugs interfering with healing

Immunosuppressant and anti-cancer drug therapies can interfere with the production of red and white blood cells as well as platelets, as described above. If the white blood count is below $2.5 \times 10^9/l$ then prophylactic antibacterial drugs should be employed to reduce the chances of postoperative infection. In patients having chemotherapy for the treatment of malignant disease, the timing of surgery is important as such regimens are given in cycles. The choice of a suitable window period should be discussed with the supervising clinician.

Healing after many oral surgery procedures is dependent on both soft and hard tissue recovery. Bisphosphonate drug therapy can affect bony healing adversely. These drugs are used in the management of osteoporosis and in the prevention of hypercalcaemia secondary to malignant disease. Patients receiving such therapy (especially but not exclusively by the intravenous route) are at risk of bisphosphonate-induced osteonecrosis of the jaw following oral surgery. The best way to avoid such a condition is to avoid surgery by using excellent preventive measures; however, if surgery is required then close follow-up with use of antibacterial regimens, especially the use of chlorhexidine oral rinses, until complete healing occurs is essential.

Further reading

British National Formulary (published biannually) BMJ Group and RPS Publishing, London (available online at http://bnf.org/bnf/).

NICE (2008) *Prophylaxis against infective endocarditis. Antimicrobial prophylaxis against infective endocarditis in adults and children undergoing interventional procedures.* Clinical guideline 64 (available online at www.nice.org.uk/nicemedia/pdf/CG64FullGuidelineShort.pdf).

Seymour RA, Meechan JG, Yates MS (1999) *Pharmacology and Dental Therapeutics,* 3rd edn. Oxford University Press, Oxford.

Chapter 6
The Operating Room, Instruments and the Surgical Team

- The operating room
- Equipment
- Instruments
- Sterilisation
- The surgical team
- Sterile technique
- The operation
- The close of the operation

This chapter discusses the dental surgery or theatre, the instruments for oral surgical operations and the preparation of the surgical team.

The operating room

The operating room in both hospital and general dental practice should be of simple design, the walls and furniture should be made of easy-to-clean materials, and the equipment normally required should be accommodated without overcrowding.

It should be well ventilated and kept at an even temperature of 18–21°C, without undue humidity. In hospital theatres this is best done by positive pressure air-conditioning, which also prevents contamination from the outside atmosphere. There should be a recovery room with experienced nursing staff where the patient may recover on a bed or trolley within easy reach of

Principles of Oral and Maxillofacial Surgery, 6th Edition. Edited by U. J. Moore
© 2011 Blackwell Publishing Ltd

surgeon and anaesthetist until the patient is fit to return to the ward or go home.

Equipment

Light

The light source should provide adequate illumination without undue production of heat, and be easily adjusted to shine into the mouth. A headlamp or fibre-optic light attached to a handpiece is recommended for operations involving the palate or deep cavities such as cysts or the antrum.

Suction apparatus

No procedure, however minor, particularly under general anaesthesia, should be attempted without suction apparatus. This must be tested before the operation starts and whenever possible an alternative form of suction should be available in case of breakdown. Electrical apparatus is very powerful but does occasionally fail. Compressed air can also provide powerful suction in a similar way. Whichever method is used, a catchment bottle must be included in the circuit so that if roots or any foreign objects are lost the bottle may be searched.

Radiographic viewing box

This should be placed such that the surgeon can see it without moving from the dental chair or operating table. It should incorporate a spotlight. Digital radiographs will require a suitable computer terminal.

The dental motor (drill)

Though the conventional dental handpiece can be sterilised, its attachment to the dental electric engine or air motor presents a problem. The surgeon may be contaminated from the cable drive unless this is covered with a sterile sleeve. Alternatively, sterilisable surgical motors and handpieces are available, but due to their high cost these are usually only found in hospital practice. For the clean and rapid cutting of the bone without overheating it is necessary that the bur be washed by a continuous stream of sterile water. Handpieces with an integral irrigation system are available and provide automatic irrigation of the bur. The air-rota is not advocated for oral surgery due to the risk of contamination of the wound with oil and the introduction of air into the tissues, causing surgical emphysema. The modern electrical motor gives very adequate speed and torque.

The dental chair

This should be of a design in which the patient can lie flat and the operator may work seated, as this is the position of choice. The light, drill and suction should be sufficiently adjustable that they can be used with a supine patient from either right or left side.

Electrical equipment

Where this is to be used in the presence of anaesthetic vapours which may form explosive mixtures of gases, the equipment, particularly the drill, must be adequately sealed and earthed to prevent sparking or a build-up of static electricity which might cause an explosion.

Diathermy

Diathermy or electric cautery can be very useful in the control of haemorrhage encountered during surgery of the soft tissues. Monopolar diathermy uses a negative electrode on the body of the patient and is usually employed under general anaesthesia in situations requiring the greater current available. This is less localised than bipolar diathermy which uses current between the beaks of the diathermy forceps to achieve ablation in areas where it is important to reduce the local damage, e.g. around nerves.

Lasers

Modern lasers give excellent control for dissection of soft tissues. Cells in the path of the cut are vapourised with little damage on either side. Their principal advantage in excisions in the mouth is the relatively small amount of postoperative pain, and a reduction in tissue swelling. Stringent safety measures must be taken during the use of the equipment to avoid damage to the patient and the operators. Laserproof glasses should be worn by all personnel in theatre at all times when the laser is in use to protect the eyes. Under general anaesthesia the endotracheal tube should also be protected to avoid inadvertent puncture, and metal instruments should be avoided to decrease possible reflection of the beam.

Cryotherapy

Cryosurgery using liquid nitrous oxide, carbon dioxide or nitrogen destroys cells by intracellular ice crystal formation which ruptures the cell membrane. Healing of the tissue damage is by regeneration of normal tissue. It is of particular benefit in the treatment of benign soft tissue lesions and fluid-filled lesions such as haemangiomas.

Operating microscope

This is essential equipment for microvascular surgery and nerve repair and is increasingly used for apical surgery. Up to 40x magnification is possible.

Instruments

The selection of hand instruments depends on the surgeon's preference. In the succeeding chapters instruments suitable for the various procedures are suggested. It is the surgeon's responsibility to check that all those needed are readily available. They should be laid up on sterile towels on a trolley.

Care and maintenance of surgical instruments

The principles of care and maintenance are:

- to clean the instruments thoroughly
- to examine them for defects
- to repair or discard those that are defective.

Mechanical cleaning

Mucus and clotted blood may harbour and protect bacteria and make it impossible for steam to reach them. The first step in the process of sterilisation is to scrub all instruments until clean with a brush under a running cold water tap. A bath agitated by ultrasonic vibrations produces a very high standard of cleanliness, especially for hinged instruments and for suction tubes and heads. The latter should have cold water sucked through them immediately the operation is finished.

Cleaning also includes stripping down, cleaning and oiling all working machinery such as handpieces.

Examination for defects

Broken or bent instruments should never be used as their breakage during surgery can result in serious damage to the patient, either directly from the fractured ends or during the retrieval of the fragment (see Chapter 10). Disposable items, burs, injection needles and scalpel blades are discarded after use.

Sterilisation

- Kills all microorganisms
- Chemical or physical methods are used
- Steam at high pressure (autoclave)
- Boiling water only disinfects.

Physical and chemical methods are both in use today. Physical methods include wet and dry heat, and gamma radiation (used commercially for sterilising packed instruments such as scalpel blades). Boiling water is no longer regarded as a safe method of sterilisation as it only disinfects and does not kill sporing organisms.

Autoclaves use steam under pressure. Some are high vacuum but all depend on downward displacement of air by steam. Steam at $2\,kg/cm^2$ pressure gives a temperature of 134°C, which will destroy all organisms and spores within 3 minutes. It is the method of choice for dressing and towels, but they must be packed loosely to allow the steam to circulate. Blunting of instruments is due to oxidation, which should not occur in a properly functioning autoclave, so it can be safely used for sharp instruments. Vapour phase inhibitor (VPI) paper can be used to wrap instruments such as burs, which tend to rust if autoclaved. Handpieces must be cleaned and oiled before being placed in the autoclave. The oil must not become oxidised or lose its oily properties at high temperatures.

Dry heat is effective in ovens that have fans to ensure even heat distribution and a door-lock that prevents opening during the sterilising period. The cycle is much slower and it takes half an hour at 160°C to destroy organisms and spores. It may be used for sharp instruments and handpieces. Both autoclaves and hot-air sterilisers are made with controlled cycles that cannot be interrupted once started, so that sterility of the instruments is ensured. The efficiency of the cycle must be checked periodically by the use of Brownes' tubes.

Chemical sterilising is not regarded favourably by bacteriologists as most of the solutions available are not considered reliable. Glutaraldehyde is effective against vegetative organisms and spores if the instruments are immersed in it for 10 hours, after which it must be washed off with sterile water as it is irritant to tissues. Because of the length of the sterilising time and the irritant properties, the use of glutaraldehyde is confined to those instruments that cannot be heat sterilised. Glutaraldehyde or hypochlorite solutions may be used to disinfect instruments potentially heavily contaminated with viruses (such as hepatitis) before these are cleaned and sterilised.

Both gamma radiation and ethylene oxide are used commercially for the sterilisation of disposables such as scalpel blades and sutures, but their toxicity precludes their use in the surgery.

To sterilise with certainty, autoclaving is the method of choice. Dry-heat sterilising is the next best and only where both of these are impossible should chemical methods be considered.

Instruments packs

In hospital practice instruments are sterilised wrapped in paper containers. These are permeable to the steam in the autoclave and, providing the latter is of an evacuating type, are dry at the end of the cycle. Packs may be made up of one instrument or a complete layout for an operation, including towels. They can be stored for up to 6 months ready for immediate use. The packs are duplicated according to the frequency with which they are used and may be prepared for local anaesthetic injections, flap preparation, suturing and so forth. This system is seldom available in general dental practice, making it necessary to sterilise and lay up instruments for each operation separately.

The surgical team

- Surgeon
- Anaesthetist
- Assistant
- Nursing staff.

The surgeon

The surgeon is responsible for checking the identity of the patient and the nature of the operation to be performed, the operation and the surgical safety of the patient. Time out procedures are now performed routinely, in an effort to eliminate wrong site operations and ensure patient safety, when the patients ID is checked against the consent form and preoperative checklist. This task is paramount and the surgeon should devote every attention and effort to it, informing and encouraging the rest of the team to assist in the endeavour. This responsibility applies to any procedure, planned or accidental, inflicted on the patient, including those carried out by assistants. The surgeon must be informed and satisfied that all instruments, swabs and packs are accounted for at the end of the operation.

The others in the team should support the surgeon and always relate information that will either alter or facilitate the outcome (Figure 6.1). In a surgical emergency, where speed and efficiency are needed, the surgeon should take the lead in managing this.

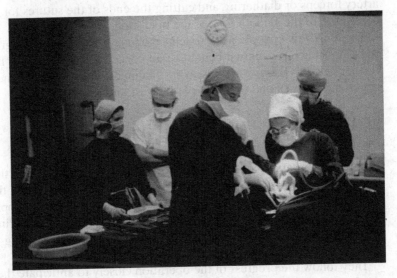

Figure 6.1   The surgical team. The surgeon is only one part of this, and cohesive working within the team promotes better care for the patient.

The anaesthetist

The anaesthetist assesses the patient's fitness for general anaesthesia, chooses the anaesthetic agent, prescribes suitable premedication and administers the general anaesthetic. He will supervise the moving of the patient to and from the ward, and on and off the operating table, as well as their recovery from the anaesthetic and such post-anaesthetic complications as may arise.

During the operation the anaesthetist is responsible for the patient's airway, which should include packing of the throat and the removal of the pack after operation. They should continually assess the patient's general condition and report any deterioration to the surgeon, so that a mutual assessment of the situation can be made. The anaesthetist's opinion about the safety of the patient is accepted and surgical procedures planned or modified accordingly.

The surgeon's assistant

The oral surgeon's assistant in the hospital theatre is either a qualified colleague or a member of the nursing staff. In the dental surgery assistance will usually be extremely effectively delivered by a dental nurse with appropriate training. The assistant will produce the patient's notes and radiographs, and help with the preparation of the patient, by cleaning and towelling up the operation area and assembling the suction and other equipment needed.

The assistant will retract tissues to give the surgeon the best possible access, clear fluid from the field of the operation with suction or swabs and remove solid debris with forceps. Assistance with haemostasis by applying pressure, artery forceps or diathermy, and cutting the ends of the sutures for instance all contribute to the smooth flow of the operation.

The longer two people work together the greater will be the degree of teamwork possible, with mutual benefit to all concerned. The surgeon may ask for further help in various ways. Involving qualified colleagues, using their previous experience, can extend their field of interest and responsibility.

The nursing staff

Before the operation begins the nursing staff will select and lay up those instruments, drugs and dressings they know to be necessary. They check the working of the dental engine and suction apparatus, and of all electrical appliances.

In the operating room they share the responsibility of ensuring that the correct patient is present and that the correct operation is being performed prior to its start.

They follow the progress of the operation closely to anticipate the surgeon's needs and inspect and clean instruments, drawing attention to any that become broken or damaged. At the beginning the end of the operation they count all swabs, packs, dressings, instruments and needles, and tell the surgeon if any are missing before the patient leaves the theatre or the outpatient surgery.

Preparation of the surgical team

Those taking part in a surgical operation must be free from infection, especially of the respiratory tract or skin, which could be transmitted to the wound. All are responsible for their own safety and must develop a sensible routine that avoids skin or conjunctiva from being contaminated by blood or saliva from patients. The use of personal protection equipment (PPE), at minimum gloves, masks and eye protection, are now mandatory.

Sterile technique

- Minimising contamination of the wound
- Wearing 'scrubs' and clogs
- Scrubbing up
- Sterile gowns and gloves
- Sterile instruments
- Preparing operation site with antiseptic solution
- Avoiding contamination during surgery.

Dress

All those entering a hospital operating theatre must change from their normal clothes into freshly laundered uniform trousers and shirt ('scrubs'). This not only reduces the risk of contamination but is cooler and more comfortable. The hair is covered with a paper cap and a mask is worn over the mouth and nose. Safety glasses should be worn to avoid splashing of blood or irrigation fluid into the eyes. Shoes are changed for rubber boots or clogs used only in the theatre.

In the dental surgery a sterile gown worn over everyday clothes is put on for each patient. A mask and protective glasses should be worn. The use of a cap is optional.

Scrubbing up

Those who have to handle sterile instruments or dressings must undertake the ritual of 'scrubbing up'. The arms are bared to the elbow and all rings and watches removed. The hands and forearms are washed under a running tap, using an antiseptic detergent solution (chlorhexidine or iodine based). They are well soaped and washed from the tips of the fingers up towards the elbow in a ritual that covers every area thoroughly. The fingernails must be kept trimmed short for satisfactory cleansing, which is done with a sterile scrubbing brush or nail scraper. The suds are rinsed away under the tap, being made to flow off at the elbow, not at the hands. This is continued for 4 minutes by the clock. The hands are then dried on a sterile towel by wiping from the hands up to the elbows. For minor procedures carried out in the dental surgery sterile gloves are put on and the operation commenced. For more extensive operations or where there is a risk of infection of staff and in theatre to conform with normal practice, a sterile gown and gloves are worn.

Gowning up

The sterile gown is lifted from its container folded in such a way that if held correctly with both hands at its neck, it will unroll and fall with the sleeves hanging away from the operator. The arms are then placed in the sleeves and a second person standing behind draws the gown over the shoulders and fastens the tapes and belt at the back. The belt avoids billowing and rubbing of the gown and is an antistatic precaution.

Surgical gloves are then put on. There is now a large selection on the market to cater for all aspects of surgery. Powder-free gloves are now the norm and alternatives for those who are latex sensitive or patients who are latex allergic are available. The gloves are taken from their envelope by the cuffs, which are folded down over the palms. The cuff of the right glove is held in the left hand and the right hand thrust in. The right hand then lifts the left glove by placing the fingers *under* the rolled cuff and the left hand is thrust in. The cuffs are turned back over the wrist to cover the sleeve. In this way at no time will the hands have been in contact with outside of either gown or gloves. From this moment if any unsterilised object is touched, the operator must gown up again.

Closed gloving further enhances the sterile technique. After gowning, both hands remain covered by the sleeves. The left glove, with its fingers directed towards the elbow, is placed with the palm surface against the left sleeve. The cuff of the glove is grasped through the material by the thumb and fingers of the left hand. The right hand (through the gown material) grasps the outer part of the glove cuff and turns it over the sleeve of the gown. The glove is drawn onto the left hand by pulling glove and sleeve up the forearm (Figure 6.2).

Preparation of the patient

In hospitals, a label carrying the patient's name, address and hospital number is attached to the wrist. The details should be checked against the patient's notes. A valid consent form must be available before the general anaesthetic is started. When local anaesthetic is being used mistaken identity may be avoided by direct questioning of the patient.

The patient's position on the table is adjusted if unsatisfactory, following which the operator then cleanses the site of operation, usually the mouth and surrounding skin, with a swab held in forceps and dipped in a detergent (chlorhexidine), care being taken to protect the eyes. The patient's body and head

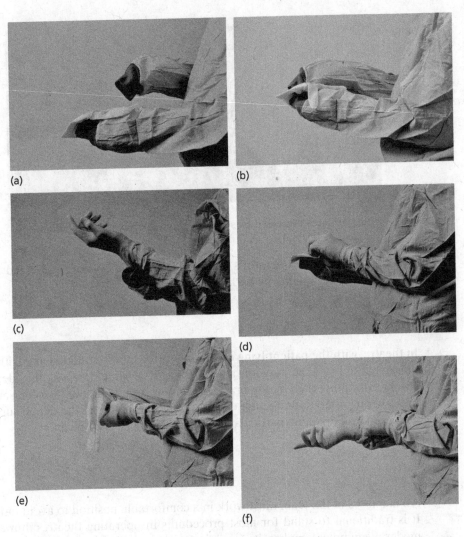

Figure 6.2 Donning gloves (closed glove method): (a) glove is placed over hand still within gown, fingers pointing up arm; (b) cuff of glove is grasped through gown by left and right hand, glove is pulled over left hand; (c) left hand is then thrust into glove; (d) left hand then positions glove on right hand; (e) and pulls glove over hand while; (f) hand emerges from gown into glove.

are then covered with sterile towels in such a way as to leave only the operation site exposed (Figure 6.3). For extraoral procedures the mouth may also be covered.

In the outpatient surgery the patient should be asked to wash the mouth thoroughly with a mouthwash and in the case of female patients all cosmetics should be removed. A sterile towel may then be pinned round the patient's neck and a sterile cap placed over the hair, to prevent contamination of the

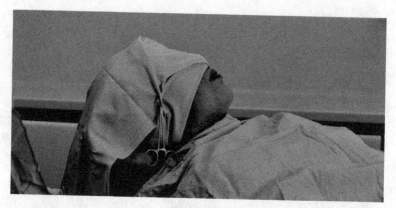

Figure 6.3   Patient is protected by sterile towels to reduce contamination.

instruments or of the operator's hands. The patient's eyes are protected from the light and instruments by dark glasses.

Preoperative check

In theatre, with the patient lying on the operating table, intubated and with the throat packed off, the surgeon and nursing team should repeat the identity checks, consulting the identity bracelet, consent form and notes as necessary to avoid wrong operations. Similar checks should take place in the dental surgery with the awake patient, particularly when sedation is to be given.

The operation

All members of the team must work in a comfortable position to avoid fatigue. It is traditional to stand for most procedures in operating theatres; however, modern equipment makes it possible for the surgeon and the assistant to work seated, which is much less tiring. With this in view the position and height of the table and chair, instrument trolleys and other apparatus are adjusted before the operation is commenced. In the dental surgery this should be done before the surgeon and their assistant scrub up.

The mouth can be held open with a rubber prop placed between the molar teeth. For operations under local anaesthesia a prop often helps the patient by resting the muscles and joints. Under general anaesthesia the mouth must not be opened by force because of the danger of fracturing teeth or damaging the temporomandibular joint.

Where the patient is given a general anaesthetic, teeth can be damaged or dislodged during induction. Special care must be taken by anaesthetists and surgeons where loose teeth are present.

The close of the operation

The surgeon refers to the notes to confirm that all the surgery planned has been completed and tells the anaesthetist of the completion of the procedure. It must be ascertained that all bleeding is controlled and that wound closure is satisfactory. Packs or drains to be left in the mouth or wound are securely sutured in place. The mouth is searched for any clot, debris or swabs and a final count is made of the teeth extracted, of swabs, needles and small instruments. With the anaesthetist's agreement the throat pack may be removed and the nursing staff should be informed also. Any debris is removed from the mouth and oropharynx, after which the patient is handed over to the anaesthetic team for the recovery phase.

The surgeon will then write up the notes of the operation. This is done immediately for the information of the ward staff and other colleagues. The value of this is particularly pertinent in an emergency.

Operation notes may be written in the following form:

Date

Name and number of patient

Time of commencement of operation

Surgeon and assistant named

Anaesthetist named

1. Anaesthetic. Local anaesthetic, general anaesthetic, type, pack used.

2. Operation described logically. Incision – reflection – bone removed – teeth extracted or fracture reduced and fixed, etc. – debridement of wound – closure of wound – sutures – dressings applied – removal of throat pack – condition of patient on finishing – time of completion of operation.

The assistant will remain with the anaesthetist to man the suction apparatus and advise about the operation site. The patient must remain under the supervision of the anaesthetist, preferably in a special recovery area, until sufficiently recovered to control their own airway. Initially the patient may be nursed on their left side in the recovery position to allow drainage of blood or saliva forwards out of the mouth, but should be fully conscious before returning to the ward.

It is usual in hospital practice for a nurse from the ward to fetch the patient from the operating theatre. The recovery nurse should hand over the patient, describing which procedures have taken place, showing the site of the operation, and giving instructions verbally and in writing for the immediate postoperative nursing. Both anaesthetist and the surgeon may be involved in this process if there are any special circumstances of which the ward should be aware.

The patient will be moved on a trolley equipped with an oxygen cylinder and mask and will be accompanied back to the ward by two people. One of these should be a trained nurse who gives undivided attention to the patient and in an emergency stays with them while assistance is summoned.

Further reading

Cottone JA, Terezhalmy GT, Molinari JA (1995) *Practical Infection Control in Dentistry*, 2nd edn. Williams and Wilkins Media, Philadelphia.

Experience of wrong site surgery and surgical marking practices among clinicians in the UK. http://qshc.bmj.com/content/15/5/363.full.pdf

Mulcahy L, Rosenthal MM, Lloyd-Bostock SM (1998) *Medical Mishaps: pieces of the puzzle*. Open University Press, Buckingham.

Sentinel events: approaches to error reduction and prevention (1998) *Joint Commission Journal on Quality Improvement* **24**(4): 175–86.

Chapter 7
Surgical Principles and Technique

Principles of:
- Painless surgery
- Asepsis
- Minimal damage
- Adequate access
- Arrest of haemorrhage
- Debridement (toilet of wounds)
- Drainage
- Repair of wounds
- Control and prevention of infection of wounds
- Support of the patient

The practice of surgery rests on certain fundamental principles which remain unchanged, though to apply them the surgeon may have to modify techniques to suit the anatomical field, the type of operation and the conditions obtaining at the time. The surgeon must have a clear and comprehensive knowledge of surgical physiology, the anatomy of the region being operated on and the pathology of the condition under treatment.

Principle of painless surgery

Today it is accepted that all surgery should be painless. This is important to avoid psychological and physical stress to the patient, which may predispose to shock, delay recovery and make surgery under local anaesthesia more difficult for the surgeon. In oral surgery, general anaesthetics are administered by a specialist in this field, whereas the oral surgeon is usually highly skilled in giving local anaesthetic injections.

Principles of Oral and Maxillofacial Surgery, 6th Edition. Edited by U. J. Moore
© 2011 Blackwell Publishing Ltd

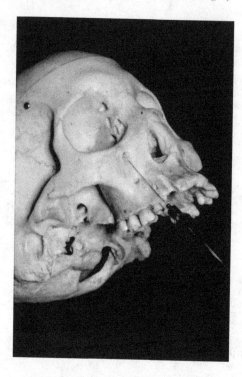

Figure 7.1 Position of needle for administration of infraorbital block. Note that this is consistent with the administration of a high infiltration above the maxillary canine.

It is outside the scope of this book to discuss the administration of local and general anaesthetics; however, the surgeon should strive to achieve local anaesthesia using block anaesthesia wherever possible, as this may save the patient considerable inconvenience (Figure 7.1). The choice between these will depend on surgical as well as medical considerations, and where doubt exists the decision should be made jointly with the anaesthetist. The patient and the anaesthetist may often have to be guided as to which is better in particular circumstances.

The indications for general anaesthesia are: first, when there is an acute or subacute infection which it is not possible to treat using regional block anaesthesia; second, where the operation involves several quadrants of the mouth, is lengthy, difficult or of an alarming nature; third, for young children and adult patients who are unable to co-operate. General anaesthetics without intubation should not be used for procedures expected to last more than 5 minutes, although use of a laryngeal mask can prolong this safely up to 20 minutes. As an outpatient procedure this is now almost entirely restricted for the treatment of children. Day-case surgery, where the patient is intubated and the postoperative period supervised by the nursing staff, is suitable for operations that can be completed within 45 minutes, allowing the patient to make a full recovery before discharge home.

Local anaesthesia is suitable for many minor oral surgical procedures. It is indicated where the patient has eaten recently and does not wish to wait and in certain medical conditions (such as chronic obstructive pulmonary disease, COPD). The combination of local anaesthesia and sedation with intravenous benzodiazepines, such as midazolam, is useful for the nervous patient. This technique requires well-trained staff and adequate recovery facilities. It should be treated in a similar fashion to a general anaesthetic and the patients prepared in the same way.

Principle of asepsis

Asepsis·is the exclusion of micro-organisms from the operative field to prevent them entering the wound. The patient's mouth, however, cannot be sterilised and remains a source of infection. A preoperative scaling and good oral hygiene practised before operation will reduce the chance of gross contamination; moreover patients seem to acquire a degree of immunity to their own oral flora.

The sterile instruments, fluids and dressings used in oral surgery are laid up on a trolley. Where pre-packed instruments are not used this must be done with sterile forceps. The surgeon and assistant should wear sterile disposable gloves and only those instruments laid on the trolley should be handled. A third person should be present to adjust the operating lights and position of the patient and obtain any further equipment required during the procedure. The patient's skin and mouth should be prepared with antiseptic to eliminate some of the bacterial load and towelled to avoid contamination from hair and nose (see Chapter 6).

Principle of minimal damage

Inexperienced surgeons often pay too much attention to the tooth, cyst or tumour to be removed and too little to the tissues left after surgery is complete. Certain radical operations may regrettably require the sacrifice of vital structures, but this does not often apply in the orofacial region, and damage or loss of function as a result of carelessness or lack of foresight is inexcusable.

The commonest causes of trauma are poorly planned operations with ill-designed flaps, a careless approach to bone removal and tooth extraction, and excessive use of force by the surgeon or assistant in dissection, retraction of flaps and in the use of elevators, burs and chisels. These practices increase postoperative pain and swelling and delay healing. They not only interfere with healing but increase the possibility of infection because they leave behind pieces of dead bone, tooth and mutilated soft tissues.

Principle of adequate access

Incision and flap

Access to the site of operation is gained by cutting the skin or mucous membrane and by dissecting through this incision to expose the underlying tissues. The site, size and form of the incision is planned to give the best possible approach with the least danger to important nearby structures. The operation completed, the flap has a second and equally important function, that of providing the first dressing to the wound. To do this it must be large enough to give easy access, be mobilised with sufficient subcutaneous tissue to give adequate support and bring with it a good blood supply. It should have healthy, clean edges that will heal by first intention. This means that, in the mouth, when the mucoperiosteum is reflected the mucosa and periosteum must not be separated. The incision must be so designed that it does not cut across the blood supply to the flap but includes the vessels that supply that area of skin or mucous membrane, otherwise the edges may slough and healing is delayed (Figure 7.2).

Where it covers a cavity in bone, it should be of such a size that when replaced the line of the incision rests securely on bone.

Incision

The scalpel is held in a pen-grip and the hand is supported against slipping. The incision is made with one firm, slow stroke of a sharp blade, which is kept vertical to the epithelial surface. The bow is used for cutting, where possible the point being kept above the skin or mucous membrane as a guide to the depth at which the incision is being made (Figure 7.3).

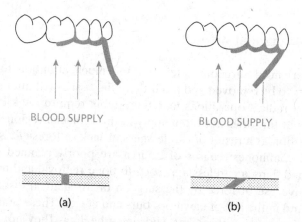

BLOOD SUPPLY   BLOOD SUPPLY

(a)   (b)

Figure 7.2   (a) Above: Correct design of the buccal flap to ensure a satisfactory blood supply to all parts. Below: Cross-section of satisfactory incision made with the scalpel blade vertical to the surface of the skin. (b) Above: Incorrect design of buccal flap. Below: Cross-section of an incision made with the scalpel blade held obliquely.

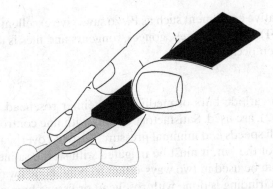

Figure 7.3   The scalpel held in the pen-grip and the bow of no. 15 blade used to make the incision. Note the fingers supported on the teeth.

The point is used at the beginning and end of the incision to ensure an even depth of cut along the whole length. Mucoperiosteum should be cut through its full thickness down on to bone at *one* stroke.

Dissection

The mucoperiosteal flap should be reflected with a periosteal elevator. An Ash or a Ward periosteal elevator may be used in this way; alternatively a Mitchell trimmer or Howarth raspatory may be used. Holding an instrument in both hands to both retract and elevate using a 'knife and fork' technique can be useful. The instrument is first inserted into the incision and, starting in the buccal sulcus where the periosteum is loosely attached, the first few millimetres at the edge of the flap are gently freed along its periphery. Thereafter, it is reflected evenly along its whole length by a clean movement, with the end of the chosen instrument pressed and kept firmly against the bone. Lifting movements are to be avoided as they tend to tear the tissues.

A skin flap is raised by separating it, with sufficient supporting tissue, from the underlying structures either by blunt dissection in a suitable tissue plane or sharp dissection using a scalpel or scissors. A combination of these techniques may also be employed. The essential point is to maintain an even depth of supporting tissue with an adequate blood supply and to avoid 'buttonholing' the flap. The deeper tissues are more usually explored by blunt dissection with either scissors or fingers, or where delicate structures are involved by separating each layer by gently packing wet gauze between them. Connective tissue, muscle and bone must be identified, laid open in turn, and all important structures identified and carefully preserved where possible.

Cutting of bone

In oral surgery the cutting of bone to give access is done with burs, the efficiency of dental handpieces and sharp burs giving superlative control. The use of innovative equipment such as Piezo saws give excellent properties of minimal damage. The use of chisels, gouges, rongeurs and files is declining but may also be used on occasion.

Burs

Tungsten carbide burs of medium size, either rosehead (Ash 7–16) or fissure (Ash 7–12), are used. Satisfactory cutting with fine control can only be attained using high speeds and minimal pressure. To avoid overheating of the tissues and clogging of the bur, it must be irrigated with sterile saline.

Burs can be used in two ways, either to grind bone away or to remove blocks of bone. Grinding is done with rosehead or fissure burs preferably used with a gentle sweeping movement over the whole length of the area concerned, thereby leaving a smooth even edge. Blocks of bone are removed using fissure burs (Ash size 7) to make cuts through the cortex into the medulla round an area that can then be freed with osteotomes.

Piezo

Ultrasonic equipment has been developed to allow minimal damage to bone while exposing an area by removal of a block of bone. This is less likely to damage teeth and soft tissues.

Chisels and osteotomes

These may be used in young patients, under 40 years of age, where the natural lines of cleavage along the 'grain' of the bone are present. In older patients (over 40 years) the use of chisels is contraindicated as the bone is brittle and the mandible may shatter in unpredictable planes. Chisels may be used either by hand or more usually with a mallet. In either case they must be supported firmly against slipping. Some resilience should be provided in the mallet, either in the handle or by use of a soft head.

The chisel may be used to plane bone away or to cut out blocks of bone. The direction in which the chisel cuts is determined by the angle of the bevelled surface. When used as a plane the bevelled face is placed against the bone and driven along at the required depth to shave off successive wafers. To remove blocks of bone the bevelled surface is usually turned towards the bone that is to be left).

Osteotomes are used to finalise cuts made with a bur or saw.

Chisels and burs

These may be combined by using a rosehead bur (size 7) to drill holes to the required depth at intervals of 3–5 mm along the planned line of the cut. The holes are then joined with a chisel and the cut deepened gradually till the bone splits off. This method is especially useful for removing large pieces of bone safely.

Rongeurs and files

These instruments are used mostly for trimming and smoothing bone edges when the operation has been completed. The rongeurs may also be used for cutting alveolar bone in alveolectomy and thin plates of bone such as those covering dental cysts.

Saws

Saws connected to either an air engine or electric motor can be used to divide the jaw in osteotomies or remove blocks of bone for grafting.

Retraction

Retraction has two objects, to provide free access for the surgeon and to protect the tissues. It is the most important task undertaken by the assistant, and if badly performed, can be a positive hindrance. The tissue layers divided by the incision and the dissection are gently held back with instruments (Figure 7.4). There should be no tugging or rough handling, for if this is necessary the incision is too small and needs to be enlarged. Retractors must not be moved without warning as they may accidentally obscure the field or deflect an instrument. To keep still for periods, without tiring, the hands must be in a comfortable position, if possible supported in some way. Thus the blade of the retractor under a mucoperiosteal flap should rest against the alveolar bone. The surgeon should pause at intervals to allow the assistant to rest and readjust their position.

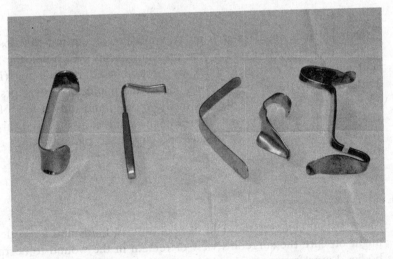

Figure 7.4 Retractors. Left to right: Kilner's cheek retractor, Bowdler-Henry rake retractor, Lack's tongue depressor, Laster's retractor for upper third molars, Ward's double ended retractor.

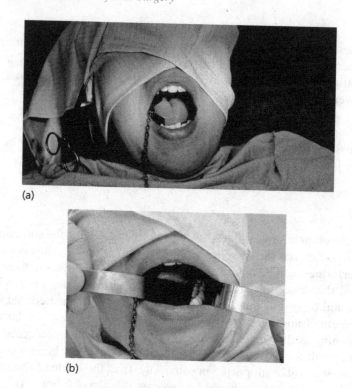

(a)

(b)

Figure 7.5 (a) Mouth prop in position between teeth with safety chain; (b) Lack tongue depressor and Kilner cheek retractor in position to allow access to left side of the mouth.

Damage may also occur from compressing or cutting the lips or cheeks against the teeth. To avoid undue pressure at any one point, the lips, tongue and cheeks are best held back by broad-bladed instruments (Figure 7.5). Unfortunately, this is more often done by the handles of retractors, the blades of which are holding back flaps in the mouth, and only a few of which are designed for both purposes. Sutures of thick silk can be passed through structures such as skin flaps or tongue and clipped to patient drapes to passively retract.

Cleansing the field of operation

The assistant cleanses the field of operation of fluids and loose debris, which might obscure the surgeon's view or remain in the wound to become foreign bodies. Large fragments should be lifted out with fine forceps as soon as they are seen, otherwise they may be lost. Blood, water and the minute debris from cutting hard tissues with the dental bur can be removed by suction. The tip of the sucker should be kept in one position, preferably at the point of dependent

drainage, as moving it continually can interfere with the surgeon's instrumentation and, if rapid, causes a visual kaleidoscope effect. At intervals sterile water
must be aspirated to prevent blood clotting in the tubing or connections. Larger
particles of bone or tags of tissue may eventually block the suction. This must
be cleared without delay as loss of suction can hinder the safe progress of the
procedure. The sucker should not be used as a retractor or to explore wounds
or sockets as it can cause damage and may encourage bleeding. The use of swabs
in similar circumstances avoids this.

Principle of arrest of haemorrhage

The natural arrest of haemorrhage and the pathological conditions that may
lead to abnormal bleeding together with their management have been discussed
in Chapter 3. At operation the arrest of primary haemorrhage may be achieved
by the application of pressure to the vessel walls, which to be effective must be
maintained for at least the time taken for the blood to clot.

Diathermy (electric cautery) or ligation with ties or metal clips can be used
on persistent haemorrhage and are particularly used in soft tissue surgery.
Haemostatis must be achieved progressively through the operation in order to
reduce blood loss to a minimum, before continuing the procedure into new
areas. Reactionary and secondary haemorrhage are discussed in Chapter 10.

Soft tissues

Digital pressure

This is particularly useful for capillary or venous bleeding and as an immediate
measure when a large vessel has been cut. It is applied either by compressing
the tissues, or the offending vessel, against bone, or in certain situations, such
as the lip, by exerting pressure between index finger and thumb. The lingual
artery may be controlled by drawing the tongue forward so that the artery is
pressed against the hyoid bone. The facial artery crosses the lower border of
the mandible where digital pressure may be applied.

Haemostats or artery forceps

Where a vessel is cut during operation it must be found swiftly and secured with
artery forceps. For small vessels the haemostats may be removed after twisting
two or three times, but on larger vessels they must be replaced by ligatures.

Ligatures

Direct ligature of a vessel is performed preferably before division. Artery
forceps are placed above and below where the cut is to be made and after
division, resorbable ligatures are firmly tied and the haemostats removed
(Figure 7.6).

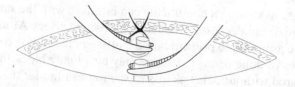

Figure 7.6   Use of haemostats. Note the position of the lower haemostats on the vessel so that after division the beaks curve upwards out of the wound (as on the upper haemostats) to facilitate passing and tying of the ligature.

In major haemorrhage from the jaws not controlled by local measures, it is on occasion necessary to ligate the external carotid artery. The collateral blood supply and anastomosis is so good in the face that it is often necessary to do this on both sides, if it is to be effective. A sufficient blood supply is still maintained by the other lesser vessels serving this area.

Packing

As a temporary measure ribbon gauze soaked in saline may be packed into operative or traumatic wounds and held under pressure for a short interval to arrest haemorrhage. Oxidised cellulose wound packs are useful to obtain haemostasis and may be left in the wounds as they are bioresorbable.

Posture

The position of the patient both during and after operation may help to reduce the blood pressure in the bleeding part. In dental haemorrhage the patient is kept sitting upright or propped up with pillows in bed unless shocked or fainting.

Electrocoagulation

This may be applied directly to the vessels or by passing the current through the artery forceps clamping the vessels. Monopolar diathermy uses an adhesive pad on the patient to complete the electrical circuit, whereas in bipolar diathermy current passes between the beaks of the specially insulated forceps.

Bleeding from bone

Capillary oozing from bone surfaces may be controlled by burnishing the bone with a small instrument or by applying hot packs prepared by soaking gauze squares in very hot water and wringing out the excess. Bone wax rubbed into the surface of the bone is also very effective in occluding small vessels, but should be removed prior to closure as it can cause foreign body reactions. Similarly, oxidised cellulose can be laid over the bone and left in situ.

Where an artery is bleeding from a bone surface it may be compressed by burnishing the surrounding bone to compress the vessel directly.

Principle of debridement (toilet of wounds)

The operation completed, the wound is prepared for closure by careful cleansing to remove debris, a major cause of postoperative infection. Pathological tissue, such as tooth follicle or sinus tracts, is excised. The bone cavity is saucerised where necessary, and the edges smoothed to leave a clean finish without sharp projections. The flaps are trimmed of all necrotic tissue or tags. Tooth chips and loose pieces of bone not attached to periosteum are removed from the wound, which is then thoroughly irrigated with saline.

Principle of drainage

Wounds need to drain freely after operation where they are contaminated or infected, where an abscess has been incised or where immediate closure is made over a dead space which may fill with blood or serum and subsequently become infected.

Fine superficial drains

These are made of pieces of rubber glove and are used in wounds of the face to allow escape of tissue exudate. They are usually removed after 48 hours (Figure 7.7a).

Larger superficial drains

Corrugated rubber or a Yeates drain is used in a dental abscess to keep the wound edges apart and allow thick pus to flow freely (Figure 7.7b). Though chiefly used for extraoral incisions and drainage, they are necessary for large collections of pus drained intraorally.

Vacuum drains

These are inserted at a point remote from the wound by means of a central sharp stylet. The stylet is then withdrawn leaving the tube drain in position. The latter is attached to a plastic bottle from which the air has been expressed. The advantages of vacuum drains are that they are inserted away from the operation wound and the negative pressure developed assists removal of fluid (Figure 7.7c and d).

Drains should be inserted into a cavity at its most dependent point and they must be fixed by a suture or some other device to prevent them falling out of, or being drawn into, the wound. They should be examined daily to ensure that they are patent and serving their function. They are removed when the discharge has ceased, usually between the third and seventh day. Long drains may be shortened before this, particularly when they are near major vessels, which they may erode.

An entry must be made in the patient's records of both when they are put in and when they are removed.

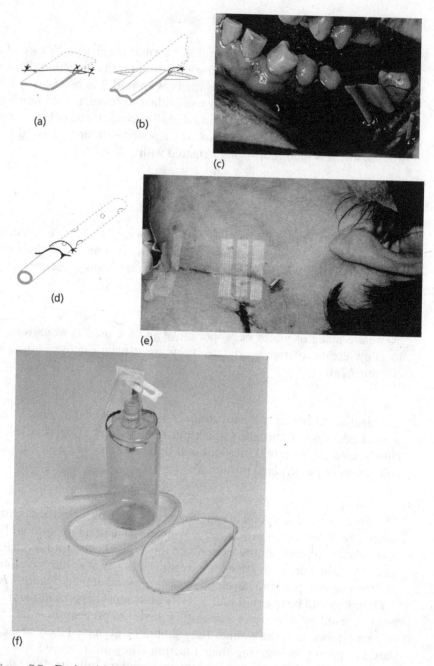

Figure 7.7 Drains: (a) rubber glove drain; (b) corrugated rubber drain; (c) drain in place after drainage of submasseteric abscess (see also Figure 12.7); (d) suction drains attached to vacuum bottles; an airtight seal must be achieved around the exit site of the drain by careful suturing; (e) vacuum drain in situ following removal of submandibular gland; (f) Readivac drain bottle with introductory stylet.

Principle of repair of wounds

Before commencing closure the surgeon makes sure that the operation has been satisfactorily completed, that bleeding is arrested and that all swabs, instruments and teeth are accounted for. Closure is carried out by suturing the wound, and many forms of needle holder, needle and suture material are available for this purpose.

Needle holder

The Kilner needle holder is commonly used in the mouth. The ratcheted handles provide a firm grip of the needle (Figure 7.8).

Needles

These may be round or triangular in cross-section; the latter are called 'cutting needles'. They may be of various shapes but the half-round or curved needle is used on the mucous membranes and skin of the face. The size of the needle should be such that it can be passed through the flap without ever holding it by either the tail or the point, where it may easily be broken.

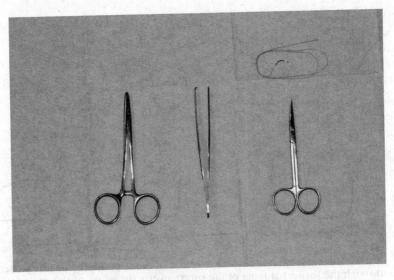

Figure 7.8 Suture kit. Left to right: Kilner's needle holder, Gillies toothed tissue forceps, suture scissors, and above, suture.

Suture materials

Manmade resorbable sutures are now most frequently used in the mouth. Vicryl® (polyglycolate) is available in conventional and 'Rapide' forms, giving support for several weeks or a few days respectively. Resorbable sutures have the advantage of not requiring removal and thus allay patient anxiety, but they can still cause some problems as they induce a mild foreign body reaction. Silk is economical and is to be preferred in the mouth if wound support is required for a precise period, although monofilament nylon sutures can be used also. Fine (5/0 or 6/0) nylon monofilament sutures are used for facial wounds.

Staples can be used for rapid closure of neck or scalp wounds but should not be used on the face.

Suturing

To suture the mucoperiosteum the edges of the wound are apposed to confirm that closure can be made without tension. Where one side is fixed to bone the first 3 mm of the margin are freed to make the passage of the needle easy. The flap is picked up and held everted with toothed tissue forceps applied at right angles to the free edge of the flap (Figure 7.9). A curved cutting needle (22 mm) with a resorbable suture (3/0) is passed through from the outer surface of the mucoperiosteum close to the tissue forceps, which splint the flap against the pressure from the needle. The suture must go through the periosteum and should be placed about 3 mm from the free edge to prevent it pulling out when tied. The other side is similarly everted and the needle passed through from the raw surface with an equal bite. To make sure that the final position will be satisfactory the margins of the wound are drawn together with the suture before

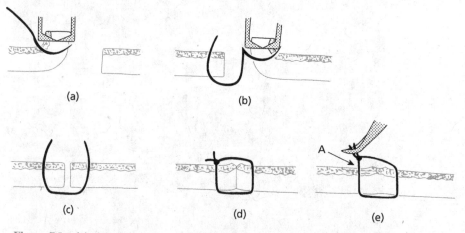

Figure 7.9   (a), (b) and (c) show eversion of the flap and the needle passed obliquely through the tissue; (d) tying of the suture everts the edges of the wound; (e) removal of sutures, by cutting at A and thereby avoiding drawing the exposed part of the suture through the tissues.

it is tied with a surgeon's knot (Figure 7.9). It should not be tied too tightly as this may cause the edges to overlap and because subsequent swelling may cause ischaemia at the wound margins. Sufficient sutures are inserted to prevent the wound gaping at any point.

Skin incisions are closed in layers, the fascial and muscle planes being identified and re-apposed with resorbable sutures such as polyglycolate, the knot of which should be tied inwards and the free ends cut very short to avoid irritation. The deep sutures should take all the necessary strain so that the skin lies in correct apposition and may be stitched without tension, which is a cause of scarring. It is very important that the skin margins are held everted with the raw surfaces in apposition to ensure rapid healing (Figure 7.9).

Types of suture

Simple interrupted sutures

Simple interrupted sutures are of almost universal application. They are inserted singly through each side of the wound and tied with a surgeon's knot (Figure 7.10). Several of these may be used at short intervals between 4 and 8 mm apart to close large wounds, so that the tension is shared and therefore not high at any one point (Figure 7.11a). When put in correctly they will evert the edges of the flap. Should one break or pull out, only this one need be replaced. The wound is free of interference between each stitch and is easy to keep clean.

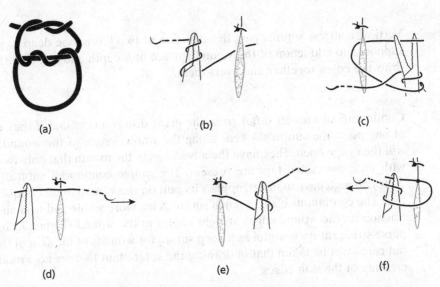

Figure 7.10 Surgeon's knot: (a) knot in detail; (b) first part of the knot made by passing suture round needle holder; (c) and (d) short free end grasped and knot slid off beaks; (e) and (f) second part of knot made by passing suture round the needle holder in the opposite direction.

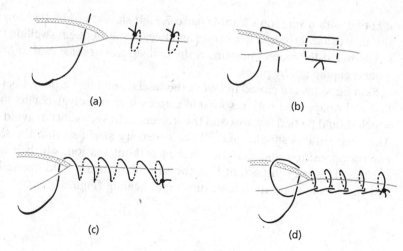

(a)

(b)

(c)

(d)

Figure 7.11   Sutures: (a) simple interrupted; (b) horizontal mattress; (c) simple continuous; (d) continuous blanket stitch.

Horizontal mattress suture

A horizontal mattress suture has the property of everting the mucosal or skin margins, thereby bringing greater areas of raw tissue into contact. For this reason it is useful for closing wounds over bony deficiencies such as oroantral fistulae or cyst cavities (Figure 7.11b).

Vertical mattress sutures

Vertical mattress sutures pass through skin at two levels, one deep to provide support and adduction of the wound surface at a depth and one superficial to draw the edges together and evert them.

Continuous sutures

Continuous sutures all suffer from the great disadvantage that if they cut out at one point the suture slackens along the whole length of the wound, which will then gape open. They have the advantage in the mouth that only two knots with their associated tags are present. The simple continuous suture (Figure 7.11c), though easy to insert, applies its pull on the wound in an oblique direction. The continuous blanket stitch suture is far more stable and firm and gives traction on the wound edges at right angles to the wound (Figure 7.11d). The purse-string suture is useful as a deep suture for wounds of the skin of the face, but care must be taken that in drawing the suture taut there is no wrinkling or creasing of the skin edges.

Knots

The knots used to tie sutures are the reef-knot and surgeon's knot. They may be tied with the fingers, but this is difficult to do in the mouth and it is important to master the technique of tying them with the needle holder as illustrated (Figure 7.10). The knot when tied must lie well on one side of the line of the wound.

Removal of sutures

Resorbable sutures in mucous membrane do not need to be removed but can be aggravating if retained for more than a week or two. In the skin, alternate stitches are often taken out about the third to fifth day and the remainder between the fifth and eighth days. A good guide is that as soon as they begin to get loose they should be taken out. They should first be cleaned and then removed as shown in Figure 7.9e.

Principle of control and prevention of infection of wounds

The incidence of postoperative infection will be reduced by careful preoperative preparation, an aseptic technique, minimal trauma and adequate drainage. Postoperatively, the tissues may be protected by the use of dressings.

In the mouth, surgical incisions are not dressed except where there is a deficiency of mucous membrane over bone, when packs are used to cover it. Small skin incisions are normally dressed with dry gauze, until the formation of serous exudate has stopped, when they are best left uncovered. More extensive wounds and abrasions may be covered with tulle-gras and dry gauze strapped into position with adhesive surgical tape. Where a drain is *in situ* extraorally, the discharge should be collected either in dressing gauze or in a stoma bag (Figure 7.7b).

Packs are used to protect exposed bone or to prevent skin or mucous membrane from closing over a wound, which should heal from its base by granulation. They can in no way serve as drains. Ribbon gauze impregnated with BIPP or Whitehead's varnish is packed firmly but not tightly into the cavity. When inserted under a general anaesthetic, packs must be sutured into place lest they come loose and obstruct the airway. They should not be changed too frequently and *both insertion and removal must be entered in the patient's notes*.

Antibacterial therapy

Views on the prophylactic use of antibiotics vary, but on no account should they take the place of an aseptic technique. In oral surgery it is impossible to obtain a sterile field and many patients present with acute or chronic inflammatory conditions such as advanced periodontal disease, pericoronitis or contaminated fractures. For this reason many oral surgeons prefer to operate under an antibiotic cover, but it should not be prescribed routinely. Each case must be assessed individually and bacterial culture and antibiotic sensitivity tests obtained wherever possible. The prescription of antibacterial drugs is discussed in Chapter 5.

Principle of support of the patient

The pre- and postoperative care and the general support of the patient have been discussed in Chapter 2.

Further reading

Cuschieri A, Grace P, Darzi A *et al.* (2003) *Clinical Surgery*, 2nd edn. Blackwell Science, Oxford.
Meechan JG (2006) *Minor Oral Surgery in Dental Practice*. Quintessence, London.

Chapter 8
Extraction of Teeth and Roots

- Examination and assessment
- Extraction of teeth
- Luxators
- Elevators
- Extraction procedure
- Extractions in children under outpatient general anaesthesia
- Fracture of the tooth
- The transalveolar approach
- Removal of roots after the socket has healed
- Arrest of haemorrhage
- Post-extraction instructions

Indications for extraction:

- Caries
- Periodontal disease
- Trauma
- Orthodontics
- Involvement in pathology
  - infection
  - cysts
  - tumours.

Tooth extraction is considered to be a straightforward procedure and in a large proportion of cases this is true; however, problems can be encountered that call for a high level of skill in order for the extraction to be carried out successfully and for healing to proceed uneventfully. Many of these potential problems can be anticipated through careful assessment.

Principles of Oral and Maxillofacial Surgery, 6th Edition. Edited by U. J. Moore
© 2011 Blackwell Publishing Ltd

Examination and assessment

After the initial history in which the justification for extraction is established, a full medical history is necessary before proceeding. Problems such as prolonged bleeding and patients whose jaws have undergone irradiation will require careful management. Other medical conditions that need special preparation, such as patients taking bisphosphonates and those with cardiac pathologies and any disease process affecting long-term healing, such as diabetes, are discussed in Chapter 3. Any previous difficulty with extractions, including postoperative bleeding or infection, is noted and if serious in extent investigated further.

Clinical examination

The patient's sex, age, general build and bone structure are significant. Heavily built men, have teeth difficult to extract, while in old age roots are brittle and the bone sclerosed, the so-called 'glass in concrete syndrome'. Access may be difficult in children who have small mouths and in patients with facial scars or trismus.

The tooth to be extracted is examined. Teeth malpositioned palatally or lingually, rotated, or inclined, or single standing teeth in occlusion, are all potentially difficult. Certain teeth frequently have abnormal root formation, particularly the upper and lower third molars. Heavily filled, root treated and dead teeth or those suffering from long-standing periodontal disease tend to become brittle. Periodontal disease predisposes to postoperative bleeding and infection. In acute ulcerative gingivitis or where the gingival condition suggests a blood dyscrasia, extractions may have to be delayed until these have been treated.

Radiographic examination

The nature of the root form and bone structure can only be determined from radiographs, and ideally these should always be taken before extraction. Radiographs are mandatory when the history or examination suggests the extractions will be difficult – this applies particularly to all lower third molars, partly erupted teeth and those that are malpositioned. Intraoral periapical views should show the whole of the crown, root and alveolus. Radiographs should demonstrate the relationship of the roots to such important structures as the maxillary sinus and the inferior dental canal (Figure 8.1). An orthopantomogram (OPG) can be a very useful scan view of the dentition but can lack some accuracy in certain areas of the mouth. Radiographs must be examined carefully as certain features, such as extra roots on molar teeth, are easily missed.

Assessment

All the findings on examination and radiography are considered, particularly the number, size, shape and position of roots and any signs of hypercementosis or resorption. The condition of the supporting bone, especially evidence of sclerosis, resorption or of secondary conditions such as apical granulomas and

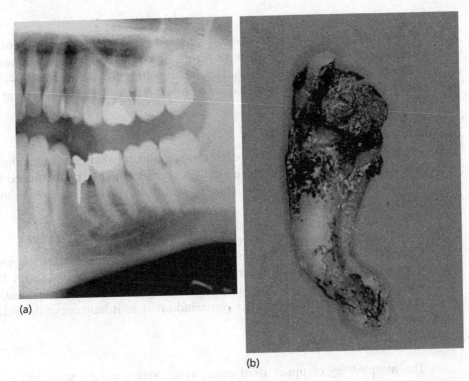

Figure 8.1   (a) Sectional orthopantomogram showing unusual curvature of lower left premolar (35); (b)the tooth was extracted by a junior student using a careful standard technique and shows that the radiographic appearance was accurate.

cysts, is noted. Where any of these complications occur the treatment plan should be modified to manage them.

Extraction of teeth

- Knowledge of tooth morphology
- Application of force related to tooth morphology
- Use of forceps
- Use of elevators to assist and facilitate
- Position of patient vital to success.

Tooth morphology

For the surgeon to extract teeth successfully it is important to understand the morphology of the roots of the tooth that is to be extracted. Only then can force be applied appropriately to remove the tooth (see Figure 8.4).

Upper incisors and canines

Upper incisors and canines have single, conical roots and are therefore rotated with a purposeful action, the forceps turning through as wide an arc as possible without damaging adjacent teeth. The upper canine, because its root is slightly flattened mesiodistally, can be extracted by an outward buccal movement if it is resistant to rotation.

Upper premolars

Upper premolars have either one strong root markedly flattened mediodistally or two fine conical roots placed buccally and palatally. They are extracted by a limited buccopalatal movement coupled with some limited rotation to avoid breaking the apices.

Upper first and second molars

Upper first and second molars both have three roots which are usually somewhat flattened. The palatal diverges strongly from the two buccal roots. They are taken buccally with a long, steady movement while the upward pressure is maintained. Palatal movement is contraindicated as it may cause the palatal root to fracture.

Upper third molars

The morphology of upper third molar roots varies widely; some are fused, others have three or more fine roots. They may be extracted in the same way as the other upper molars, but access can make them more difficult and the use of elevators obligatory.

Lower incisors and canines

The roots of lower incisors and canines are flattened mesiodistally and as the buccal plate of bone is very weak they are extracted with an outward buccal movement.

Lower premolars

Lower premolars and canines have conical roots and are therefore rotated.

Lower first and second molars

The roots of lower first and second molars are flattened mesiodistally. They should be extracted by a buccal movement while the downward pressure is maintained.

Lower third molars

A wide variation occurs in the root form of lower third molars and in their position in the mandible as they are often misplaced or inclined. Radiographs should always be taken before extraction, which may require an open or transalveolar approach.

Deciduous teeth

The upper and lower incisors and canines are extracted with the same movements used for their permanent successors. The molar teeth, however, have divergent roots that enclose the follicle of the developing premolar teeth and it is possible to remove or damage the latter when extracting a deciduous molar. Great care must be taken in using the forceps, which should not be driven too far up the periodontal membrane. They are applied to the tooth *root*, avoiding the bifurcation under which the permanent tooth germ nestles.

Where, owing to caries or a fracture of the tooth during surgery, a deciduous molar root is retained which cannot be grasped with the forceps, it may be extracted by applying a right-angled Warwick James elevator to the mesial aspect of mesial roots or distal aspect of distal roots to elevate them gently along their natural curvature. Should there be a risk of damaging the underlying permanent tooth, then the retained root is best left and the patient's parent told the reason.

Forceps

(See Figure 8.2)

Forceps are designed to apply appropriate forces to the teeth. They have two blades with sharp edges to cut the periodontal fibres. The blades are wedge-shaped to dilate the socket and are hollowed on their inner surface to fit the roots. They are made to various designs, and a range should be available so that a pair that is designed to fit snugly round the roots and have even contact with the cementum over a wide area may be selected. One- or two-point contact is bad and prevents the tooth being gripped firmly. They should engage only the roots and never the crowns of the teeth.

The blades are hinged, which allows them to close and grasp the root. The handles act as a lever, which gives the operator a mechanical advantage. The farther from the blades the surgeon grasps the handles the less effort they will have to make to apply force to the tooth. In order to drive the forceps blade straight up the long axis of the tooth, the shape of the handle is varied. Lower forceps have handles at right angles to the blades, upper forceps are straight for anterior teeth and cranked for the posteriors. For the upper third molars the beaks as well as the handles are bent.

Grip of forceps

The ergonomic use of force in tooth extraction relies on a good grip of the forceps. The hand positions shown in Figure 8.3 are guides and the operator must find a grip that allows free movement of the joints of the hand, arm and shoulder while maintaining the maximum amount of feedback from the forceps themselves. The forceps are perhaps to be considered as 'steel fingers' and the sensory feedback from the finger and thumb gripping the forceps is crucial in developing a progressive and sensitive technique.

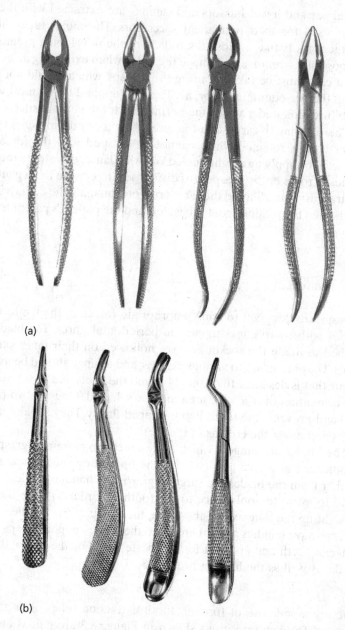

(a)

(b)

Figure 8.2 Extraction forceps. (a) Left to right: Upper straights, upper premolars, upper molars, bayonets; (b) side view of the same forceps to show increasing curvature to allow access to teeth further back in the mouth; (c) lower roots, lower premolars, lower molars, cowhorns. Note that only the beak design changes.

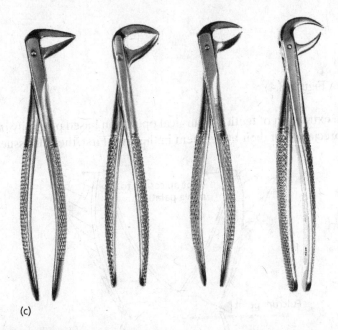

(c)

Figure 8.2 (Continued).

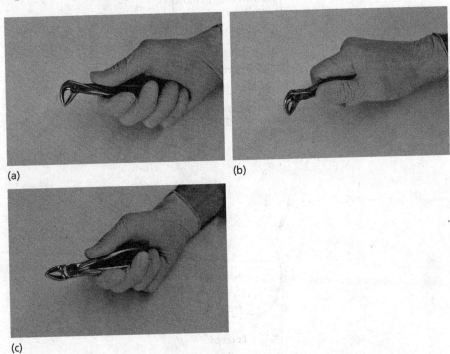

(a)

(b)

(c)

Figure 8.3 Holding the forceps. Note grip and position of finger and thumb opposed across handles to give maximum feedback during the extraction. (a) Method of holding lower forceps with thumb on top allows more directed pressure through long axis of tooth; (b) with thumb on side of handles it is easier to perform rotatory movements on operator's contralateral side, i.e. on teeth in lower left quadrant for right-handed operators. (c) Method of holding upper forceps. Palm is turned upwards to give most ergonomic and safe method of applying force buccally.

111

Extraction of teeth with forceps

(See Figure 8.4)

The extraction of teeth is a surgical operation based primarily on an anatomical appreciation of their attachment in the jaws. First, the soft tissues of the gingival

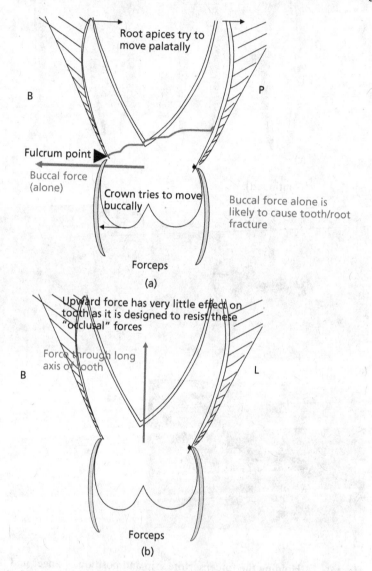

Root apices try to
move palatally

B   P

Fulcrum point

Buccal force
(alone)

Crown tries to move
buccally

Buccal force alone is
likely to cause tooth/root
fracture

Forceps

(a)

Upward force has very little effect on
tooth as it is designed to resist these
"occlusal" forces

Force through long
axis of tooth

B   L

Forceps

(b)

Figure 8.4 Movements in the extraction of teeth: (a) buccal movement; (b) force through long axis; (c) combined equal forces; (d) increased upward force; (e) lower molar; (f) teeth with round roots, rotational force by itself; (g) combined forces in round-rooted teeth; (h) upper premolars have unpredictable root pattern. Two-rooted variants can be extremely difficult to remove without fracture. A progressive steady technique must be applied using a constant upward force coupled with small rotatory or buccal forces.

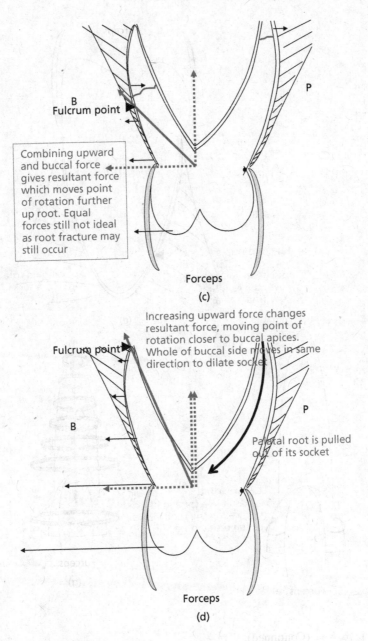

B
Fulcrum point

Combining upward
and buccal force
gives resultant force
which moves point
of rotation further
up root. Equal
forces still not ideal
as root fracture may
still occur

P

Forceps

(c)

Increasing upward force changes
resultant force, moving point of
rotation closer to buccal apices.
Whole of buccal side moves in same
direction to dilate socket

Fulcrum point

B

P

Palatal root is pulled
out of its socket

Forceps

(d)

Figure 8.4 (Continued).

attachment and periodontal membrane are cut to separate the tooth from bone.
Next, the socket is dilated either by applying a force to the bone with instruments, such as luxators (Figure 8.7) or Coupland elevators (Figure 8.7), with
wedge-shaped blades that are driven along the periodontal membrane, or by
applying force to the root, which then expands its bony socket. Finally when the

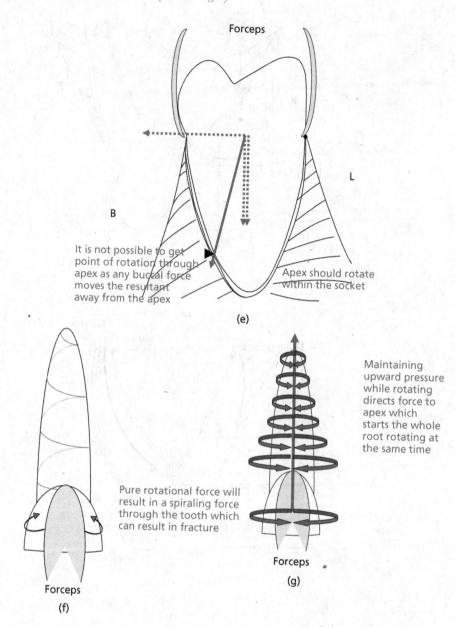

Forceps

B

L

It is not possible to get point of rotation through apex as any buccal force moves the resultant away from the apex

Apex should rotate within the socket

(e)

Pure rotational force will result in a spiraling force through the tooth which can result in fracture

Forceps

(f)

Maintaining upward pressure while rotating directs force to apex which starts the whole root rotating at the same time

Forceps

(g)

Figure 8.4   (Continued).

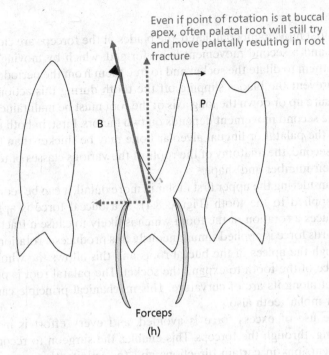

Even if point of rotation is at buccal apex, often palatal root will still try and move palatally resulting in root fracture

B

P

Forceps

(h)

Figure 8.4   (Continued).

tooth is loose it may be drawn out of the alveolus. When completed with forceps, extractions are performed in two movements.

First movement

This is the same for all the teeth of both jaws. The forceps are applied on the buccal and the palatal or lingual aspect of the tooth, regardless of whether it is normally or abnormally positioned in the arch. For multirooted teeth the blades may engage on a root, or the bifurcation depending on the design. The blades are passed carefully under the gingival margin of the tooth avoiding damage to the soft tissues, and driven up or down the roots (according to the jaw concerned) in the same plane as the long axis of the tooth to penetrate as far as possible. This can only be done successfully if the forceps blades are held sufficiently apart that initially they do *not* grip the tooth root.

Considerable force is used, particularly in the upper jaw. In the lower jaw this must be limited to that which the operator can counteract by supporting the mandible with his free hand. While driving up the root in this way the blades should be in contact with the root surface but not gripping it. This movement cuts the gingival attachment and periodontal membrane and also uses the wedge-shaped blades to dilate the socket. Conical roots may sometimes be extracted by this movement alone.

Second movement

The first movement completed, the blades of the forceps are closed to grasp the root and a second movement is performed, which by moving the tooth roots uses them to dilate the socket and to free them from the periodontal membrane. To prevent the blades slipping off the tooth during this action, a firm vertical pressure up or down the long axis of the root must be maintained. The character of the second movement depends on two factors. First, in both upper and lower jaws the palatal or lingual alveolar bone may be thicker than the buccal bone, and second, the anatomy of the roots of the various classes of teeth differs both in their number and shape.

Considering the upper first molar in more detail, it can be seen that two forces are applied to the tooth (Figure 8.4). If a buccal force is applied alone this produces a rotation of the tooth which is likely to cause a fracture. If a greater upwards force is applied simultaneously this produces a rotation approximately through the apices of the buccal roots and this allows the whole of the buccal surface of the tooth to expand the socket. The palatal root is pulled out of the socket along its arc of curvature. This mechanical principle can be applied to lower molar teeth also.

The use of excess force is avoided, and every effort is made to develop 'feeling' through the forceps. This enables the surgeon to recognise resistance to excursions in certain directions and to exploit other movements that the tooth will follow more easily, and so to extract always along the line of least resistance. During the operation the second movement is always slow, steady and purposeful, and not a series of short, jerky, shaking gestures which are both ineffective and unpleasant for the patient.

Difficult extractions

The ultimate aim of the surgeon is to acquire the ability to assess the tooth to be extracted and to modify the technique accordingly to achieve success.

Should there be complete resistance to the forceps when the usual pressure is applied the operation is stopped and a new assessment made from radiographs. Further use of luxators to expand the buccal bone may be required, but where necessary the roots are freed through a transalveolar approach by raising a flap, removing bone and dividing the tooth, rather than by exerting more and more force until the tooth breaks.

Luxators

Luxators (Figure 8.5) are designed to luxate either tooth or bone, by which it is meant that the instrument will displace the object to which it is applied. They have design features that make them ideal for this purpose, being very thin and quite fine at their working end. In contradistinction to elevators, they are not designed to lift the tooth out of the socket and must not be used for this purpose

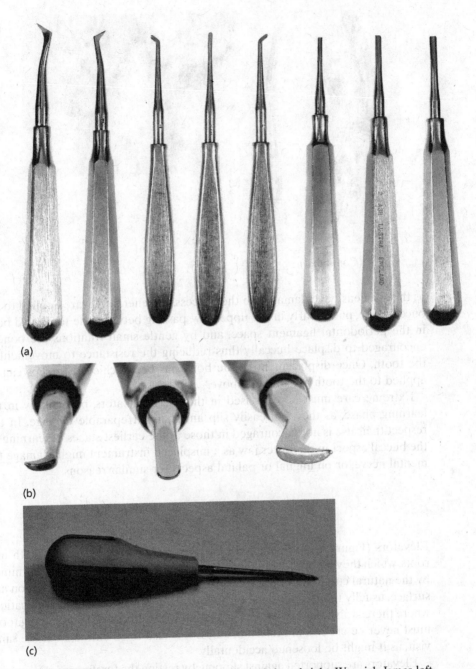

Figure 8.5 Elevators. (a) Left to right: Cryer left and right; Warwick James left, straight and right; Coupland 1, 2 and 3. (b) The blades of all the elevators have the curved surface and working edge in common. (c) Luxators. (d) Forceps and elevator design. Coupland and blade of forceps designed for single teeth are very similar. (e) Luxators have a similar design to Coupland but are thinner and thus more delicate.

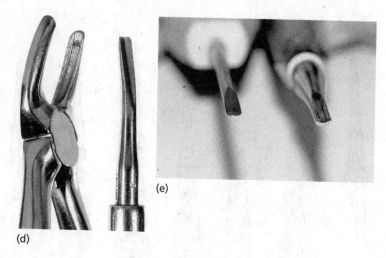

(e)

(d)

Figure 8.5   (Continued).

as they can easily be damaged in the process. In general they are applied to the buccal bone, particularly in the upper jaw, passing between the tooth and bone in the periodontal ligament space, and by gentle small rotations the bone is encouraged to displace buccally thus reducing the resistance to movement of the tooth. Once displacement of the bone has been achieved forceps can be applied to the tooth as outlined above.

Extreme care must be exercised in the use of luxators, particularly in the learning phase, as they can easily slip and cause irreparable damage. In this respect their use is not encouraged in those at the earliest stages of learning on the buccal aspect in the lower jaw as a misplaced instrument might damage the mental nerve, or on lingual or palatal aspects for similar reasons.

Elevators

Elevators (Figure 8.5) are single-bladed instruments for extracting teeth and roots, which they do by moving them out of the sockets along a path determined by the natural curvature of the roots. They are applied to the cementum on any surface, usually the mesial, distal or buccal, at a point (the point of application) where there is alveolar bone to provide them with a fulcrum. An adjoining tooth must never be used as the fulcrum, unless it is also to be extracted at the same visit, as it might be loosened accidentally.

Elevators are supported against slipping by resting the forefingers of the working hand on an adjacent tooth or the jaw They may be pushed firmly *between tooth and bone* to engage the point of application, but when elevating the tooth the force used is carefully controlled and should not exceed that which can be applied by rotating the instrument between finger and thumb (Figure 8.6). Where

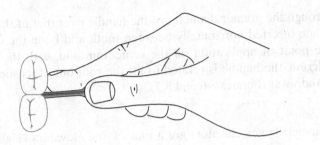

Figure 8.6 Application of an elevator to a lower right molar tooth viewed from above. Note the palm grip and the index finger used as a support.

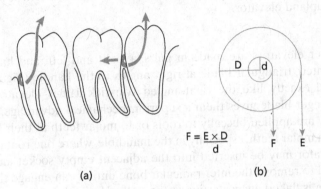

$$F = \frac{E \times D}{d}$$

(a)   (b)

Figure 8.7 (a) Left: Correct point of application between tooth and bone. Right: Incorrect application between tooth and tooth. (b) The force applied at the elevator handle (E) is multiplied by the ratio of the diameter of the handle (D) to the diameter of the blade (d) at the point of application.

this is insufficient to move the tooth, other measures such as removal of bone or division of the tooth may be necessary. An elevator should never be used as a class 1 lever, that is like a crowbar, as bone will be crushed and the mechanical advantage is such that the jaw may be fractured (Figure 8.7).

Throughout elevation its effects on the tooth to be extracted and on the adjacent teeth is carefully watched so that ineffective or damaging movements are avoided. Where a tooth is standing distal to the one to be extracted, every precaution must be taken not to transmit injurious forces to it.

Many elevators have been designed to exert more than finger and thumb pressure, but these should not be used to extract teeth. A description follows of some elevators which are safe to use, provided the above principles are obeyed.

Coupland elevator

Coupland elevators are made in three sizes; each has a single blade not unlike that of the forceps (Figure 8.5d). They may be used as a wedge to dilate the socket when driven vertically up the periodontal membrane. More commonly they are used as a pulley lever, the mechanical advantage being obtained through the greater diameter of the handle over that of the blade (Figure 8.6). When inserted horizontally between tooth and bone the sharp blade engages the point of application on the cementum and, with the alveolar bone as a fulcrum, the handle is rotated to lift the root out of its socket along its line of withdrawal (Figures 8.6 and 8.7).

Warwick James elevators

Warwick James elevators are a pair of fine elevators (Figure 8.5a). The blade may be driven into the periodontal membrane to engage the root mesially, distally or buccally, and the handle rotated to lift it from its socket. A straight Warwick James elevator is also available and used in a similar way to the Coupland elevator.

Cryer elevators

Cryer elevators are made in pairs, a right and left, and have a short, sharp-pointed, triangular blade at right angles to the handle (Figure 8.5a). They are used exactly like the right-angled Warwick James elevators but the larger, stronger blade gives them a superior mechanical advantage, particularly when they are applied buccally to roots or to molar teeth at their bifurcation.

In molar teeth, especially in the mandible, where one root is retained a Cryer elevator may be inserted into the adjacent empty socket and the sharp point used to remove the inter-radicular bone until it can engage the cementum. The bone is flaked away starting at the occlusal margin of the septum and working down towards the root apex.

The combined use of forceps, luxators and elevators

The combined use of these instruments will enable the operator to exploit the best qualities of all and thereby develop a gentle, progressive technique. For example, the first instrument to be applied in the upper jaw should be a suitable luxator driven vertically up the long axis on the buccal side. This will cut the periodontal membrane and dilate the bony socket on the buccal aspect and indicate if undue resistance is present. As soon as there is some response to the luxator, forceps may be applied. For upper third molars, in contrast, it can very difficult to control the application of luxators and thus a curved Warwick James elevator may be applied mesially to move the tooth distally before applying bayonet forceps.

Extraction procedure

The supporting hand

The responsibility for seeing that the jaws are adequately supported rests with the operator, and their free hand is used for this purpose. This is particularly important in the mandible, where the downward force must be resisted. Under local anaesthesia a prop may be inserted and the patient can help by biting

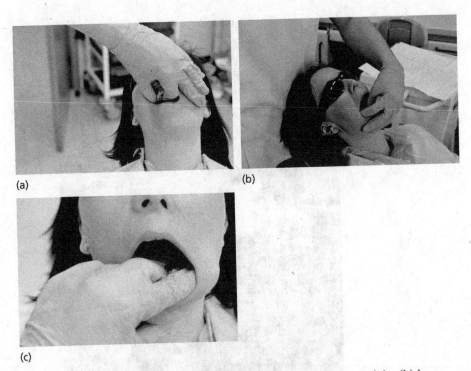

(a)   (b)

(c)

Figure 8.8 · Position of supporting hand: (a) for extraction in upper right; (b) lower right; (c) lower left. Note: finger and thumb used where possible to give sensitive feedback on tooth movement. Lower jaw must be adequately supported.

firmly on this. Under general anaesthesia the assistant may support the mandible at the angles. Satisfactory support is equally important when using forceps or elevators (Figure 8.8).

The other function of the supporting hand is to retract the cheeks and tongue and to protect the tissues. This is done by placing a finger and thumb (or two fingers) one on each side of the gum on the buccal and the lingual or palatal aspects of the tooth. At the same time the operator is able to feel that the blades of the forceps are indeed under the mucous membrane and correctly applied to the tooth. During the second movement of extraction, the watching fingers can feel any slipping of the forceps on the tooth or any tendency of adjacent teeth to move, or alveolar bone to fracture. When working on the maxilla the free fingers of the supporting hand should be kept closed to avoid the fingers causing accidental damage to the patient's eyes.

Stance

The right-handed operator stands facing the patient to the left of the chair but not too close as this makes lighting difficult. The stance has been compared to that of a boxer about to deliver a blow. The left foot is advanced, the weight

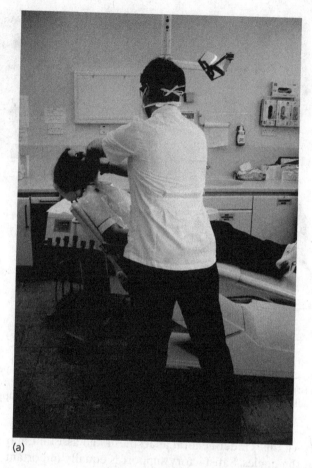
(a)

Figure 8.9   Position of operator: (a) for extractions in upper jaw; (b) lower right; (c) lower left.

balanced on both feet, with the arms slightly bent. The left hand is put forward to support the jaw while the right grasps the forceps. This position is adopted for the extraction of all upper teeth and for those in the left mandible (Figure 8.9).

Teeth in the right mandible are extracted from behind the patient. The feet are approximately shoulder width apart, and the left arm is placed round the patient's head to support the lower jaw (Figures 8.8 and 8.9). Ideally the axis of the tooth should lie on the operator's centre line.

Chair position

The chair should be adjusted to allow force to be applied correctly without compromising the operator's spine (Figure 8.9). Considerable force may be

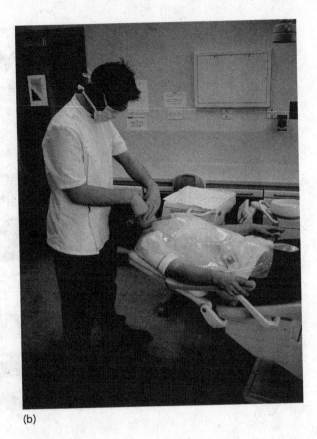

(b)

Figure 8.9 (Continued).

applied, and if this is not done ergonomically, significant damage can be inflicted on the operator's back, neck or arms. The patient should be seated comfortably with the buttocks well back in the chair and the head supported with the neck slightly extended. The angle and height of the chair is adjusted so that the operator has a clear view of the tooth without bending or twisting of the spine. A good posture should be maintained at all times. In general the chair is higher for extractions in the upper jaw and lower for those in the lower jaw. Further information on maintaining a healthy working position can be found at the Rapid Upper Limb Assessment (RULA) website.

Order of extraction of teeth

To prevent blood from the sockets of extracted teeth obscuring the field of operation it is usual to remove lower teeth before uppers, and posteriors before anteriors. Unnecessary movement to and fro about the chair is avoided

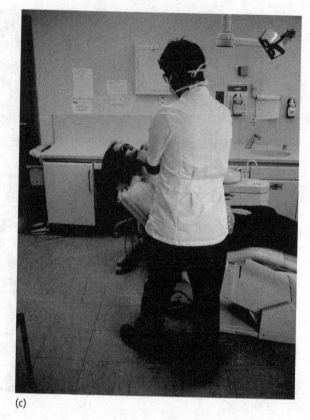

(c)

Figure 8.9   (Continued).

by starting multiple extractions with those from the right mandible, which are the only ones done from behind on the sitting patient.

It is wise to begin with the most painful tooth when undertaking multiple extractions lest any surgical or anaesthetic difficulty prevents the completion of the operation. Similarly, when working under local anaesthesia only one quadrant of the mouth should be injected at a time. When the surgery in this area has been successfully completed a new quadrant may be injected. It is better to take out teeth from one side of the mouth only at one visit, thereby leaving the other comfortable for chewing.

The extraction of a great many teeth at one outpatient sitting is contraindicated as it may upset the patient and the blood loss can be considerable. It is not possible to state a figure for the number of teeth, as much will depend on the surgical difficulty and the patient's health and morale, but between four and eight would seem reasonable. Where it is necessary to do more at one visit the patient should be kept in the recovery room for at least half an hour postoperatively and then accompanied home by a relative. Alternatively, the patient should be admitted to hospital.

Extractions in children under outpatient general anaesthesia

The preoperative preparation for general anaesthesia is discussed in Chapter 2.

Outpatient general anaesthetics are now restricted to facilities that are in close proximity to critical care and are reserved for children under 16. Use of sedation in the form of relative analgesia is becoming more common. Adults requiring a general anaesthetic are listed as day cases, or if necessary as an inpatient.

Control of the airway is paramount in this situation and the guidance of the anaesthetist, whose responsibility it is, is crucial in this respect. A laryngeal airway is more frequently used as this may improve the security of the airway. This can compromise the access in small children but does give the opportunity for a more prolonged procedure.

The surgeon checks the patient's name, the teeth to be extracted and that there are no loose teeth in the mouth. The patient is treated in the supine position. With the anaesthetist's agreement, a prop, the smallest that will keep the mouth open widely, should be placed as far back in the mouth as possible. The prop must be inspected before it is put in place to ensure it is in good condition and that there is a chain firmly attached to it which can be left hanging out of the mouth (see Figure 7.5).

When induction is complete the mouth must always be packed with a length of gauze, even if a laryngeal airway is employed. The pack is inserted into the lingual sulcus to lift the tongue against the soft palate and thus occlude the oral airway. This should safeguard the nasal airway, which the anaesthetist uses to maintain the anaesthetic. Care must be taken not to over pack. While the teeth are being extracted the surgeon must not obstruct the airway, particularly by failing to support the lower jaw. They should beware when extracting from the upper jaw of damaging the lower lip by trapping it between forceps and lower teeth. All broken tooth fragments are removed from the mouth immediately and, together with the extracted teeth, are placed in a special receptacle, care being taken not to carry them back into the mouth by accident.

On finishing the operation the prop and pack are removed by the person who put them in place, and the patient is turned on their side with the lower jaw held forward to allow blood to drain out of the mouth. The mandible is pushed into occlusion to check that the condyles are not dislocated (see Chapter 17). The teeth are counted and all apices checked.

Extractions with the surgeon seated

The chair is adjusted with the patient supine and the surgeon seated on a mobile chair capable of moving in an arc about the patient's head (Figure 8.10).

The extractions are performed using the same principles described previously in this chapter. Some slight modification of the supporting hand is necessary when working on the upper jaw. It must be emphasised that there are hazards

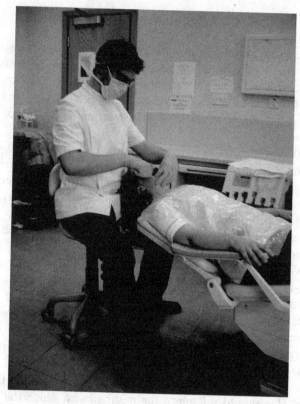

Figure 8.10   Extractions with operator seated. Note: chair should be adjusted to allow a stable spine position.

in operating on a supine patient as displaced teeth, roots or fillings may fall back into the pharynx and the dental surgeon must take adequate steps to prevent this. Gauze may be placed to catch parts of the tooth dislodged during the extraction. The conscious patient can be asked to co-operate by turning their head well to one side during the operation. Further, the assistant should have high-power suction and a suitable instrument immediately available for grasping any displaced object. Under general anaesthesia the throat must be adequately packed off.

Ambidexterous extractions

Once the techniques have been learned with one hand they can be extrapolated to the other, less dominant hand to facilitate extractions from only one position. All forces applied will be the same regardless of which hand is used. For instance, some operators may favour the use of only one pattern of lower right-angled premolar forceps for all extractions in both upper and lower jaws by sitting behind the patient and using both hands. The upper and lower teeth on the right side are extracted with the right hand, those on the patient's left with the left hand.

Fracture of the tooth

Fracture of the tooth during extraction occurs frequently, though its incidence may be reduced by a conscientious assessment and a careful progressive technique. Where the fracture is at or above the level of the margin of the alveolar bone and is thought to be due to brittleness or caries and not to excessive resistance, then the extraction may be continued using forceps and elevators as for standing teeth.

In other cases if the fracture is below the level of the alveolar margin or there appears to be undue resistance, the situation should be reassessed with radiographs. The retained portion may vary in size from a whole root to a tiny apex. It may have broken either before or after there was movement of the tooth. The first decision to be made is whether the root should be left or extracted. There is little doubt that all pieces over 3 mm in length, or those that are non-vital or loose in the socket and might behave as foreign bodies, should be removed. This procedure may be contraindicated if the root lies near some important structure that could be damaged, or if there are special medical considerations. Fractured roots of teeth extracted for orthodontic treatment should be removed. Where the orthodontist wishes to move teeth into the extraction site, every effort must be made to conserve alveolar bone for this purpose. Whenever it is thought unnecessary or unwise to extract the roots they should be radiographed, the fact noted in the records and *the patient must always be told of their presence.*

Some roots can be seen by direct vision and the operator may decide they can apply elevators or forceps to them successfully through the socket, but often the very limited access makes this difficult and such manipulations can cause considerable trauma to bone and soft tissues. Where the retained fragments cannot be seen by direct vision it is bad surgical practice to attempt them 'blind' and an open or transalveolar approach is required.

The transalveolar approach

This is used to facilitate the extraction of retained roots or teeth that are considered difficult to extract or prove resistant to normal application of forceps or elevators. The surgeon must make a step-by-step plan for this operation, analysing carefully the size of flap, amount of bone removal and the point of application required to deliver the tooth or root satisfactorily.

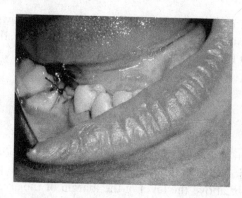

Figure 8.11 Incision for flap for transalveolar approach. Distal relieving incision avoiding the mental nerve. The flap has been repositioned with sutures. Further flap designs are shown in Figure 9.8.

A mucoperiosteal flap is raised to expose the alveolar bone enclosing the retained root. The incision should start at least the width of one tooth away from the root, and where standing teeth are present it is made in the gingival crevice. From either end the incision is then cut obliquely and up or down into the buccal sulcus to create a two-sided flap with either a mesial or distal relieving incision (Figure 8.11). It is designed to avoid dividing the interdental papilla between standing teeth and should lie firmly supported on bone after the root has been removed. Another oblique relieving incision may be required to provide adequate access (three-sided flap). The use of a distal relieving incision in the more anterior regions of the mouth may improve the aesthetics of the scar and further posteriorly in the lower jaw it can usefully avoid damage to the mental nerve.

Bone is then removed to expose the root by a few millimetres to provide a new point of application for an elevator mesially, distally or buccally, and to obtain an unobstructed line of withdrawal. An elevator can be used to remove the root. For larger roots a Cryer elevator can be satisfactorily applied buccally by drilling a hole into the root with a fissure bur at the level of the remaining alveolar bone. This is directed towards the apex at an angle of 45° to allow the elevator a greater range of upward movement; however, this may result in a fracture of the root requiring further bone removal (Figure 8.12d). Sometimes, where there is hypercementosis or an apical hook, bone may have to be removed down to the apex to free it, care being taken not to expose the roots of neighbouring teeth.

Palatal roots of upper molars do present a problem. When approached buccally it is necessary to remove both the outer alveolar plate and the interradicular bone on the buccal aspect of the palatal socket. This gives good access and is a safe approach if the maxillary sinus does not dip down between the roots, but is very extravagant of alveolar bone. A palatal approach is advocated by some, but it is more difficult to see into the wound and the bone is quite thick over the apical third of the root. An intra-alveolar approach is probably the best, the interseptal bone between palatal and buccal roots being slowly removed with burs till the root is exposed and an elevator can be used to draw it down.

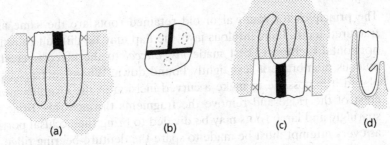

Figure 8.12   (a) Division of roots of a lower tooth. (b) and (c) Division of upper molar roots. (d) Hole cut to apply Cryer elevator to buccal aspect of a tooth. Note the angle of the cut to give maximum 'lift' to the root.

Where the whole of a difficult tooth or all the roots of an upper or lower molar tooth are retained, the buccal bone should be removed at least to the level of the bifurcation to allow division or forceps and elevators to be used. A Cryer elevator may be applied buccally at the bifurcation to lift the roots. In many cases the radiographs will show them to have an unfavourable curvature, which requires them to be divided and to be extracted separately (Figure 8.12). This may be done with a fissure bur. Teeth must not be divided unless they have been exposed sufficiently to leave an adequate point of application on what remains of the roots after division.

A strong word of warning is necessary on two matters. First, the use of elevators on single retained roots that are in close relation to the maxillary sinus or floor of the nose. *Upward pressure must not be used* even to gain a point of application, as this may cause the root to be displaced into one of these cavities. Bone should be gently removed to expose the root on one surface and downward movements only employed to extract it. In the mandible the inferior dental canal may present a similar hazard. Second, wherever flaps are being raised or bone removed near to the mental foramen the mental nerve must always be found, and protected. In this respect bone cutting should be severely limited in the vicinity of this structure.

Removal of roots after the socket has healed

The dental surgeon may be required to extract buried roots as a preparation for dentures, or because they are believed to be a source of pain or sepsis.

Localising roots

Once more, diagnosis and assessment is all important if minimal damage is to be inflicted on the alveolar bone. The first step is to localise the root accurately. Two radiographs at right angles to each other are sometimes required; either an orthopantomogram (OPG) or long cone periapical and occlusal views would be suitable.

Removal of roots

The principles for removal of old retained roots are the same as for newly fractured teeth. In edentulous jaws the flap may be difficult to reflect and the horizontal incision is best made *just buccal* to the alveolar crest where the mucous membrane is less tightly bound down. Where root apices are deeply placed it is possible to make a curved incision in the alveolus away from the crest of the ridge and remove the fragments through this. Bone is removed sparingly and large roots may be divided to bring the occlusal portion apically as every attempt must be made to spare the denture-bearing ridge.

Arrest of haemorrhage

After extracting teeth haemorrhage is arrested by asking the patient to bite gently but firmly on a rolled-up gauze swab placed over the socket. The buccal and lingual gingival margins of the sockets must not be displaced outward by the swab as this may lead to more bleeding. Should this not stop after 10 minutes, digital pressure is applied to the margins of the socket to localise the bleeding point and to confirm that it can be stopped by pressing the gum against the bone. Where this is effective, simple interrupted or horizontal mattress sutures are placed across the socket to draw the buccal and lingual alveolar mucoperiosteum together. Though sutures closing an incision should not be tied tightly, an exception is post-extraction haemorrhage, where the soft tissues must be firmly drawn against the bone. Tight suturing of this kind is contraindicated where a defective clotting mechanism (as in haemophilia) may result in large haematomas forming in the tissue spaces if the blood is prevented from escaping into the mouth.

Agents assisting haemostasis

Vasoconstrictors such as adrenalin (epinephrine) are commonly in local anaesthetic solutions and can give good control of post-extraction haemorrhage. However, once the local effect has worn off it is not unusual to have a reactionary haemorrhage.

Certain agents assist the physiological clotting mechanism. The most important is thrombin, which acts on fibrinogen to form fibrin. Either human or bovine varieties are available and may be applied topically, either as a powder or as an aqueous solution on gauze. Tranexamic acid mouthwash (5%) is advocated and helps to prevent fibroinolysis. It has been used successfully to maintain haemostasis in patients taking warfarin (see Chapter 3).

Mechanical agents, which include fibrin foam, gelatin foam, oxidised cellulose and oxidised regenerated cellulose, are substances that form a water-wettable meshwork and assist clot formation. In general surgery they appear to be readily absorbed from wounds. In oral surgery the use of oxidised cellulose can give effective clot support and is resorbed with only few complications.

Post-extraction instructions

The incidence of post-extraction haemorrhage may be reduced by clear post-extraction instructions (see Box 2.1). The patient must be warned not to use a mouthwash for the first 24 hours and thereafter normal oral hygiene may be resumed. Very hot or cold foods, alcohol or exercise are best avoided over the same period. Should bleeding occur the patient must sit upright and bite on a rolled-up handkerchief. Where after half an hour these measures fail, professional advice is required and the telephone number and address at which the surgeon can be contacted must be given with the instructions. Where extractions were performed under a local anaesthetic the danger of biting or burning the anaesthetised lips or mouth should be stressed, particularly to children.

Further reading

Meechan JG (2006) *Minor Oral Surgery in Dental Practice*. Quintessence, London.
Rapid Upper Limb Assessment, www.rula.co.uk/

Chapter 9
Extraction of Unerupted or Partly Erupted Teeth

- Diagnosis
- Treatment
- Extraction of the impacted lower third molar
- Extraction of the upper third molar tooth
- Extraction of the unerupted maxillary canine
- Extraction of maxillary supernumerary teeth
- Other unerupted teeth

Teeth fail to erupt for many reasons. Evolutionary and hereditary factors that result in a disproportion in size between teeth and jaws are important. Local causes include retention or premature loss of a deciduous predecessor, the presence of supernumerary teeth, abnormal position of or injury to the tooth germ. Tumours and cysts may also prevent teeth from erupting. Certain conditions such as cleft palate, cleidocranial dysostosis, hypopituitarism, cretinism, rickets and facial hemiatrophy predispose to delay or failure of eruption.

The teeth most commonly concerned are the mandibular and maxillary third molars, and the maxillary canine. Others not infrequently seen are the mandibular second premolar and canine, the maxillary central incisors, and supernumerary teeth in both jaws. Many unerupted teeth are impacted – that is, prevented from erupting completely by other teeth or bone. Thus the lower third molar tooth commonly impacts against the second permanent molar.

Reasons for treatment

The majority of unerupted teeth are extracted because they give rise to symptoms of pain or become foci of infection. Other indications for removal are involvement in pathology such as cysts or tumours, evidence of causing resorption of roots of adjacent teeth and interference in lines of osteotomies or fractures. Infection is less commonly seen in patients over 30 years old. The National Institute for Health and Clinical Excellence (NICE) has published accepted guidelines for the removal of lower third molars which stress that the removal

Principles of Oral and Maxillofacial Surgery, 6th Edition. Edited by U. J. Moore
© 2011 Blackwell Publishing Ltd

of asymptomatic unerupted teeth is not justified due to the possible sequelae of the surgery. Of particular importance is the potential damage to the inferior dental and lingual nerves. Symptomless unerupted or partly erupted teeth should be monitored at intervals to detect the development of complications as outlined above.

Diagnosis

The diagnosis of unerupted teeth is based on the history, clinical examination and radiographs.

History

In the absence of infection the patient often has no complaint other than that a tooth is missing. The crown may cause a symptomless swelling under the mucosa. Where pain is thought to be a symptom from a completely buried tooth, every effort must be made to eliminate other possible causes, particularly pulpitis from another tooth.

Where infection is present, more acute symptoms supervene. Inflammation about the crown of an unerupted or partly unerupted tooth is known as pericoronitis and is particularly serious when it arises from a lower third molar owing to the tendency of the infection to spread into the neck (see Chapter 12).

Examination

The dentition is accurately charted for missing permanent teeth, retained deciduous teeth, caries and periodontal disease. Caries in a neighbouring tooth can often be the actual cause of the patient's symptoms of pain or infection, or may influence the plan of treatment where extraction of the carious tooth may allow the unerupted one to come into the space. Vitality tests of all doubtful teeth are essential. The unerupted tooth may displace, loosen or resorb the roots of adjacent teeth against which it impacts. A cyst may form in association with the crown of the buried tooth. The mouth is examined for signs of infection such as swelling, discharge, trismus and enlarged tender lymph nodes.

Radiography

The object is to show the whole of the unerupted tooth, the size of its crown and the shape of its roots together with the direction in which they curve. The presence of hypercementosis or widening of the root particularly in the apical third is noted. In multirooted teeth the number of roots and whether they are fused or divergent is important. The position of the tooth in the jaws and its

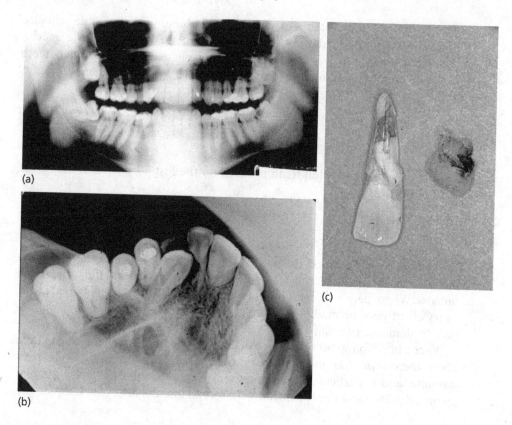

Figure 9.1   (a) Impacted third molars; caries in lower left third molar and lower right second molar; (b) impacted canine causing resorption of lateral incisor; (c) retained deciduous canine and resorbed lateral incisor.

relationship to other teeth, including the degree of impaction, are an indication of the difficulty of the operation. Secondary conditions such as caries, an increase in the size of the follicle or resorption of adjacent tooth roots or of bone will all affect the treatment plan (Figure 9.1).

Radiographs in two planes at right angles to one another are required to show clearly the position of the tooth and the degree of impaction (Figure 9.2). The orthopantomograph (OPG) is useful as a whole mouth scan where multiple unerupted teeth may be present.

Mandibular teeth

In the mandible, localisation of unerupted teeth must show the whole tooth, its relationship to the inferior dental neurovascular bundle, its buccolingual position, and the relationship to adjacent teeth and the lower border of the mandible. The OPG is useful to show the position of the inferior dental neurovascular bundle and the depth of the mandible. For lower third molars this may be

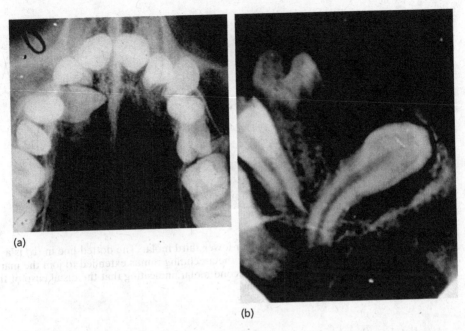

(a)

(b)

Figure 9.2   Radiographs in two planes showing position of unerupted upper right canine. Occlusal view shows crown is palatally placed.

supplemented by an intraoral periapical film which shows more accurately the morphology of the tooth and its relationship to the second molar. To be of clinical value the radiograph must be correctly taken. The periapical film is placed with the upper border level and parallel with the occlusal plane of the second molar. The central ray is directed so that the buccal and lingual cusps of the second molar are superimposed one upon the other. The contact point between the first and second molars should be clearly shown without overlapping if the central ray has been correctly directed. This ensures that the film shows the true situation at the contact point between the third and second molar teeth, particularly how heavily the former is impacted. The distal bone over the crown of the unerupted tooth should be included. An occlusal film will show the buccolingual positions of buried teeth. It is indicated for those teeth that lie across the arch, such as premolars. It is a difficult radiograph to take for third molars.

Deeply placed teeth or those lying in the ascending ramus cannot be seen on intraoral films and if not clearly seen on the OPG, lateral oblique extraoral views may be indicated. These may also be used where there is an extensive secondary condition such as dentigerous cyst or where the mandible is very thin, as in elderly edentulous patients.

Where the crown of the third molar tooth has not obviously erupted clear of bone, it may be difficult to see on the radiographs exactly how the crown and distal bone are related. If the line of the anterior border of the ascending ramus

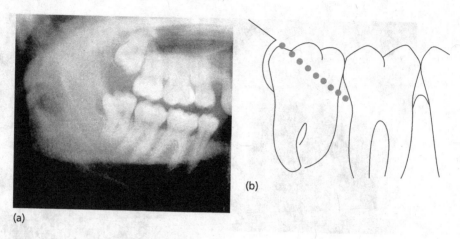

(a)

(b)

Figure 9.3   Projection of bone over lower third molar. The dotted line in (b) is a projection of the anterior border of the ascending ramus extended to join the margin of the alveolar bone distal to the second molar, indicating that the distal cusp of the third molar is just covered by bone.

distal to the third molar is projected to join the margin of the alveolar bone round the second molar, it will give a fair indication of the depth of overlying bone (Figure 9.3).

Maxillary teeth

Intraoral periapical and occlusal films are both used in the diagnosis of unerupted maxillary teeth. The maxillary canine may need several periapical films to cover the whole of its length and its relationship to the adjacent teeth. Its position relative to the dental arch is important as it may be placed palatally, buccally or, more rarely, across the arch. The only radiograph that will establish the true position of the canine in this respect is the vertex occlusal view taken with the central ray passing through the long axis of the incisor teeth (Figure 9.2). This film will also show how close the unerupted canine lies to these teeth and may reveal curvatures of its root not obvious on the periapical view.

Alternatively, the parallax method of Clark is used. In this, two periapical radiographs are taken with the films in the same position but with the X-ray tube moved horizontally 3 cm in a known direction between exposures (that is from 1.5 cm behind the normal centring point to 1.5 cm in front of it). Where two teeth lie in different planes the one that appears to move in the same direction as the X-ray tube lies furthest from it, that is palatally. In analysing these radiographs the relationship of the crown and the root of the buried tooth to the roots of the standing teeth must be considered separately.

The true position of the unerupted tooth in the vertical dimension is not accurately shown on a periapical film because of the angle at which the ray is directed onto the maxilla. The OPG may provide a more satisfactory answer and will show unerupted teeth high in the maxilla related to the maxillary sinus. In teeth lying buccal to the arch, a tangential view of the maxilla may be of assistance. Other unerupted maxillary teeth, supernumerary teeth and mesiodens are examined radiographically in much the same way.

Summary of findings

From these investigations the dental surgeon should know the following facts about the patient and the unerupted tooth.

- The patient's age, general development and the state of the dentition.
- The size and form of the crown of the unerupted tooth.
- Whether it is resorbed or, in partly erupted teeth, carious.
- The form of the roots, fused or divergent, straight or curved mesially or distally.
- The position of the tooth in the bone, whether it is lying vertically, horizontally or inverted, how deeply it is buried in bone and its buccolingual or palatal relation to the arch.
- The relationship of the tooth to other teeth and to vital structures such as nerves, the nose and the maxillary sinus.
- The size of the follicle, which may have atrophied, making extraction more difficult, undergone cystic change or have become infected.
- The texture of the bone, signs of osteosclerosis or in edentulous patients the degree of resorption of the mandible.
- The state of the adjoining teeth, whether caries, periodontal disease, apical areas or root resorption are present.

With these facts established treatment may now be considered.

Treatment

Treatment may be conservative, to bring the tooth into useful occlusion in the arch, to remove it or to leave the tooth *in situ* but keep it under review.

Conservative treatment

Conservative treatment should be considered for patients where the tooth might be brought into occlusion. The advice of a specialist orthodontist is necessary as orthodontic treatment may be required prior to surgery to create space in the arch for the unerupted tooth. A conservative approach is particularly important where a neighbouring standing tooth is carious or heavily filled. In some cases eruption may not take place without exposure of the tooth and the use of traction.

Exposure of teeth

To expose teeth a mucoperiosteal flap is made and bone is removed with burs to free the crown down to its greatest circumference. For incisors and canines the cingulum must be exposed, as must the incisal edge. Every precaution should be taken to avoid dislodging the tooth accidentally. Where the orthodontist wants a bracket, or other device to apply traction, this is placed at operation. For palatally placed teeth the soft tissues are then excised round the crown and the dead space packed with Coepack or Whitehead's varnish on gauze. These are removed after 10 days when the patient should be referred back to the orthodontist. Care must be taken with exposure of buccally placed teeth because there is evidence that excision of the soft tissues back to non-keratinised mucosa results in an unsatisfactory epithelial cuff around the erupted tooth. Many orthodontists prefer to apply a bracket to such teeth with a gold chain or wire brought out through the wound for traction. The mucoperiosteal flap is then sutured back into position.

Transplantation

In transplantation the tooth is carefully extracted and placed in a surgically prepared socket. It is immobilised with a splint for about 4 weeks, when it is usually firm. Good results are obtained with young patients, but resorption of roots is a complication after 2–5 years and occasionally leads to loss of the tooth. Early endodontic treatment may help to prevent this. The teeth most frequently transplanted historically were unerupted maxillary canines replanted into their correct position and third molars used to replace carious first molars; however, the technique has been mostly supplanted by improved use of orthodontics to enable guided repositioning as described above.

Extraction of unerupted teeth

NICE has considered the removal of symptomless lower third molars and given guidelines as to when it is appropriate to remove them. The main reasons are related to pathology, e.g. pericoronitis and caries, which make the decision easier. Many other teeth are unerupted and the clinician has to make the decision as to whether it is in the patient's best interest to leave them or remove them. Unerupted teeth can cause damage without causing symptoms and often need careful monitoring (Figure 9.1). If the decision has been made to remove an unerupted tooth this is best accomplished before it is complicated by sclerosis of bone, atrophy of the follicle, which reduces the free space round the crown, or by the presence of infection. The roots when fully formed frequently develop hooked or bulbous apices and in adults the impaction of the crown against adjoining teeth is often severe.

Ideally, the tooth is removed when the roots are two-thirds complete; before this the crown may be difficult to elevate as it tends to turn in its socket like the ball in a ball-and-socket joint. Removal of a symptomless tooth is best postponed if it is acting as a buttress for the root of an adjacent tooth, which may be simultaneously bereft of support and denuded of bone.

It is also contraindicated where vital structures such as the inferior dental nerve may be damaged in the course of the operation. In acute pericoronitis around lower third molars, surgery may have to be delayed due to difficulties in opening the mouth, but otherwise surgery will be the quickest route to relief of symptoms.

Planning the operation

This is best done by considering first the position of the tooth in the jaw, second its natural line of withdrawal, third the obstacles to its extraction and how these may best be overcome, fourth the points of application for elevators, and finally access by removing bone and raising the flap sufficient to allow the necessary procedures to be performed.

Thus the plan is made in the reverse order to that in which the operation will be performed, as obviously the size and form of the flap depends on bone removal and this in turn is related to the position of the tooth and any manoeuvres required to disimpact it.

Natural line of withdrawal

This may be shown on radiographs by projecting the line along which the tooth would move if it followed the course dictated by the curvature of its roots. Teeth are most easily extracted by moving them out of their sockets or out of bone along this pathway. Where the tooth would come through the alveolus into the mouth unimpeded, except by alveolar bone, it is said to be favourably placed, but where it would go deeper into bone or impact against another tooth it is classified as unfavourable.

Extraction by moving the teeth along their line of withdrawal is done with elevators, using a gentle touch and always watching the effect of the forces applied to the tooth or roots. Heavy levering either to disimpact the tooth or lift it from its socket may have serious consequences such as fracture of the bone or displacement of the tooth into the soft tissues or the maxillary sinus. Where the roots of mandibular teeth are near the inferior dental canal, this nerve may be damaged. Resistance to elevation should be foreseen and plans made to overcome it.

Obstacles to elevation of a tooth

These may occur along its natural line of withdrawal and may be 'intrinsic', that is due to the shape of the tooth, such as hooked or bulbous apices, roots curving in opposite directions or a constriction at the neck of the tooth, all of which may anchor the tooth in bone. As many of these difficulties are found in the apical third of the root considerable bone removal may be necessary to free the tooth.

The obstacles may also be 'extrinsic', that is due to bone, adjacent teeth or vital structures such as the inferior dental nerve or the maxillary antrum. The depth of the tooth in bone is a major factor in assessing difficulty, presenting problems of access, increasing the time of operation, and requiring foresight and experience to avoid excessive bone destruction.

Where the unerupted tooth is impacted against other teeth that are not for extraction, its disimpaction is usually a simple problem in geometry. The tooth may be extracted whole by removing sufficient bone to allow it to be rotated, and this is often possible (Figure 9.4a). Where the impaction is severe (Figure 9.4e) or the root curvature adverse (Figure 9.4b), it must be divided and extracted in pieces. This is a less traumatic and safer method than forceful levering to disimpact the tooth and preserves bone that may later form part of the edentulous denture-bearing ridge. Division may be horizontal (crown from roots, Figure 9.4e) or vertical (down the long axis of the tooth, Figure 9.4d). Both are preferably done with a large fissure bur, to leave an appreciable space between the divided parts. A hole is made through the centre of the root below the amelocement junction with a No. 7 fissure bur. To divide the crown from the roots the cut is extended mesially and distally through the whole thickness of the tooth. The angle of cut is important and should be made to favour the

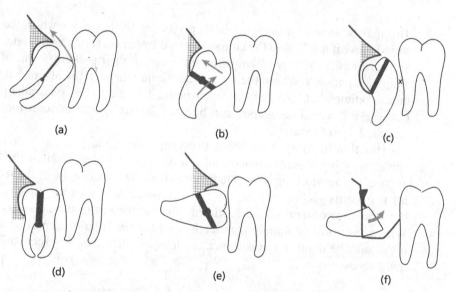

(a)   (b)   (c)

(d)   (e)   (f)

Figure 9.4 The distobuccal bone to be removed is shown by cross-hatching. (a) Mesioangular impaction with favourable roots. The tooth may rotate about the distal apex but may require division as shown and the roots elevated separately. (b) Mesioangular impaction with unfavourable roots requiring division. (c) Distoangular impaction with oblique division to maintain mesial point of application. (d) Vertical impaction with separate roots may require vertical division. (e) Horizontal impaction: note angle of division of crown to allow removal of divided fragment. (f) The roots can then be elevated forwards.

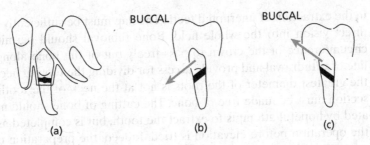

Figure 9.5 Impacted second premolar: (a) bone removal, and division of tooth; (b) correct buccolingual angulation of the dividing cut; (c) incorrect angulation as crown cannot disimpact from the first molar.

line of withdrawal of the crown (Figures 9.4 and 9.5). Wherever the tooth is related to any important structure, a thick layer of dentine is left intact and the last portion cracked through by rotating an elevator in the cut. Division with an osteotome is less satisfactory as it produces a hairline crack, often at the wrong angle, which makes disimpaction of the crown very difficult. When it is used, the tooth must be firmly supported in bone and not loose; the osteotome is applied to the cementum and given a sharp blow with the mallet.

Division vertically is reserved for molar teeth, particularly those with divergent roots, and is very effective in certain impactions (Figure 9.4d). The bifurcation must be clearly identified and the fissure bur is used to cut from the bifurcation through the crown. It is obviously ineffective where the roots are fused or the cut misses their bifurcation. Removal of part of the crown must leave a convenient point of application for an elevator, which is crucial for success in distoangular impaction (Figure 9.4c).

Point of application for elevators

Dental elevators when properly used are very sensitive instruments through which even the slightest resistance to movement of a tooth or root can be felt. For this reason they are the most satisfactory instrument for extracting buried teeth. It must be decided at the planning stage at which points it will be necessary to apply an elevator to lift the tooth, or after it has been divided the crown and then the roots, out of the socket. Bone may have to be removed with the sole object of obtaining satisfactory access or a fulcrum for the elevator. Tooth division must be planned so that after removal of the crown enough root is exposed to enable elevators to be applied easily. No tooth should be divided until an adequate point of application on the fraction that is to be left in bone has been prepared and tested, otherwise the operator's difficulties may be greatly increased by this injudicious action.

Access

Only after all the above factors have been considered can the full extent of bone removal be calculated. Inadequate access is the commonest cause of difficulty in the extraction of unerupted teeth. The flap must be sufficiently large to allow direct vision into the whole field. Bone removal should permit the greatest circumference of the crown to pass freely out of the bone along the planned line of withdrawal and provide access for dividing the tooth if necessary. Where the greatest diameter of the roots is not at the neck of the tooth, the bulbous section must be made free of bone. The cutting of bone should not be punctuated by hopeful attempts to extract the tooth, but is completed as one stage of the operation before elevation is tried. Indeed, the preparation of satisfactory access for elevators and of a fulcrum on firm bone offering them adequate support is an important part of planned bone removal.

The size and shape of the flap in its turn depends on the extent of the operation as it must provide access without subjecting the soft tissues to tension or trauma. The flap must extend beyond the area of bone removal so that the line of closure rests on bone (Figure 9.6).

Teeth in edentulous jaws

These often present in older patients when the bone is sclerotic and the periodontal space very narrow. The principles of removal are similar to those described, but it may be necessary to cut a point of application for an elevator

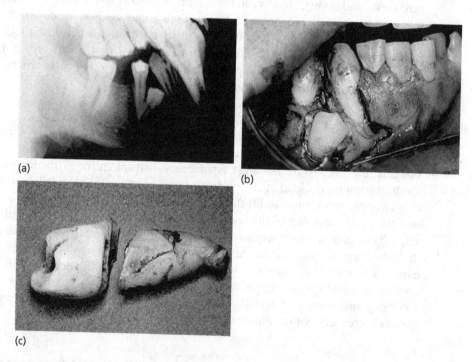

(a)

(b)

(c)

Figure 9.6   Unerupted lower first premolar: (a) radiographic appearance; (b) buccal mucosa reflected to reveal position; (c) division required to remove tooth.

and very gentle forces should be applied as the bone is brittle. Special care is taken to preserve the alveolar ridge by making an accurate assessment and removing minimal bone. Where gross resorption of the mandible has taken place, and there is danger of fracturing the jaw, the patient should be warned and a suitable plating kit should be available (see Chapter 14).

Closure

Debridement is completed in the normal way and the flap reapposed. Sutures, which may be resorbable, should be kept to a minimum. If the design of flap allows primary closure of the wound then this should be achieved as long as the flap is not under tension.

Extraction of the impacted lower third molar

Assessment

Position of the tooth and its line of withdrawal

The position of the unerupted lower third molar may be vertical (Figure 9.4d), horizontal (Figure 9.4e), mesioangular (Figure 9.4a) or distoangular (Figure 9.4c). The crown usually lies nearer the lingual than the buccal plate. Occasionally it is inverted or lies across the mandible, with the crown facing either buccally or lingually. Very rarely it is found in the ascending ramus or at the lower border of the mandible. Where the tooth lies below the inferior dental canal an extraoral lower border approach is indicated.

The natural line of the tooth can only be determined by a study of radiographs showing the form of the roots, which may be fused, divergent, straight or curved to favour or prevent extraction of the tooth.

The difficulty of the extraction is increased if access is difficult. This may occur if the mouth is small, where the space between the anterior border of the mandible and the distal aspect of the second molar is narrow or when the tooth is deeply buried in bone.

Obstacles to extraction

Bone

All or part of the crown may be covered by bone (Figure 9.3). How deeply the tooth is buried is calculated by measuring the vertical distance from the cervical margin of the second molar to the mesial cervical margin of the tooth, except in distoangular impactions where the distal cervical margin is used. Where this distance is more than 4mm the tooth should be regarded as deeply buried. Vertically placed buried teeth may only need bone to be removed from over the whole of the occlusal and buccal surfaces of the crown for them to be luxated distally and then elevated upwards with a Coupland elevator, or delivered buccally with a curved Warwick James. Alternatively, the tooth may be elevated up and out with a Cryer elevator applied to the buccal aspect of the root.

This situation must, however, be distinguished from the tooth that is distally impacted against the bone of the ascending ramus. These are the most difficult of all impacted third molars to extract. They should always be approached with great caution, especially where they are deeply placed, lie far back in the ascending ramus or the roots have a distal curvature (Figure 9.4c).

After removal of buccal and occlusal bone to clear the crown, the tooth should be divided obliquely to leave the mesial part of the crown intact with a mesial application point. The tooth may then be rotated distally and elevated up from the buccal side. Alternatively, the crown may be removed, and using a point of application on the buccal aspect of the roots they are elevated into the space created. However, the loss of the mesial application point can leave the surgeon with a very difficult problem if the roots lie very close to the second molar.

Where the roots are curved distally this may still prove difficult until further bone has been cut to free them distally, or the roots are sectioned again. If the roots are separate, vertical division is often useful.

The inferior dental neurovascular bundle

This may be damaged by direct trauma from burs or elevators, or indirectly when the tooth is elevated or rotated, as the root can crush or tear the neurovascular bundle.

The relationship of roots, particularly of the lower third molar, to the inferior dental canal may be deduced from radiographs. It may clearly lie below the roots or appear to cross them. In the latter relationship it is probably grooving the roots if the radiolucent band of the canal is seen to cross them above their apices. Where the root is deeply notched, the white lines representing the cortical plates lining the canal converge, are diverted or are interrupted (Figure 9.7). This is a warning that heavy or repeated elevation may compress the nerve

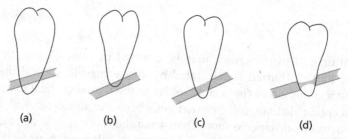

(a)   (b)   (c)   (d)

Figure 9.7   Relationship of the third molar roots to the inferior dental canal as seen on radiographs: (a) root lightly notched; (b) apical notch; (c) deeply notched; (d) the canal perforates the root.

against bone to cause hypoaesthesia or paraesthesia. Such damage can be avoided by planning the operation so that sufficient bone is removed and, where indicated, the tooth divided to allow the roots to be lifted out with a single, gentle movement.

Perforation of a root by the canal contents is suggested where the radiolucent band crosses the root and shows the loss of both white lines with maximum constriction of the radiolucent band at the middle of the root (Figure 9.7d). The tooth must then be divided and removed from around the nerve, taking care not to damage the neurovascular bundle.

Lingual nerve

The lingual nerve can be closely associated with the crown of the impacted third molar and may lie above the level of the lingual bone before passing downwards and forwards into the floor of the mouth and the tongue.

Nerve repair

When the inferior dental nerve or lingual nerve are damaged and sensation is lost or dysaesthesia (unpleasant sensation) occurs, nerve repair should be considered. This is best undertaken by an experienced operator using a microscope and fine sutures (10/0 gauge). Some return of sensation may occur but the patient must be warned that this may not happen.

Impaction against a tooth

The third molar may impact against the second molar either in the mesioangular (Figure 9.4a) or in the horizontal position (Figure 9.4e). The impaction may be overcome in one of three ways.

Extraction of the second molar can be justified by gross caries or periodontal disease. It is often advised where the third molar is heavily impacted against the distal root of the second molar without any apparent intervening alveolar bone. This should not be necessary if the surgeon avoids damaging the second molar roots and the soft tissue round the neck of that tooth. Usually the second molar is sound and the operation must be planned to protect it from damage during the extraction of the buried tooth.

Rotation of the impacted tooth, particularly if it is in a favourable mesioangular position, may allow it to be turned bodily away from the second molar. This can be planned on radiographs. The apex of the distal root of the third molar is taken as the centre of a circle through which the tooth might be rotated. A radius is drawn to the mesiobuccal cusp and if the arc of this circle passes clear of the second molar, then the third molar should disimpact without difficulty, providing sufficient bone can be removed distally to allow it to turn (Figure 9.4a). This technique is often satisfactory for mesioangular impactions, but would require extensive bone removal for horizontal impactions. When assessing the tooth for rotation, the relationship of the apex of the distal root to the inferior dental canal should be examine, as rotation may force this apex downwards and if the canal is immediately below, the neurovascular bundle may be crushed with resulting anaesthesia or paraesthesia.

Division of the impacted tooth is indicated where the impaction is heavy, the curvature of the roots is unfavourable or where a large amount of bone would otherwise have to be removed. In horizontal impactions bone is removed from the buccal and upper surface of the crown and coronal third of the root. The tooth is then divided through the neck, using an oblique cut (Figure 9.4e) so that the crown may be easily disimpacted by sliding it up and back along the distally inclined plane on the root. The roots are then brought forward using a Cryer elevator on their superior surface. Where the roots have a mesial unfavourable curvature or are divergent, difficulty may be experienced and further division of the roots may be necessary.

Operative technique

(See Figure 9.10)

The flap

The incision for partly erupted third molars is commenced in the distal part of the gingival crevice and carried buccally around the crown of the tooth to just behind the crown of the second molar (where the tooth is buried the incision starts on the alveolar crest, distal to the second molar). It is then carried around the distal papilla of the second molar and continued down and forwards to the depth of the reflection. The distal end of the incision is extended at a similar angle out towards the external oblique ridge; care must be taken not to extend distally as the lingual nerve may be encountered well into the operculum. The length of this extension depends on the extent of the eruption of the crown. Using a sharp periosteal elevator, such as the Ash, the edge of the flap is freed, starting in the buccal sulcus exposing the underlying bone. This plane is established using the Howarth periosteal elevator in the left hand and the two instruments work distally in a 'knife and fork' technique. The gingival margin is usually quite easily lifted from the bone but distally some fibrous tissue may be encountered, which makes this area problematic, particularly if there have been frequent episodes of pericoronitis. The flap may then be retracted to expose the buccal bone from the external oblique ridge to the mesial root of the second molar (Figures 9.8a and 9.8b).

The envelope flap

The incision is carried forward in the gingival crevice of the second and first molar teeth and relieved distal to the third molar towards the external oblique ridge as in the description above. Initially the flap is raised along the gingival margin with a suitable fine instrument such as an Ash, a flat plastic or a curved Warwick James elevator to avoid damage to the margin (Figures 9.8c and 9.8d).

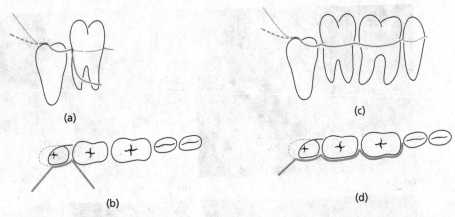

Figure 9.8   Flaps for removal of unerupted third molar: (a) and (b) standard flap with distal relieving incision following external oblique ridge; (c) and (d) envelope flap with same distal extension as standard; further flexibility can be gained by lengthening the ginvial margin incision.

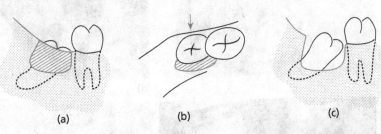

Figure 9.9   Distobuccal bone removal for third molar removal: (a) bone should be removed vertically around the crown (shaded area); (b) from above it can be seen that bone should not be removed toward the disto-lingual aspect; (c) at the end of bone removal the bifurcation area should be exposed. This will facilitate division of the tooth as indicated in Figure 9.4.

Both of the above flaps should give adequate access to remove bone from the buccal aspect only. Lingual retraction is not advocated as it may cause damage to the lingual nerve. If a lingual flap is necessary this should be raised with extreme care distal to the third molar ensuring the instrument is below the periosteum to avoid damage to the lingual nerve.

Bone removal

With the improvement in high-speed drills incorporating water-delivery systems, bone removal is now almost universally achieved using burs. Bone can quickly be removed by grinding using a tungsten carbide rosehead bur.

Sufficient bone should be removed to allow the tooth to be elevated without the use of undue force. In general the whole of the buccal aspect of the crown as far as the bifurcation should be exposed (Figure 9.9). This facilitates tooth

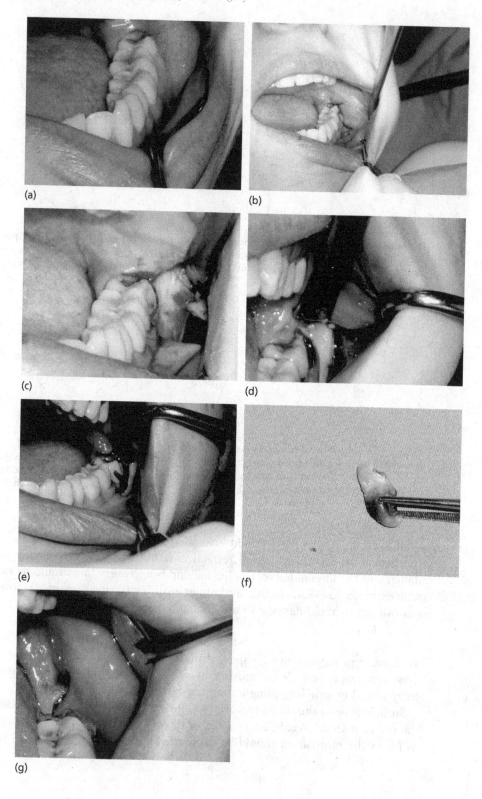

(a)

(b)

(c)

(d)

(e)

(f)

(g)

Figure 9.10   Surgical removal of lower left third molar: (a) preoperative appearance of partly erupted 38; (b) three-sided flap designed and incision made; (c) flap raised to expose buccal aspect of tooth and bone; (d) buccal bone removed to expose whole of crown and bifurcation; (e) distal tooth division was necessary as 38 was mildly distoangular; (f) appearance of tooth after removal showing distal part of crown divided and removed. Note that mesial application point has been maintained; (g) closure of wound with one suture distal to 37.

division, which, as discussed previously, may be essential to enable the tooth to be elevated more easily. Care should be taken not to destroy the application points for elevators by injudicious division, particularly when distal angulations are encountered.

Elevation

The use of elevators or luxators as described in Chapter 8 is the most likely way in which the tooth will be delivered. Horizontally impacted teeth may be divided, whereas mesioangular teeth are disimpacted using a No. 1 Coupland elevator or a straight Warwick James elevator placed mesially at the neck of the tooth, and rotated to move it distally and buccally; it is then lifted out of its socket with a suitable elevator used mesially or buccally in the bifurcation of the roots. If division of the roots has been achieved these can be elevated individually, the direction of elevation being decided by the curvature of the roots. Distal angulated impactions require the most skill and care as the natural elevation point at the mesial aspect of the third molar is compromised by the lack of space between it and the second molar. A luxator can help to displace the third molar distally before elevation commences. The greatest care must be taken to preserve this mesial elevation point as injudicious division of the crown can lose this and leave an extremely difficult situation (Figure 9.4c). The learner will need to explore the potential effect of elevators placed mesially or distally to a root to discover the most efficient movements.

Debridement

The wound must be cleansed of debris and the follicle of the tooth removed by grasping it firmly in tissue forceps and drawing it gently off the bone. Where it is attached to the flap, this may be gently dissected off with a Mitchell trimmer, but great care should be taken on the lingual side as the lingual nerve may be inadvertently damaged.

Any rough edges of bone due to elevation should be smoothed using a large round bur or a hand instrument such as a Mitchell trimmer.

At the end of debridement the socket and under the flap should be irrigated with either saline or chlorhexidine. Care at this stage can help to facilitate the healing process.

Closure

One suture placed distal to the second molar, taking the papilla over to the lingual mucosa, is usually sufficient to hold the flap in position. This usually protects the socket well and helps to re-establish the gingival margin distal to the second molar. The flap should not be placed under tension to achieve this as it will tend to break down. Resorbable sutures are used as these do not need to be removed.

Extraction of the upper third molar tooth

Assessment

Upper third molars seldom give trouble while buried and in view of this there is a strong argument for leaving those that are symptomless to erupt. If a decision is made to remove an unerupted upper third molar it is important to understand that access is made difficult by the position of the upper third molar behind the second molar, the presence of the malar buttress and the way in which the coronoid process comes forward when the mouth is open. Fortunately, the majority are buccally placed and covered by only a thin layer of bone.

Their roots vary widely in form but they are often small and fine and fracture easily. The roots, and sometimes the whole tooth, are commonly in close relation to the maxillary sinus, into which they can be displaced. Deeply placed distoangular teeth can easily be pushed into the soft tissue behind the maxillary tuberosity. Erupted upper third molars that are functionless may be extracted at the same time as the lower third molar, but this is by no means an indication for extraction.

The flap

The incision is made from the distal aspect of the maxillary tuberosity forward to the middle of the distal aspect of the second molar crown. This part of the incision should be kept over towards the palate to expose the third molar without raising a second palatal flap, which is often difficult to retract and may cause retching in some patients. The incision is then carried obliquely forward into the buccal sulcus in a similar fashion to the design of the lower third molar. The flap is reflected and held back with the periosteal elevator (Figure 9.11) or Laster retractor (see Figure 7.4).

Bone removal

The bone over this tooth is usually quite thin and can be removed with burs or with a sharp chisel used with gentle pressure by hand to avoid accidentally pushing the tooth into the maxillary sinus. When the occlusal, buccal and distal aspect of the crown have been exposed, an elevator (Warwick James or Cryer) may be applied to the mesial surface of the tooth to bring it *backwards, downwards and outwards*. Mesioangular impactions may be disimpacted from behind

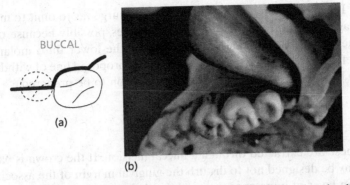

BUCCAL

(a)

(b)

Figure 9.11   (a) Design of buccal flap for upper third molar. Note that the distal extension of the incision over the tuberosity is carried well over towards the palatal side. (b) Laster retractor positioned behind upper third molar to expose it and stop the tooth displacing posteriorly into the pterygoid or infratemporal space.

the upper second molar with an elevator. In either case a Howarth raspatory or Laster retractor must be placed distally to prevent the tooth being luxated backwards into the soft tissues (Figure 9.11).

Extraction of the unerupted maxillary canine

Assessment

The unerupted maxillary canine may lie palatally, buccally or across the dental arch between the roots of the standing teeth. In this last case the root apex or the crown may be palpated in the buccal sulcus. Some are deeply placed high up in the maxilla or in the floor of the nose. The tooth may be in vertical, mesio-angular, distoangular or horizontal impaction; rarely it is inverted. Many unerupted canines have curved roots, often sharply hooked in the apical third.

Radiographs in two planes must be carefully examined to localise the tooth, to determine its relationship to the dental arch and to detect the site and direction of any curvature of the roots (Figure 9.2). The relationship of the canine to the standing teeth is most important, particularly for palatally placed canines, which may in fact have caused so much resorption of alveolar bone that they are supporting the teeth against which they are impacted. Wherever the impaction is close, or the standing teeth have been moved or show signs of resorption by the canine, vitality tests should be carried out and splints prepared beforehand to support the standing teeth during and after operation.

In those canines lying in the arch between the roots of the standing teeth, tangential views of the maxilla are important in determining the position of the incisal tip, whether it is lying palatal or buccal to the arch. Where it has passed buccally between the roots of the teeth it is necessary to expose the crown buccally even though the tooth may have to be approached palatally as well.

It is a common fault for inexperienced surgeons to omit to make a stage-by-stage operation plan for unerupted canines, possibly because the approach to these teeth is less standardised than for the lower third molar. It is essential before starting to be quite clear about the proposed line of withdrawal, the bone to be removed and the points of application to be prepared.

Buccally placed canines

These are extracted through a buccal incision. If the crown is palpable the flap may be designed not to disturb the gingival margin of the associated teeth. The thin layer of bone over the tooth is often easily removed and the tooth gently eased outwards with a Cryer elevator and, when it is disimpacted, extracted with forceps. If the crown is not palpable then a full buccal flap should be raised to give adequate access for its discovery and removal.

Palatally placed canines

The flap

As the approach is through a palatal flap, the field of operation is best seen if the surgeon works from the opposite side, that is the patient's left, for a tooth on the right. The incision is made in the gingival crevice round the necks of the standing teeth. For a tooth on the right side it extends from the upper left canine to the upper right first molar. The flap is reflected carefully to lift the mucoperiosteum containing the palatine artery without damaging that vessel. The structures passing through the incisive foramen may have to be divided as they restrict access (Figure 9.12).

Where two canines are to be extracted the flap is best made from first molar to first molar. The flap can be held back with a retractor, a hook or by passing a suture through it tied to the teeth on the opposite side.

Bone removal

This should be done very accurately with a medium-sized rosehead bur (5–9) keeping to the *palatal side* of the buried tooth. Bone is removed until the crown is found; it is then cleared of bone, particularly over the incisive tip and the

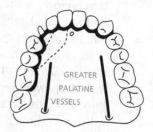

Figure 9.12 Design of a palatal flap for extraction of a buried canine. Note the position of the incisive foramen and the palatine vessels.

coronal third of the root. Every effort must be made to *leave the supporting bone over the roots of the standing teeth* and to avoid accidentally cutting into their roots. Special care is needed where the canine lies across the arch.

Extraction

Many vertical canines with straight roots will elevate downwards once the crown is cleared. Others, particularly those in a horizontal position impacted against other teeth, should be divided and the crown extracted first. Elevators are best applied to the palatal side of the tooth or up its long axis. Occasionally, elevation from the buccal side is unavoidable. In these circumstances the fingers of the watching hand are placed over the standing teeth to detect even the slightest movement in them, and where a splint has been constructed this may be put over the teeth to support them and removed after the extraction.

Division of the crown may be required to allow disimpaction of the crown. The root can then be elevated into the space created.

Great difficulty may be found when the apical third of the root is curved or hooked, particularly if this curvature is unfavourable and turns the tooth into the dental arch, making it necessary to remove bone from over its whole length to free the apex. Many canines are closely related to the maxillary sinus, into which they can be displaced by forceful or misdirected application of elevators. Should a root apex that is known to be near the antrum fracture, it is wise to consider leaving it.

Those teeth that lie across the dental arch with the crown in the palate and the root apex in the buccal sulcus may require a flap made both palatally and buccally. Where the apex of the root is hooked, division may be necessary to extract the apex bucally, and to allow the crown to be removed palatally, which can often be done by firm pressure exerted through the buccal approach.

Closure

The palatal flap when replaced will require only one or two sutures to hold it. The knots should be tied buccally.

Osteoplastic flaps

Canines in edentulous jaws are often lying along the arch so that their removal may destroy the bony ridge and damage the denture-bearing area. The ridge can be preserved by the use of an osteoplastic flap. Two buccal, vertical incisions are made just beyond the estimated position of the root apex and the incisal tip of the tooth. These are joined by an incision along the crest of the ridge. The margin, 3 mm only, of the buccal flap is reflected to admit a chisel or fissure bur which is used to make cuts through the bone parallel to the vertical and horizontal incisions. The latter must be on the crest of the ridge and cut up to the tooth. A Howarth periosteal elevator is placed in this cut and rotated outwards so that the buccal bone fractures and, still attached to mucoperiosteum, is raised buccally (Figure 9.13). The canine can then be seen and removed with

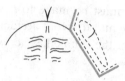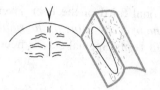

Figure 9.13 Osteoplastic flap. Left: Continuous dark line indicates the incision through mucoperiosteum along the alveolar crest and extended obliquely upwards in the buccal mucoperiosteum anteriorly and posteriorly. Dashed line indicates limited extent of reflection of the flap to allow bone incision to be made. Right: Mucoperiosteum and bone flap reflected to expose canine tooth.

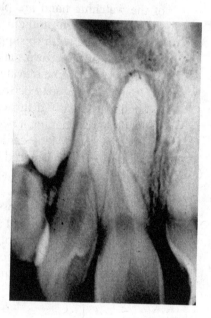

Figure 9.14 Upper midline supernumerary (mesiodens). Note rotation of left central incisor.

an elevator. The osteoplastic flap is carefully replaced and the mucosa sutured. The bony ridge is thus preserved and the patient can often continue to wear the denture within alteration.

Extraction of maxillary supernumerary teeth

Supernumerary teeth in the incisor region of the maxilla are of common occurrence. They are diagnosed and operated in much the same way as unerupted maxillary canines. Where the supernumerary is associated with an unerupted incisor it is best extracted as soon as possible to avoid causing delayed or arrested eruption. It is essential to expose clearly and identify the permanent teeth and the supernumerary *without doubt* before any form of elevation is started. Patients should be made aware of the potential damage to the permanent incisors in the consent (Figure 9.14).

Other unerupted teeth

Other unerupted teeth in the maxilla and mandible will present their own problems to the surgeon which must be solved by applying the principles described above to each new situation.

Further reading

Dimitroulis G (1997) *A Synopsis of Minor Oral Surgery*. Wright, Oxford.

Meechan JG (2006) *Minor Oral Surgery in Dental Practice*. Quintessence, London.

NICE guidelines www.nice.org.uk/nicemedia/live/11385/31993/31993.pdf.

Robinson PP, Smith KG (1996) Lingual nerve damage during lower third molar removal: a comparison of two surgical methods. *British Dental Journal* **180**(12): 456–61.

Rood.JP, Nooraldeen Shehab BAA (1990) The radiological prediction of damage to the inferior alveolar nerve during the extraction of mandibular third molar. *British Dental Journal* **109**: 335.

Chapter 10
Complications of Tooth Extraction

- Pre-extraction
- During extraction
- Post-extraction

Pre-extraction

Difficulty in achieving anaesthesia

Where breakdown in pain control is encountered during extraction, careful diagnosis of the nerve distribution in which pain sensation remains is essential. In the maxilla, use of the superior posterior alveolar and infraorbital nerve block should become part of the surgeon's practice. The presence of collateral nerve supply must be anticipated and appropriate techniques such as periodontal ligament injection employed. Tooth extraction under local anaesthesia should be possible in almost all co-operative patients and the surgeon should strive to perfect techniques that ensure the procedure is painless (see Figure 7.1).

Difficulty in co-operation

This may be encountered at any time during the procedure, especially in those patients not amenable to reasoning, but careful preoperative assessment should alert the surgeon to such problems. The surgeon should on no account force any patient to accept treatment and an alternative method of achieving the extraction should be sought with as little delay as possible. This might involve the use of sedation or general anaesthesia.

Principles of Oral and Maxillofacial Surgery, 6th Edition. Edited by U. J. Moore
© 2011 Blackwell Publishing Ltd

Difficulty of access

Trismus

Limitation of opening may be due to intrinsic causes (abnormalities in the temporomandibular joint) or extrinsic causes (facial scars and inflammatory swellings). In chronic cases it may be possible to improve the opening with exercisers, but forcing the jaws open when trismus is due to infection will break down the pyogenic membrane and cause spread. The acute phase may be treated with antibiotics and drainage and the extractions delayed until the opening is sufficiently improved, but if there is a risk to the airway there should be no delay in removing the cause and instituting drainage. In this situation admission to hospital for a general anaesthetic and high doses of intravenous antibiotics is often required.

Reduced aperture of the mouth

This may be due to congenital malformation (microstomia) or to scarring, making it difficult or even impossible to apply forceps or elevators to the teeth. In extreme cases a surgical approach through the angle of the mouth may be necessary.

Crowded or misplaced teeth

These frequently make it difficult to apply forceps or elevators without the risk of loosening adjacent teeth. This may be made easier by using a surgical technique to divide and elevate the tooth to be extracted.

During extraction

Abnormal resistance

Where there is no obvious clinical cause for abnormal resistance, such as the position of the tooth or the thickness of the alveolar bone, the operator should make steady and repeated efforts to loosen the tooth, avoiding too much force in one direction. After a reasonable attempt, if there is no movement, a radiograph, if not already available, is taken before proceeding further. This may show abnormalities of the roots in number or in form such as twisted, divergent, bulbous or hypercementosed roots. In age or chronic periodontal disease there may be sclerosis of the alveolar bone. Isolated teeth in occlusion are renownedly difficult to remove owing to narrowing of the periodontal membrane. Unerupted teeth impacting against the roots of the tooth to be extracted (lower third molar against second molar roots) can be a source of difficulty only discovered on a radiograph.

In all cases of abnormal resistance it is advisable to plan removal of the tooth through a transalveolar approach to reduce trauma to bone and soft tissues and avoid fracturing the tooth.

Damage to other teeth

Extraction of the wrong tooth

This is a common source of litigation and is indefensible because it is avoidable if the proper precautions are taken. Extractions should never be started without checking *immediately* before operation the patient's name, address and age, the teeth to be removed and any radiographs available. This applies equally to patients operated on under local or general anaesthesia. The patient or, in the case of children, the parent is asked to confirm which teeth are to be extracted, and any doubts must be settled before the anaesthetic is given.

The notes should be placed so that the operator can see them throughout the operation and can make a final check just before the forceps are applied to the tooth. Should an error occur, the patient must be informed and the surgeon must proceed to extract the right tooth to complete the operation. A decision then has to be made whether to reimplant the wrongly extracted tooth immediately or to accept the situation.

Dislocation of adjacent teeth or of restorations in adjacent teeth

Careless application or movements of forceps and elevators may cause this mishap. Forceps can accidentally engage part of the next tooth and so loosen it, or when drawing a lower tooth from its socket without sufficient control they may bang against the upper teeth. Elevators, misused either as class I levers or by employing a neighbouring tooth, and not bone, as the fulcrum, can do similar damage. The watching fingers of the supporting hand can assist in preventing this by feeling that the forceps are in a good position and detecting even slight movement in adjacent teeth. Where misplaced or mildly impacted teeth occur in the arch, a surgical approach may be required to allow extraction without transmitting pressure or force to neighbouring teeth.

The permanent premolars may be luxated when extracting the deciduous molars due to the root formation of the deciduous teeth, which may closely approximate the crown of the permanent tooth, or to infection, which may cause fibrosis or even ankylosis between them. More often it is due to the misapplication of instruments in the extraction of deciduous molars or injudicious attempts to remove their retained roots.

Fracture of teeth

Where normal extracting methods are used the teeth may frequently be fractured due to advanced caries or large restorations which weaken the crown. In devitalised teeth, in periodontal disease and in the aged, the roots may become brittle, and it is unfortunate that the last two conditions are also characterised by sclerosis and loss of elasticity of the alveolar bone thereby causing undue resistance to add to the difficulties.

Another common cause is ill-fitting forceps, which impinge on the crown or do not fit the root accurately. Forceps may be misapplied, particularly on rotated, inclined or misplaced teeth. The use of excess force or short, jerky movements prevents the surgeon feeling which way the tooth wants to come and frequently results in fracture.

The management of retained roots has been discussed in Chapter 8. However, if certain principles are neglected the attempted removal of such roots may lead to more serious complications. It is essential that a radiograph is available to judge the presence of vital structures such as the antrum or mental nerve. Except where the crown has fractured at or above the level of the alveolar margin, it is bad practice to use forceps up the socket as the limited access makes it difficult to open the beaks sufficiently to grasp the root. If forceps are applied knowing that one or both blades are outside the alveolus, this bone will be severely damaged in order to deliver the root. The use of luxators may further expand the alveolus to allow elevation or safe application of root forceps.

The transalveolar approach must always be used wherever the root is not clearly visible or supporting tissues will be damaged. It is safe, leaves the tissue in good condition and, if regularly practised without delay, is economic in time.

Loss of tooth or roots

As the teeth and roots are extracted they should be carefully placed in a special container, and care should be taken not to carry them back into the mouth by accident. At the end of the operation, particularly under general anaesthesia, they should be counted and the number checked against the chart.

Where during extractions a tooth or root is lost, the surgeon should stop operating *immediately* and conduct a systematic search.

The mouth

All the recesses of the mouth, under the tongue and recent sockets are examined. In patients under general anaesthesia, the posterior aspect of the tongue and oropharynx are searched too. After this has been done the superficial layers of the throat pack may be drawn forward lest it be lying there. The pack should not be removed completely till the end of the operation.

Spittoon and suction apparatus

The spittoon should always have a trap, and the suction apparatus a bottle in the circuit to stop fragments of tooth disappearing down the drain. The suction tip, tubing and other connections should be washed through as they often trap root apices.

Alimentary tract or lungs

Roots or teeth may be swallowed or inhaled. Whenever it is suspected that this may have happened, radiographs of the chest should be taken to ensure the tooth is not in one of the bronchi (usually the right). Swallowed fragments seldom give cause for anxiety as they should pass through the gut without incident, but if inhaled into the lungs the patient must be referred, without delay, to a thoracic surgeon for removal by bronchoscopy.

Under the mucoperiosteum

Roots and occasionally teeth can be displaced under the periosteum, particularly in the posterior maxilla, or the mandible where there has been gross recession of alveolar bone or flaps have been raised past the reflection of the mucous membrane. A finger should be placed at once below the root and kept there to prevent it going deeper. A flap may be raised to expose the root, which can then be lifted out using a blunt hooked instrument. Attempts should not be made to grasp it with forceps as if they fail to grip the root they may drive it deeper into the space.

The tissue spaces

In the mandible, roots or teeth can be lost in the tissue spaces of the floor of the mouth either above or below the mylohyoid muscle. The lower third molar roots can be pushed down lingually through the bottom of the socket if this is deficient, as does occasionally occur; the root then lies below the mylohyoid. During the extraction of the unerupted lower third molar it can be elevated lingually into the tissue spaces. In all these cases the grave danger is that the tooth will pass into the deeper planes of the neck as a result of gravity and movements of the muscles. Without delay a finger must be placed either extra- or intraorally to stop the tooth moving. A flap may then be raised to explore the tissue space when the tooth may be 'milked' out or removed as described for those under the periosteum. When the tooth is lying superficial to the mylohyoid, removal is better delayed to allow an extraoral approach, followed by a blunt dissection up to the tooth.

The unerupted upper third molar can be elevated distally into the soft tissue space behind the tuberosity of the maxilla to lie in the pterygomandibular space. This is explored through an incision made down the anterior border of the ascending ramus of the mandible.

Bone cavities

The roots of the maxillary second premolar, first, second and third molars, and occasionally the first premolar are related to the maxillary sinus, into which they can be displaced during extraction. Unerupted and supernumerary teeth may be related to the floor of the nose. Lower apices can be pushed into the inferior dental canal. In both jaws roots can be driven into pathological cavities such as cysts or abscesses. Where it is suspected that a root is lost in a bone cavity the operation is stopped and radiographs are taken in two planes at right angles to each other in an effort to localise the lost root or tooth.

Roots displaced into the inferior dental canal are removed by a transalveolar approach, care being taken not to damage the inferior dental nerve. They should not be left as they may give rise to infection or pressure symptoms of paraesthesia or anaesthesia. Roots pushed into the nose, if they lie under the mucous membrane, are usually easily recovered through the socket, or through the anterior nares if they are lying in the nasal cavity.

Oroantral communication

The relationship of the apices of the maxillary premolar and molar teeth to the maxillary sinus is variable and depends on individual anatomy and the age of the patient, as pneumatisation of the sinus continues throughout life. Often the antrum dips down between the roots of the molar teeth, which virtually form part of the antral floor.

Occasionally the uncomplicated extraction of a tooth may fracture the thin floor of the sinus and cause an oroantral communication (OAC). Apical infection can destroy the bone over the apex, bringing an apical granuloma into contact with antral lining, which is then torn by the extraction of the tooth. Infection in the maxillary sinus may also predispose to the establishment of a fistula. More commonly the communication is produced by attempts to remove retained apices so that the antrum floor is perforated or the apex displaced into it. An oroantral fistula (OAF) is established if the communication becomes epithelialised (Figure 10.1).

Signs and symptoms

The patient will complain of air passing from the nose into the mouth and the operator will be able to see this bubbling through the communication, particularly when the patient is asked to breathe out. Blood from the wound and mouthwashes used to rinse the mouth may pass through the sinus into the nose. A blunt probe passed very gently into the socket will be found to penetrate into the maxillary sinus. This last test should rarely be performed as it may create a communication. Established fistulae tend to reduce in diameter but the track from mouth to sinus frequently fails to heal spontaneously and becomes epithelialised. When this is large the patient complains that drinks pass from the mouth into the nose, that cigarettes are inhaled with difficulty, and that air passes into the mouth. As the hole shrinks it remains a pathway for infection,

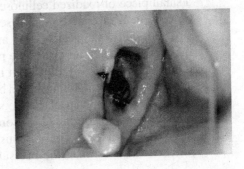

Figure 10.1 Oro-antral fistula.

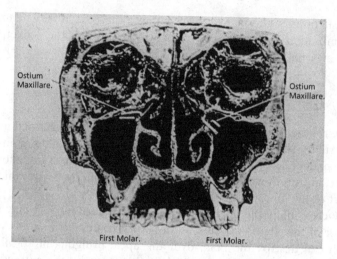

Figure 10.2   Section through the maxillary sinus. Ciliated mucosa allows rapid movement of mucus to give efficient drainage despite ostium being close to the root of the sinus.

but fails to provide adequate drainage for the sinus so that often the symptoms of acute sinusitis are superimposed on those of a fistula. The aim of treatment is to re-establish the normal drainage pattern of the sinus (Figure 10.2) by closing the communication either by use of a splint or surgically.

Treatment

Immediately on diagnosing a communication the tooth should be checked to ensure that it has been completely extracted. All pieces of loose bone that might form sequestra are then gently removed. The buccal plate of alveolar bone is trimmed if a flap has been raised, but is otherwise left alone. Irrigation is best avoided. The mucous membrane over the socket is gently drawn together with simple interrupted sutures and every effort made to obtain a sound clot in the socket.

Under no circumstances should the socket be packed with any material that will prevent healing. Thus ribbon gauze should be avoided at all costs. However, a small piece of oxidized cellulose (Surgicel®) to help to stabilise the clot may be of benefit in encouraging a seal. Impressions are taken and a splint constructed with a flange to cover and protect the socket (Figure 10.3). Before taking the impressions a sizeable piece of foil should be placed over the socket to protect the clot and to prevent the impression material being forced into the communication. The splint should be produced quickly as an emergency measure and, if possible, put in place the same day. Antibiotic therapy is commenced immediately and continued for some 5 days as a prophylactic measure whether or not there is a history of previous sinusitis. The patient is instructed that under no circumstances must the pressure in the nose be raised by blowing it until

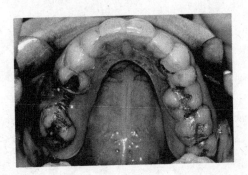

Figure 10.3   Splint for oroantral communication (OAC). Soft splint covering defect at upper right molar.

healing has taken place. Such energetic measures immediately applied will in most cases result in satisfactory healing by first intention.

Where the above measures fail and the fistula remains patent after 6 weeks, but there are no signs of maxillary sinus infection, a surgical repair should be undertaken without delay. This may be done under general anaesthesia as an inpatient or local anaesthesia as an outpatient, but always under an antibiotic cover started before operation. There are two commonly described methods, using a buccal or less commonly a palatal flap to cover the defect. In both cases the operation commences by excising the fistula cleanly and curetting out the tract from the socket. The deeper part of the fistula adjoining the antrum may be left undisturbed where there is no evidence of infection.

Buccal advancement flap

This is the operation of choice. The flap is raised by making an incision along the buccal edge of the socket concerned and two vertical incisions from the cervical margins of the adjacent teeth obliquely up into the buccal sulcus. The flap is carefully raised well past the reflection. Normally this would not cover the socket because the periosteum is still attached, beyond the reflection, to maxillary bone. To overcome this the periosteum *only* is divided by a long horizontal incision made well *above* the line of reflection of the mucosa. It will then be found that the flap can be drawn down over the socket without tension (Figure 10.4). Buttonholing of the buccal flap must obviously be avoided. The palatal mucoperiosteum can be trimmed so that the line of closure will be supported by palatal bone. This margin is raised slightly to permit eversion of its edges when suturing. Haemorrhage is carefully arrested, as a haematoma could prevent the flap taking, and closure is effected with mattress sutures. A splint may be worn over the wound to protect it. The only disadvantage of this operation is that it may reduce the depth of the buccal sulcus opposite the socket concerned, but this is usually only temporary.

Palatal flap

The palatal flap is rarely used except in the repair of oronasal fistulae. It is a pedicle flap that derives its blood supply from the palatine artery and therefore

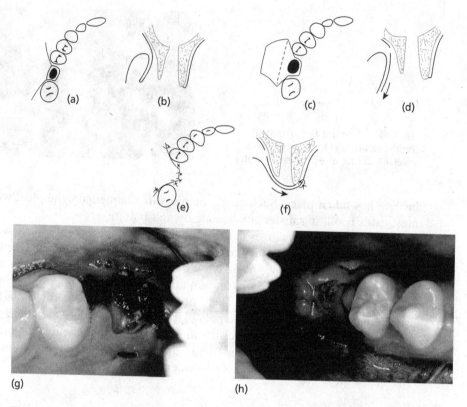

(g)   (h)

Figure 10.4   Closure of oroantral fistula (OAF) using a buccal flap. (a) Shows excision of fistula and buccal incision through mucoperiosteum. (b) Flap raised; note palatal mucosa trimmed back to expose ledge of palatal bone. (c) Dotted line shows incision through *periosteum only* above line of reflection of mucosa. (d) Mucosa extended once periosteum is divided. (e) and (f) Closure effected with buccal flap resting on palatal bone. An OAC closed by buccal advanced flap (g) and after suture removal (h).

has its base over the greater palatine foramen. It is raised by making an incision in the palate parallel to the cervical margins of the teeth but about 5 mm above them. This extends from the second molar to the lateral incisor and is then taken back almost down the midline of the palate. The flap is carefully raised with the periosteum to include the palatine artery. This must be preserved because if its function is impaired the flap will be deprived of its blood supply and die (Figure 10.5). A second hazard to the artery occurs when the flap is rotated to cover the fistula, because if it is twisted too sharply, the blood supply may be cut off. Indeed this fact limits its use to the second premolar and first molar sockets. The buccal flap is trimmed back to a clean edge and, if possible, supported on bone, though often loss of the buccal alveolar plate at the time of extraction makes this difficult to achieve. The flap is sutured into place with mattress sutures and the bone deficiency in the palate covered with a dressing (Figure 10.4b). It has the advantage that the palatal flap is very thick and tough and is

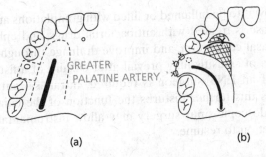

GREATER
PALATINE ARTERY

(a)   (b)

Figure 10.5 Oroantral fistula. (a) Design of palatal flap for closure of the fistula showing the palatine artery in the flap and the excision of the fistula. (b) Closure showing rotation of the palatal flap and pack sutured over the area of bare bone.

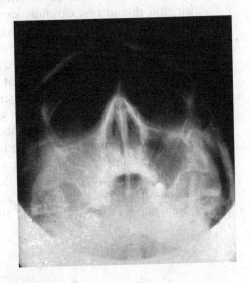

Figure 10.6 Opacity of right antrum.

of sufficient length to cover the whole socket; however, patients report this flap as being extremely uncomfortable.

Infected maxillary sinus

Where the maxillary sinus is infected closure must not be attempted until this has settled.

Acute sinusitis

In acute sinusitis the patient complains of pain together with a feeling of weight in the cheek on the affected side, especially on bending down. Discharge from the maxillary sinus is often described as 'catarrh' on that side, especially in the morning. Examination often shows the cheek over the infected sinus to be red, there is tenderness on pressure in the canine fossa and pus may be seen and smelled in the nostril. Transillumination and radiographs show opacity and, if pus is present, a fluid level (Figure 10.6). Careful examination of the fistula will often show it to be inflamed or filled with granulations and discharging pus. The acute phase is treated with antibacterial drugs, and ephedrine nasal drops to reduce nasal congestion, and improve drainage through the ostium. Persistent symptoms of sinusitis may prevail after closure of a fistula. In these cases the opinon of an ENT surgeon is required. Intranasal antrostomy is rarely performed as this further disturbs the function of the ciliated epithelium of the sinus. Endoscopic sinus surgery may allow instrumentation to enable normal sinus function to resume.

Root in antrum

When a root is believed to have been pushed into the maxillary sinus the surgeon should first carefully examine the socket and mouth as well as any gauze that might have been used, and any adjacent sockets in case it should have been displaced there. He then considers whether the root is lying below the antral lining or has penetrated it to enter the sinus. Presence of an oroantral communication is strong, but not conclusive, evidence that the root is in the antrum. Radiographs, long cone periapical or dental pantomograph, are required (Figure 10.7). It is usual to take a second set after shaking the head to see if the root has moved. If it has it is probably lying free in the sinus cavity. The root if fixed may be jammed under the lining, though this is not certain as it can be lying in the antrum anchored by a blood clot.

In the immediate period after the root has been displaced, before the socket has healed over, a transalveolar approach is used to identify and remove it. A buccal flap is raised as described above and the socket enlarged to allow access

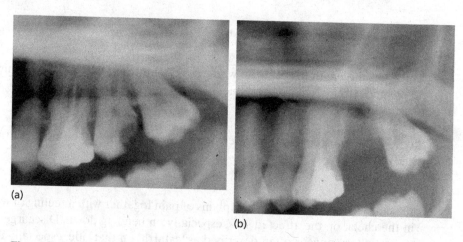

(a)

(b)

Figure 10.7   Tooth root in left antrum. (a) Preoperative radiograph showing close proximity of upper teeth to antrum; (b) socket of upper left second molar and apical part of root in antrum. This was displaced during attempts to retrieve the root during routine extraction.

to the sinus. Careful exploration often reveals the root. This can be retrieved using artery forceps, but the use of irrigation and good suction is also extremely helpful. The buccal flap is then advanced by division of the periosteum to close the defect. Antibiotics and judicious use of nasal decongestants is advocated postoperatively.

Once the socket has healed the Caldwell–Luc extranasal antrostomy is preferable. For this latter operation the patient is admitted to hospital and, under general anaesthesia and an antibiotic cover, an incision is made in the mucous membrane of the canine fossa at its reflection into the cheek. A flap is reflected to expose the anterior wall of the antrum. The infraorbital nerve must not be damaged, particularly by stretching when retracting the flap during the operation. With chisels or burs a round hole about 1.5 cm in diameter is cut through the thin anterior wall, above the roots of the teeth and near to the lateral wall of the nose. All spicules of loose bone are carefully removed and the interior inspected using a headlamp. Suction should be used very carefully to avoid damaging the delicate lining. The root is lifted out with sinus forceps and the sinus cleared of any infective material. The mouth wound is then closed.

Damage to soft tissues

The chief cause of damage to soft tissues is carelessness by the operator. The gingivae can be torn by misapplication of dental forceps, pulling on teeth to which gingival margins are still attached instead of dissecting them free, and by attempting the removal of roots without adequate access. When extracting upper teeth the lower lip can be trapped between the forceps and the lower teeth.

During surgery the drill can easily inadvertently damage the buccal tissues or lips due to trauma from the shaft of the bur and, if this is noticed by the assistant, should be brought to the attention of the operator.

The cheek, tongue, floor of mouth and palate can be damaged by instruments that slip because they are not properly supported. This applies particularly to luxators, elevators and burs. Burns may be caused by hot instruments from the steriliser, overheating of burs or handpieces and antiseptic solutions.

Nerves

The inferior dental nerve can be damaged during the extraction of buried teeth or retained roots. Its relationship to the third molar has been discussed (see Chapter 9). When a flap is raised for operations in the lower premolar area the mental nerve should be identified and preserved. Stretching of nerves when retracting flaps can produce paraesthesia ,which may be very painful and of long duration, and this can occur with the mental and infraorbital nerves. The lingual nerve where it lies in the lingual mucoperiosteum of the mandible opposite the third molar can be damaged when this tooth is being extracted.

Fracture of alveolar and basal bone

The buccal and lingual alveolar plates

These can be fractured during the extraction of teeth, particularly if as a result of chronic periodontal disease the tooth is ankylosed to the socket wall. The buccal plate in the molar region is most frequently involved but is usually firmly attached to periosteum, which provides it with a satisfactory blood supply. This bone can be retained if it is repositioned by gently compressing the socket between finger and thumb after completing the extractions.

Loose fragments not attached to periosteum must be removed to avoid the formation of sequestra, suppuration and delayed healing.

Occasionally extraction of a tooth causes a horizontal fracture of the alveolus, which may carry other teeth. This occurs classically in the maxilla during an attempted extraction of single standing upper molars, especially the third molar, and may cause fracture of the tuberosity. This will be felt during the extraction by the movement of bone rather than the tooth, and a radiograph should be taken to confirm the presence of a fracture. Where the portion of bone attached to the tooth is small, bone and tooth should be dissected out by blunt dissection through a buccal flap, taking every precaution to prevent tearing of the mucous membrane. The antrum is frequently opened following this manoeuvre, but if the flaps are healthy it can be closed satisfactorily. The surgeon may wish to retain a large piece of bone or one with other teeth, not for extraction, attached to it. It is very difficult to hold the bone still and complete the planned extraction. So long as any pain from the tooth can be alleviated, the fragment can be splinted for a month until it is firm. The tooth may then be extracted by a transalveolar approach and gentle elevation. This procedure is seldom justified unless sound teeth in occlusion are to be saved.

Basal bone

The predisposing causes of fracture of the body of the mandible are general bone diseases (osteogenesis imperfecta, osteopetrosis), weakened bone owing to age, osteomyelitis, cysts, tumours, teeth with large or misplaced roots and buried teeth. The immediate cause is misapplication of instruments or the use of undue force, particularly with elevators. As soon as the operator realises that a fracture has occurred they should complete the operation if this can be done without causing further damage. Radiographs must be taken to confirm the position and extent of the injury, and the patient referred immediately for treatment by reduction and fixation (see Chapter 14).

Dislocation of the temporomandibular joint

This occurs most frequently following the extraction of lower teeth under general anaesthesia, but may happen even under local anaesthesia in those patients who have a lax capsule and weak supporting muscles.

Dislocation may be prevented by supporting the mandible firmly and never exerting more force in the primary downward movement than can be opposed by the supporting hand. During extractions under local anaesthesia, a prop placed on the opposite side of the mouth gives the patient something to bite on and thereby support their jaw.

At the close of operations under general anaesthesia the jaws should be brought together with the teeth in occlusion at the time the prop and pack are removed from the mouth. The jaw, if dislocated, may be reduced before the patient returns to full consciousness (see Chapter 17).

Post-extraction

Haemorrhage

Prolonged haemorrhage is a common complication following extraction of teeth and occurs as primary (see Chapter 7), reactionary and secondary haemorrhage. The most important aspect of treatment is prevention. The systemic causes have been discussed in Chapter 3, but local factors are more often responsible for postoperative haemorrhage. These include infection, excessive trauma and local vascular lesions.

Infections include gingival conditions, which should be treated by scaling and instructions in oral hygiene. To be effective, scaling should be completed a week before operation and mouth-brushing conscientiously undertaken by the patient. This preparation should be done for all but emergency extractions, and the dental surgeon must stress the importance of a clean mouth as many patients tend to neglect oral hygiene on the ground that they are about to lose their remaining teeth. The use of chlorhexidine mouthwash before and after surgery may reduce infection. Where there is an apical or pericoronal condition, the use of antibiotics may be indicated, not only to prevent a flare up but to protect the blood clot from destruction by bacteria.

Reactionary haemorrhage

Reactionary haemorrhage occurs within 48 hours of the operation or accident when a local rise in blood pressure may force open divided vessels insecurely sealed by natural or artificial means. It is common in patients recovering from shock and in those treated under local anaesthesia when the effect of the vaso-constrictor wears off. It is arrested by one of the methods described below and, for excited patients, by administration of a sedative.

Secondary haemorrhage

The cause of secondary haemorrhage is infection, which destroys the blood clot or may ulcerate a vessel wall. It starts about 7 days after operation, usually with a mild ooze, which is a serious symptom in wounds near major vessels because, if the vessel is not found and ligated, a massive haemorrhage may ensue. In the more mild capillary form such as from a tooth socket it will be more trouble-some than dangerous. Bleeding is arrested by local measures and antibacterial drugs are prescribed to combat the infection.

Treatment

A practitioner who is called to a post-extraction haemorrhage should first take a *rapid* history from the patient, or a relative, which must include the number of teeth extracted, the duration of bleeding (the volume of the loss is unreliable as it is invariably diluted by saliva) and whether there has been any similar previous occurrence or known blood dyscrasia. The patient's general condition is then rapidly assessed and, if they appear shocked and ill, arrangements must be made at once for transfer to hospital. Meanwhile local measures should be applied to arrest the bleeding.

It is never a waste of time to clean the patient, for much of the distress and fear associated with bleeding is due to the sight of blood on the face, sheets and clothes. The mouth is then examined in a good light with adequate suction apparatus, if available. The latter should only be used to remove blood from the floor of the mouth and not be applied to the sockets since aspiration will disturb stable blood clots and encourage further bleeding. A local anaesthetic contain-ing adrenaline should be administered and the patient encouraged to bite on a damp gauze while this takes effect. Pressure is then applied by placing a finger on each side of the alveolus to find the bleeding point. If this is successful in arresting the haemorrhage it indicates bleeding from soft tissues, and sutures may be placed across the socket. Where pressure fails to arrest the haemorrhage, bleeding is from the bony socket and an oxidised cellulose pack may be placed in the socket. When local measures have controlled the bleeding, the patient's general condition should be more accurately assessed by recording their pulse and blood pressure. They should receive supportive treatment including warmth, administration of fluids by mouth, and drugs to relieve anxiety and pain.

Surgical emphysema

Surgical emphysema is a collection of air that has been forced into the tissue spaces through the extraction wound and forms a swelling which characteristically crackles on palpation. It results from increased air pressure in the mouth from using an air spray, or blowing a trumpet or a balloon. Surgical emphysema seldom gives rise to discomfort and settles without treatment as the air is slowly absorbed.

Delayed healing and infection

Normally a tooth socket heals by second intention, the blood clot becoming organised as capillaries and fibroblasts grow into it from the bony or soft tissue periphery. The blood clot may fail to form if there is little bleeding owing to sclerosis of the bone forming the tooth socket, the action of the vasoconstrictor present in the local anaesthetic solution or packing of the socket to arrest haemorrhage. Infection may rapidly supervene if the extracted tooth was septic or contamination takes place from the mouth. Even where a satisfactory clot does form, this can be destroyed by bacteria either present in the socket or introduced by imperfectly sterilised instruments. Lacerated or bruised tissues, loose pieces of bone or retained tooth fragments also favour secondary infection.

Dry socket

Early loss of the blood clot produces an acutely painful condition in around 5% of normal extractions. The socket contains either remnants of the blood clot or food debris. The aetiology of this condition is unclear, although infection has been mooted. The blood clot fails to organise and healing is subsequently delayed, on account of which the socket may become secondarily infected. A decrease in blood supply to the healing socket may be one of the factors and a higher incidence has been seen following the use of local anaesthetic containing adrenaline. Smoking also seems to increase the chance of developing dry socket. Treatment is aimed at protecting the socket during the production of granulation tissue over the exposed socket walls. Packing materials that contain some analgesic and sedative properties together with an antiseptic are used once the socket has been irrigated with warm saline or chlorhexidine to remove any debris. Various materials are available such as Alvogyl®, an iodoform dressing that does not need to be removed, and bismuth, iodoform and paraffin paste (BIPP®) on ribbon gauze. This dressing may have to be removed and replaced on occasions until the socket has epithelialised after about 3 weeks.

Infection

Post-extraction infection may take another form in which exuberant granulations and a discharge of pus localised to the socket appear a week or so after the extraction. Frequently bone sequestra are the cause, and when they are removed healing takes place rapidly. This condition is relatively painless and the granulations make packing difficult. Treatment is first by hot mouth baths, but if these fail to settle the socket radiographs are necessary to confirm the local nature of the infection. The socket is then opened up, sequestra and granulations removed, and the cavity packed open. Forceful curettage is contraindicated as it may spread the infection.

Truly infected sockets are a rare but serious condition, which, if neglected, may progress to osteomyelitis or to a severe cellulitis of the face and neck (see Chapter 12). Suspicion should be raised if the infection arises in an otherwise healthy individual as this may be the first presentation of an underlying medical condition (Figure 10.8).

Damage to other organs

Faulty or careless handling of instruments may result in damage to other organs. Under general anaesthesia the eyes, if not suitably protected, can be damaged by caustic fluids, instruments and the operator's fingers.

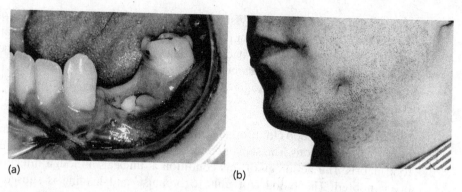

(a)   (b)

Figure 10.8   Infected socket in previously undiagnosed type 1 diabetic. The socket was colonised by candida. (a) The appearance of the socket. Note whitish appearance of candida in socket; (b) discharging sinus associated with the infected socket.

Pain

Post-extraction pain may result from incomplete extraction of the tooth, laceration of the soft tissues, exposed bone, infected sockets or damage to adjacent nerves. Treatment is by eliminating the cause and symptomatic by prescribing analgesic drugs.

Swelling

Swelling or oedema following surgery is part of the inflammatory reaction to surgical interference. It is increased by poor surgical technique, particularly rough handling of the tissues, pulling on flaps to gain access and inadequate drainage. There is also a wide individual variation in the response to trauma that does not seem to be related to any of these factors.

Trismus

Trismus may occur as the result of oedema and swelling, in which case opening improves as the swelling resolves. Damage to the temporomandibular joint due to excessive downward pressure or to keeping the patient's mouth open wide for a long period may lead to a more chronic, painful condition with symptoms of the pain dysfunction syndrome (see Chapter 17). The injection for the inferior dental nerve block may cause a painless trismus without swelling, which has variously been ascribed to trauma to the medial pterygoid muscle causing spasm, or to penetration of a small blood vessel and formation of a haematoma. As the haematoma organises so the trismus becomes apparent, often starting 2–3 days after the injection. It will recover with time, usually 6 weeks, but may be improved more quickly by gently opening the mouth using wooden spatulas in a progressive manner (see Chapter 17).

Broken instruments

All instruments should be carefully examined after use and any that are defective immediately discarded or sent for repair. Should one break, a search is made at once for the fragment and if it is not recovered radiographs are taken to locate it. If the instrument is sterile and the piece small, such as the point of a suture needle or a tiny portion of a dental bur, this may be left and the patient informed (Figure 10.9).

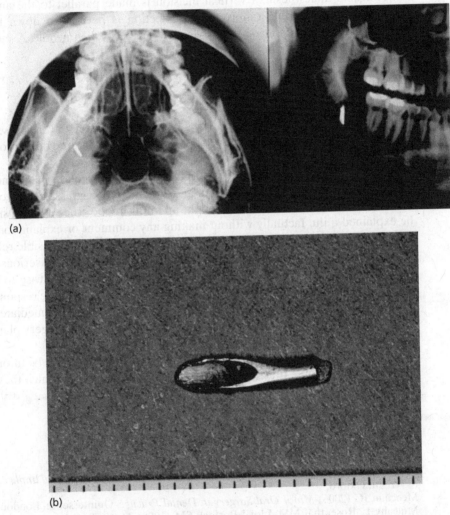

(a)

(b)

Figure 10.9 Broken instrument: (a) a fragment can be seen in the lingual tissues adjacent to the third molar socket; (b) the retrieved fragment: the end of an elevator that fractured during the removal of the lower third molar. The patient suffered temporary loss of sensation in the lingual nerve.

Broken local anaesthetic needles occur chiefly when giving an inferior dental nerve block. The needle should never be inserted up to the hub but one-third of its length must be kept clear of the tissues. A pair of artery forceps should always be close at hand to grasp the fragment immediately before it disappears if the patient moves or swallows.

Removal of broken needles from the pterygomandibular space is a difficult operation. First the needle must be localised by taking radiographs in two planes (lateral oblique and posterior anterior views of the mandible), preferably with a second needle in position to serve as a marker. At operation, performed under endotracheal anaesthesia, a vertical incision is made parallel to the anterior border of the ascending ramus, blunt dissection is performed down to the marker and a search is made in the vicinity for the broken needle. A metallic foreign body detector can be of great assistance.

Mishaps

The patient or a relative should always be warned beforehand if any serious difficulty or complication is envisaged and this should be entered on the consent form signed by the patient.

When a mishap has occurred it is important to keep quite calm and not become emotionally involved. The patient is often upset, aggressive and vociferous, and the surgeon must not get caught up in this mood. The situation should be explained quite factually without making any comment or explanation that might imply liability. If the patient is nervous it is best to tell a sensible relative or, failing that, the patient's medical or dental practitioner. In any serious accident, such as a fracture of the jaw or a root in antrum, it is very wise to hand the case over to a colleague, preferably a specialist, as thereafter the responsibility is shared. It is also wise when treating a mishap to limit the immediate care to putting it right, and not to attempt the completion of all the surgery planned, as a new disaster may occur elsewhere in the mouth.

In any case of doubt the practitioner's protection society should be informed at the earliest possible time and asked for advice and guidance, which they will willingly give.

Further reading

McGowan DA, Baxter PW, Jones J (1993) *The Maxillary Sinus and its Dental Implications.* Wright, Oxford.

Meechan JG (2006) *Minor Oral Surgery in Dental Practice.* Quintessence, London.

Mulcahy L, Rosenthal MM, Lloyd-Bostock SM (1998) *Medical Mishaps: pieces of the puzzle.* Open University Press, Buckingham.

Robinson PP (1998) Observations on the recovery of sensation following inferior alveolar nerve injuries. *British Journal of Oral and Maxillofacial Surgery* **26**: 177.

Chapter 11
Preparation of the Mouth for Prostheses

> - Preservation of alveolar bone
> - Surgical preparation for tissue-borne prostheses
> - Surgical preparation for endosteal implant-borne prostheses

The surgical preparation of the mouth for prostheses begins at the time the first permanent tooth is extracted. At this and at all subsequent operations the oral surgeon must try to leave the soft and hard tissues in satisfactory condition to support a tissue, tooth or implant borne prosthesis. For more complex cases it is helpful for surgeon and prosthodontist to plan the case together. Even for simpler cases, it is always important that the practitioner considers the future prosthodontic requirements when selecting any surgical procedure. Joint planning of surgery for prostheses should give the surgeon a clear treatment plan and a transparent rationale to work to. Joint planning should also ensure the retention of potentially restorable teeth either to assist denture retention or bridge construction, or to retain overdentures, which will help maintain alveolar bone height.

As a general rule those who require tissue-borne prostheses, for example complete dentures, should not be subjected to surgery to improve the stability, comfort or aesthetic appearance of their dentures without the opinion of a specialist prosthodontist or restorative dentist. This is largely due to the advancement in prosthodontic techniques that may mean surgery can be avoided altogether, or that less extensive surgery can be carried out.

This chapter will outline some general principles on the preservation of alveolar bone and discuss some of the preparatory surgery for tissue-borne prostheses. However, it will largely concentrate on the implant-borne prosthesis. This is due the increasing importance of implants in prosthodontics. The surgical techniques discussed throughout the chapter such as torus removal, bone grafting, etc., are equally applicable to tissue-borne, tooth-borne and implant-borne prosthesis.

Principles of Oral and Maxillofacial Surgery, 6th Edition. Edited by U. J. Moore
© 2011 Blackwell Publishing Ltd

Preservation of alveolar bone

Atraumatic extraction

This is a contradiction in terms; however, the principle it tries to communicate is sound and appropriate for all oral surgeons. It should always be borne in mind that alveolar bone is precious and once lost cannot easily be replaced. This is even more important since the advent of dental implants. Alveolar bone, possibly more than any other tissue, suffers from instrument mismanagement, and a conservative approach with a careful surgical technique will help to reduce prosthetic difficulties later.

During extractions the alveolar bone may be damaged or fractured by the use of excessive force or worse, by the inclusion of the socket wall within the forcep blades. The commonest site of alveolar fracture is the buccal plate of the upper molars. The surgeon should always strive to avoid the fracture and loss of the maxillary tuberosity as this may interfere with retention of the upper denture by making the peripheral seal at this point inadequate. Alveolar bone, if still attached to periostium, may be preserved and pressed back into place, but if detached from its blood supply it should be removed to avoid sequestration and delayed healing.

Consideration should be given to the initial use of periotomes to cut the periodontal ligament, followed by luxators to begin the widening of the tooth socket, prior to application of elevators and forceps (see Chapter 8). Sectioning multirooted teeth before extraction and the use of piezoelectric instruments, harnessing ultrasonic forces to sever the periodontal attachment and remove bone, may facilitate minimally traumatic extractions. Alveolar bone may also be conserved by the immediate placement of implants directly into healthy extraction sites.

Difficult extractions may be best completed through a planned transalveolar approach to avoid accidental alveolar fractures that may lead to more widespread loss of bone. Sharp burs and copious irrigation should be used to help prevent overheating of the bone and subsequent necrosis.

Access to deeply buried roots or teeth can often be made through the lateral aspect of the alveolus, leaving the ridge intact. Indeed, this principle holds true for access to cystic or granulomatous tissue at apices. This approach attempts to maintain ridge height for any prosthesis planned. In all such operations bone cutting should be limited to one side, leaving the lingual or palatal plate and its mucoperiostium untouched. Osteoplastic flaps, as described in Chapter 9, are an alternative to lateral access to deeply buried roots or teeth. Piezoelectric saws now allow minimal trauma to both hard and soft tissues when creating such flaps. Sometimes it is more appropriate to leave a buried root to be removed at the time of preparing the bone for a dental implant.

Edentulous jaws can prove a difficulty, as the bone in such jaws is often dense and brittle. Compounding this is the resorption of the alveolar ridge, which makes the bone less strong. Under such conditions the extraction of buried teeth and roots can be difficult. Those teeth and roots that are symptomless need not be extracted if they are covered by bone and are unlikely to come to the surface during the life of the denture or to affect any planned implant placement. Those lying superficially, close to implant sites, or that are associated with secondary disease such as cysts or granulomas, should be removed. Roots and teeth must be accurately localised and tooth division carried out to reduce the amount of bone removed. This is confined as far as possible to the buccal aspect, and osteoplastic flaps are used to preserve the ridge where teeth are lying in it.

Socket preservation

This involves minimising the trauma of the extraction by the methods described in previous paragraphs followed by the placement of autogenous (from the same individual), allogenous (from another individual of the same species, e.g. cadaveric bone) or xenogenous (from another species, e.g. cow) bone, or alloplastic substances (synthetic or naturally derived material, e.g. calcium triphosphate or hydroxyapatite) into the empty socket. Either a mucosal graft or a biological membrane is then used to cover the inserted material.

The principles behind this technique are dependent on the material placed within the socket but the aim is to reduce to the absolute minimum the amount of local alveolar resorption. Potentially it can provide:

- osteogenesis – only autogenous bone has this potential
- an osseoinductive stimulus – autogenous and allogenous bone
- an osseoconductive scaffold to facilitate bone formation – alloplasts, allogenous and xenogenous bone.

Practitioners should be wary of placing any type of material into recently infected sites as some new bone should be formed irrespective of whether or not a material is placed into the socket following extraction.

Bone recontouring

It is advisable to do the minimum recontouring of the bone at the time of extraction and wait for at least 3 months to reconsider the situation once healing and remodelling has taken place, as some natural resorption always takes place and it is impossible to tell how extensive this will be. A conservative approach is particularly important where periodontal disease has already caused appreciable bone loss. Indications for minor surgery at the time of the extractions include the following.

- Jagged or irregular alveolar margins and septal bone, which are treated by dividing the buccal interdental papillae from the lingual along the ridge and exposing the bony edges of the sockets just enough to smooth the bone with a bur or file, after which the mucosa is closed over the ridge.
- Minor local deformities, such as fibrous bands, bulbous tuberosities and undercuts, which may be removed.

Surgical preparation for tissue-borne prostheses

Surgery for complete immediate dentures

Where a complete denture is to be provided, consideration can be given to removing all the posterior teeth first. Sufficient teeth can be left in the premolar region to maintain the vertical dimension of the occlusion while the molar sockets are healing. Three months later the rest of the teeth are removed and the denture(s) inserted.

When an anterior flange cannot be worn either because it would cause the lip to be over supported in an unsightly way, or there would be an undercut preventing flange insertion, an open-faced denture with the anterior teeth socketed into the alveolus is provided as a temporary measure until natural resorption has taken place. In certain cases, however, it is obvious that some alveolectomy is necessary at the time the teeth are extracted.

Where the patient must be admitted to hospital for a general anaesthetic, the less satisfactory procedure of fitting an immediate complete denture can be performed.

Hard tissue irregularities

Torus

A large palatal torus can be prosthodontically acceptable if smooth, but when nodular or irregular in shape it may need to be removed. Tori, often bilateral, are sometimes found on the lingual aspect of the mandible in the premolar region and can cause pain from denture contact or interfere with the path of insertion.

The torus palatinus is excised through a Y-shaped midline sagittal incision and the bony prominence removed with burs, chisels or a piezoelectric saw. A full denture or cover-plate lined with a periodontal dressing is immediately fitted to hold the flap in place and prevent formation of a haematoma (Figure 11.1).

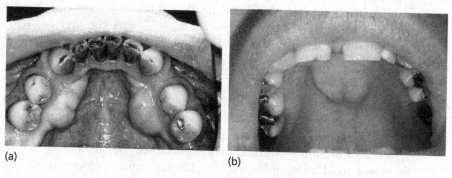

(a)   (b)

Figure 11.1   Tori. (a) Mandibular tori would cause problems when denture is worn. (b) Palatal torus.

Mandibular lingual tori are removed where they cause a hindrance to the design of tissue- or tooth-borne prostheses or when they are continually traumatised by a denture. A lingual mucoperiosteal flap is raised and an instrument (e.g. a Howarth periosteal elevator) is passed below the torus to isolate it. Burs or a piezoelectric saw can be used to section the majority of the distance through the torus and final fracture is achieved with an elevator. The torus is removed and the operation site, smoothed, debrided and toileted.

Tori in either arch can provide an excellent source of bone for grafting and should be one of the considerations when bone is required elsewhere in the arch.

Alveolectomy

This is the operation used to smooth irregular ridges and remove undercuts. Radiographs must be studied to determine the extent of the antrum and the position of the mental nerve. Plaster casts of the ridges may be used to assist planning so that the procedure is completed with minimum unnecessary destruction of alveolar bone.

A horizontal incision is made on the buccal aspect of the alveolus through fixed mucoperiosteum just short of non-keratinised mucosa so that this is not disturbed by the operation. Two vertical incisions are taken over the crest of the alveolus and on to the lingual or palatal mucosa. The flap is reflected to expose the alveolar crest. The bone may be trimmed with a large rosehead bur or rongeurs and smoothed with a bone file. The operator then replaces the flap and runs their finger over the ridge to check it is smooth. The wound is thoroughly irrigated with saline and if much reduction has taken place the flap is trimmed conservatively. The mucoperiosteal flap is closed without tension.

Feather edge ridge

This condition typically occurs in the lower anterior region. The patient complains of inability to wear the denture for more than 1 or 2 hours owing to soreness. The ridge is usually very narrow and covered with thin atrophic mucosa, which is inflamed and tender to palpation. Radiographs show an uneven resorbed ridge with a feathered appearance due to spicules of bone standing vertically.

Surgery should be considered only when all prosthetic techniques to reduce the load (selective compression impressions, narrow teeth and resilient linings) have failed.

Genial tubercles

These sometimes become prominent in the floor of the mouth owing to alveolar resorption. They are best left, as genioglossus is attached to them. Occasionally, the upper part of a prominent genial tubercule may require excision to facilitate denture wearing.

Mylohyoid ridge removal

Where the mandibular alveolus has undergone gross resorption, the mylohyoid ridge may be at the level of the resorbed alveolus and, if sharp, be a source of pain under the lower denture. Its removal, by cutting off the attachment of the mylohyoid muscle, does deepen the lingual sulcus of the mandible and may assist denture retention.

An incision is made along the alveolar crest and reflected lingually to expose the mylohyoid muscle, which is detached from the bone. The prominent bony mylohyoid ridge is then separated from the mandible with burs. Bleeding is meticulously arrested and the incision closed. This procedure may be carried out in combination with sulcus deepening in the anterior mandible (see later in this chapter).

Soft tissue irregularities

Mobile ridges

Ideally, denture-supporting alveolar mucosa should be firm and closely adherent to the ridge, but especially after the extraction of teeth for periodontal disease, hyperplastic tissue may remain to form a mobile ridge. Often such ridges are found in the anterior region of the maxilla when a full upper denture is opposed only by the natural lower anterior teeth. The occlusal forces from the natural lower dentition against the complete upper denture is thought to cause localised resorption of the maxillary bone, leaving a thick mobile fibrous ridge of soft tissue. The thick mobile ridge offers unstable support for the denture. However, as this may be better than the alternative of a completely flat surface left by surgery, the prosthodontist often prefers to manage this problem with special impression techniques and denture design. An alternative approach is to augment the underlying bone with alloplastic substances to try and provide support for the soft tissue.

Reduction of tuberosities

With careful denture design and construction techniques, large maxillary tuberosities with deep sulci can assist retention, but if too large they may encroach on the interocclusal space available for dentures. Many also have appreciable bony undercuts on their buccal aspects, which, if unilateral, can be used to improve denture stability, but when present bilaterally, interfere with the path of insertion. Radiographs before surgery are necessary to identify unerupted upper third molars, to establish the relationship between soft tissue and underlying alveolar bone, and to determine the extent of the maxillary antrum.

Treatment

A fibrous tuberosity may be reduced by making palatal and buccal incisions down to bone to excise a wedge of mucous membrane, fibrous tissue and periosteum from the crest of the ridge. To facilitate closure the incisions are carried

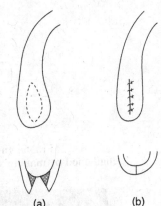

Figure 11.2   Reduction of the tuberosity. (a) Above: Elliptical incision over tuberosity. Below: Cross-section of excision showing deep portion secondarily excised (shaded) to allow flaps to be apposed on bone without tension. (b) Closure.

forward to meet in the first molar region. The raw edges are then undermined and the underlying fibrous tissue removed to produce a reduction in the height of the ridge and to allow satisfactory closure (Figure 11.2). The space available for denture(s) between upper and lower ridges at the approximate occlusal vertical dimension is checked before the wound is sutured.

Where only the bone is to be reduced in height or a buccal undercut removed, the approach is made through a buccal mucoperiosteal flap. Care is required not to perforate the antral lining when cutting bone in this region. Usually both bone and soft tissue are to be reduced and the elliptical incision is used to expose the ridge by reflecting the edges of the wound. Buccal undercuts in this area are often found high above the crest, making a vertical incision at the anterior buccal edge of the ellipse necessary.

Fraenectomy

A fraenum is a musculofibrous band attached to the alveolus and inserted into the muscles of the face or tongue. The most important of these are the labial fraena in the midline of the upper and lower jaw, the buccal fraena in the premolar region and the lingual fraenum of the mandible. During movements of the facial muscles or tongue, fraena can lift the dentures and so reduce their stability. The denture can usually be relieved around the fraenum in question, but where the ridges have resorbed and the fraenum approaches the crest of the ridge, this may greatly reduce the possible depth of the flange and even weaken the denture, making treatment by excision necessary.

Treatment

The maxillary labial fraenum is excised as follows. First the extent of its attachment to the maxilla is found by drawing the upper lip forward to put the fraenum on tension. This causes the base to blanch and it is frequently seen to extend palatally into the incisive papilla. The whole length of the fraenum and the mucosa over it is removed but the periosteum is left intact. A

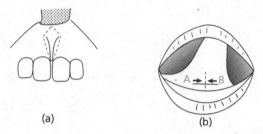

Figure 11.3   Fraena. (a) Incision for excision of labial fraenum. (b) Lingual fraenum lengthened by making a horizontal incison A–B and suturing it vertically.

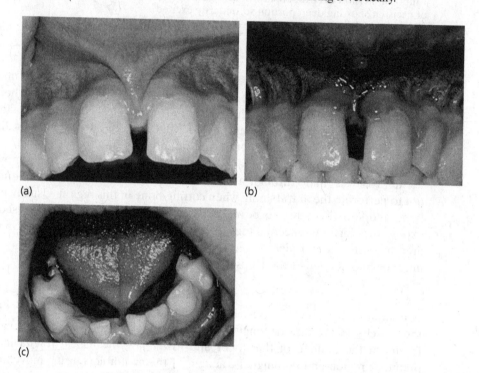

Figure 11.4   Fraenectomy. (a) Tight labial fraenum. (b) Following fraenectomy. (c) Tight lingual fraenum.

diamond-shaped incision is made round the margins of the band sufficiently deep to allow it to be dissected out and for the portion in the lip to the superficially excised (Figure 11.3). The mucosa is undermined before suturing. The effect of suturing the lateral edges of the diamond-shaped incision together is to lengthen the wound and this allows a greater depth of sulcus to be achieved.

Fraena may be lengthened by making a *horizontal* incision across the middle of the band which passes through the *whole depth* of the fibrous tissue it contains. The mucosal edges are undermined and the incision is sutured *vertically* (Figures 11.4 and 11.5).

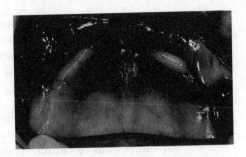

Figure 11.5   Denture hyperplasia.

Denture irritation hyperplasia

This is a fibroepithelial overgrowth in response to chronic trauma. The cause is an overextended denture flange, which transmits the masticatory forces to the soft tissues. This situation often occurs with continued use of a denture following resorption of the ridges (Figure 11.5).

The denture hyperplasia may present as one fold or a series of folds like the leaves of a book, which lie in the buccal sulcus either between the alveolus and the denture or along the periphery of the flange.

Treatment

First the irritation is removed by leaving out the denture or easing back the flange. The patient is reviewed after one month and if satisfactory recession has not taken place, the hyperplasia should be excised.

A single hyperplastic fold can be removed by excision at its base with either a blade or laser. The edges of the resultant wound are then undermined and sutured without altering the depth of the buccal sulcus. Large multi-leaved hyperplasias require excision. If a multi-leaved hyperplasia is excised with a laser then the resultant open wound will present less pain while healing and can be left to heal by secondary intention. If a blade is used to excise a multi-leaved hyperplasia consideration should be given to covering the resultant raw area with a split thickness skin graft or a mucosal graft from the cheek or palate to help reduce contracture and pain. Removal of a multi-leaved hyperplasia may be combined with sulcus deepening if necessary.

Cryosurgery has also been used to remove multi-leaved hyperplasia and does leave a satisfactory sulcus, but has the disadvantages that no tissue is obtained for biopsy and that the area can be very sore and swollen after operation.

Papillary hyperplasia

This presents typically in the hard palate as multiple small elevations of fibroepithelial hyperplasia, often associated with chronic candidosis. Treatment may be with antifungal agents and, where indicated, surgery. Where the lesion is extensive or there is doubt about its benign nature, the area is excised and sent for histological examination. In less severe cases the small hyperplasias can be removed by crysosurgery, laser ablation or by shaving off the elevations using rotary abrasives.

Sulcus deepening

Widespread use of dental implants has meant that these procedures are now performed much less often than was the case.

The dimensions of denture flanges can be increased by deepening the sulci, providing there is adequate underlying bone. Retention and transverse stability for the lower denture would often benefit from deepening of the sulci, particularly where muscle attachments have come to lie near the crest of the ridge. Anteriorly the mentalis muscle, laterally the buccinator muscle and lingually the mylohyoid muscle are involved. To deepen the sulci effectively, these muscles must be detached from the mandible and the mucosa made to heal with a new reflection at a lower level. This last is the most difficult part of the operation. It is complicated by the presence of the mental nerve, which must be located and preserved from accidental damage.

The procedures available can be considered in four groups.

1. *The mucosa is separated from underlying muscle (submucosal vestibuloplasty)*
An example of this group is Obwegeser's operation. The procedure is usually performed in the maxilla. Two vertical incisions 1 cm long are made in the buccal sulcus of the canine regions or a single incision in the midline. Scissors or a scalpel are then passed between mucosa and periosteum. The muscle attachments on the buccal aspect are cut, as far back and upwards as possible, to free the mucosa. The new sulcus is maintained by using a denture lined with gutta percha. One or two bone screws in the palate retain the denture for 2 weeks. Obwegeser's operation has the disadvantage that it is performed blind and if a haematoma occurs the new sulcus may be obliterated.

2. *Skin is transplanted to line both sides of an extended sulcus (buccal inlay)*
In this operation a pouch is made in the mandibular buccal sulcus, which is lined with a split-thickness skin graft from the patient's arm or thigh. A mucosal incision is made in the mandibular labial sulcus and a pouch dissected to the required size leaving the periosteum intact and attached to bone. An acrylic splint with a gutta percha mould, larger than will eventually be required, is made. Where the skin graft and mucous membrane meet, the mould is grooved so that on healing the scar contracts into the groove. The mould is chilled and the skin graft attached to it with the raw surface outwards. This is then placed in the pouch and the splint secured to the mandible with bone screws for 2 weeks.

3. *Skin is transplanted to line one side of an extended sulcus (lower labial vestibuloplasty)*
An incision is made along the mandibular alveolar crest from canine to canine. The incision goes through the mucosa as above. The mucosal flap is dissected

off periosteum and muscles. Care must be taken not to tear the mucosa. Dissection is continued past the reflection, just short of the inner margin of the lip. The mentalis muscle is then divided with a scalpel close to the periostium, which is left undisturbed. The muscle will retract into the deeper tissues. The mucosal flap is repositioned to cover the labial side of the new sulcus and held in position by sutures through the periosteum. A split-thickness skin graft is placed against the raw area of the periostium with a gutta percha mould on a splint. In this way, the labial aspect of the new sulcus is lined with mucosa, and the periosteum with the skin graft.

4. *Lowering of floor of mouth and vestibuloplasty*
This operation combines a buccal vestibuloplasty and skin graft with a vestibuloplasty on the lingual aspect of the ridge which heals by secondary intention. In all vestibuloplasty procedures, the splint or modified denture must be maintained in place for 2–3 weeks to allow initial healing. During this period, a high standard of oral hygiene is vital. Following removal of the splint, there is a marked tendency for the sulcus to contract. To reduce this, the denture must be modified to extend into the full depth of the sulcus and be worn continuously for several weeks.

Surgical preparation for endosteal implant-borne prostheses

It is beyond the scope of this book to describe implant dentistry in detail; many excellent texts already exist on this subject. This section will aim to provide:

- an overview of the phenomenon of osseointegration
- a generic explanation of endosteal implant systems, their terminology and basic components
- an overview of considerations for implant-based treatment planning
- an overview of the surgical procedures in implant surgery.

Prosthodontic aspects of implant dentistry will not be covered.

Over the past decade there has been a dramatic rise in the development and use of endosteal (within bone) root form implants for rehabilitation of the edentulous and partially dentate patient. This is in part due to increasing success rates; in healthy patients the success rate of endosteal root form implants can often exceed 90%. The consequent increase in number of implant manufacturers has also had several effects:

- improvement of implant surfaces increasing the rapidity and reliability of achieving osseointegration
- simplification of implant systems
- reduction in the price of implant systems
- increasing numbers of courses aimed at training the general practitioner in implant dentistry.

Osseointegration

The term osseointegration was first used by Branemark in 1969. This phenomenon, fundamental to all successful endosteal implants, is defined as a direct connection between living bone and a load-bearing endosteal implant when viewed at the light microscopic level. The main factors necessary to achieve osseointegration are as follows.

- A totally biocompatible implant material
  - The implant must not cause any form of foreign body reaction as this will lead to a weaker bone–implant bond and possible rejection. Titanium is in common usage as on contact with air it forms titanium dioxide, an extremely stable compound, as a microscopically thin layer on the surface of the implant providing the bioactive surface which enables osseointegration to occur.
- Precise adaptation of the implant to living bone
  - This is achieved using a series of drill sizes matched to implants to minimise the distance between the bone and the implant.
- A minimally traumatic surgical technique
  - Overheating of bone during preparation of the implant site causes intrabony alkaline phosphatase to be denatured with consequent reduction of alkaline calcium production. This is controlled by the use of copious irrigation and low-speed high-torque drilling with sharp burs.
- A period of unloaded healing
  - The provision of a very close bone–implant interface and features such as screw threads help to prevent movement during the establishment of osseointegration (primary stability). New bone forms on the surface of the implant (contact osteogenesis) and bone is laid down on the surface of the drilled osteotomy (distance osteogenesis). The two new bone layers merge and the initial woven bone is gradually remodelled into mature lamellar bone. Movement at the bone–implant interface in the early stages of healing beyond a certain level, due to excessive loading, may prevent osseointegration and lead to a fibrous interface. The first month following placement is the most critical.
  - Immediate loading: It should be noted that in general, despite modifications in design, immediately loaded implants still have lower success rates than those allowed a period of unloaded healing.

Soft tissue integration

As well as osseointegration, soft tissue integration is also established around a healthy dental implant as it emerges through the mucosa. This is similar to the dentogingival complex around teeth, comprising a superficial epithelial attachment and an underlying connective tissue attachment providing a protective physical attachment, and a selective chemical and microbial barrier.

Endosteal implant systems and terminology

Generally an endosteal implant system can be designed in one of two ways:

- One-piece permucosal design: this design has an endosseous portion with a permucosal extension that protrudes through the gingiva (by varying amounts) immediately after (non-submerged) placement.
- Two-piece system that consists of an endosseous (inside the bone) component and a *separate* transmucosal (protruding through the gingival or mucosa) component. This allows the endosseous component to be placed and kept subgingival during 'first stage' surgery and initial osseointegration. A 'second stage' surgery can then be undertaken to expose the endosseous component and connect the transmucosal component to restore the edentulous space(s).

One-piece systems with long supragingival extensions are designed for immediate loading. They do not, however, easily allow significant alteration of the angle of the component protruding through the gingiva as this is almost wholly dependent on the angulation of the endosseous portion. The angulation of an endosseous component is dictated by a number of factors and may not be in alignment with the ideal position for the supragingival prosthesis. The two-piece system offers the advantage and flexibility of fabricating or selecting differentially angled transmucosal components (Figure 11.6). The two-piece system can also be used for immediate loading by simply placing the transmucosal component directly onto the endosseous component at the time of implant placement if sufficient primary stability of the endosseous portion is achieved.

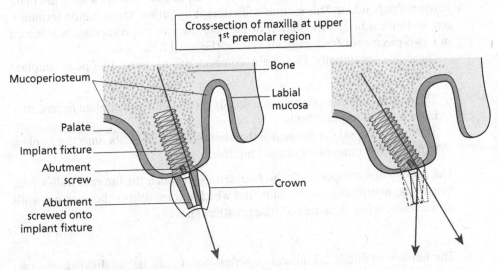

Figure 11.6 Schematic representation of altering the emergence angulation of a two-piece endosseous implant using differentially angled abutments.

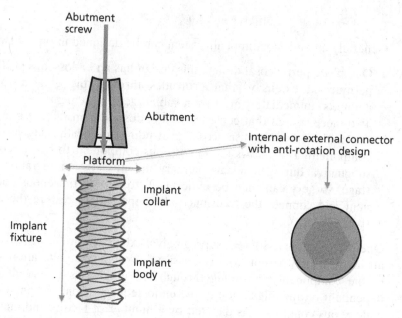

Figure 11.7   Schematic diagram of implant system.

Two-piece systems

The rest of this chapter will concentrate on the two-piece design, but in the main the terms and considerations for the two-piece system can equally be applied to the one-piece system.

Two-piece systems have many different components that are somewhat manufacturer dependent. This section will attempt to outline the common terminology and give a brief explanation of the relevance of the components involved in a two-piece root form implant system (Figure 11.7).

There are essentially two main components to most two-piece implant systems:

- The endosseous component – previously often called the implant fixture, now known as the implant body.
- The transmucosal component – the abutment, which seats onto the implant fixture at the implant–abutment interface.

The endosseous component is the foundation on which the internal walls of the house (the abutment) can be built, and which in turn allows the external walls of the house to be constructed (the prosthesis).

The endosseous implant

The implant is either cylindrical or screw-like. It can be subdivided into two regions: the implant body and the implant collar. Debate continues on how to retain bone around the implant collar: machined versus polished collars; submergence of implant collar versus implant collar at tissue level.

Most modern implants now no longer have polished or 'machined' surfaces at the collar. (The term 'machined' is frequently used in relation to turned, milled or smooth surfaces. It can, however, also refer to surfaces produced by electro discharge, sandblasting, etc.; Esposito *et al.*, 2002.) The collar is now effectively subsumed into the body and is surface treated or coated using the same specialised techniques as for the body. The shape of the implant fixture can be either root form (tapered) or parallel sided, and the implant collar may taper or flare.

The surface of the implant body/collar has progressed dramatically over the past two decades from the original 'machined' implant body with or without polished collar, to the current surfaces available. The current surface of an implant will vary depending on which implant system the operator uses, but all have similar features that aim to enhance primary stability and encourage rapid osseointegration. These features can be described as macro or microtopographies (Stanford, 2008). Some of the currently available features of implant body/collar are summarised in Table 11.1.

Implants are available in a plethora of lengths and diameters. The size used is determined by a number of factors including: likely functional load on implant; size of tooth to be replaced, proximity of adjacent structures. etc.

Implant–abutment interface

At the emergence of the two-piece design implant body at bone level, there needs to be a interface with the suprabony transmucosal abutment. This interface occurs on the top of the implant body. The area at the top (head) of the implant is known as the platform. The platform will have a geometric connecting feature incorporated that allows connection of the abutment to the implant. This connecting feature may sit within the implant body (internal connector, Figure 11.7) or protrude from the implant body (external connector, Figure 11.7). The connector surfaces vary in design depending on the manufacturer but will usually contain an anti-rotation feature to prevent rotation of the abutment, for example a hexagon male and female connector (Figure 11.7).

Table 11.1 Potential macro and microtopographies of implant body/collar (data from Stanford, 2008)

Macrotopography of implant body	
Advancement of implant	Self-tapping versus tapping
Threading design	Threaded versus non-threaded Differing thread pitch and density
Microtopography of implant body	
Surface modifications (Esposito *et al.*, 2002)	'Turned, blasted, acid-etched, porous-sintered, oxidised, plasma-sprayed, hydroxyapatite coated surfaces, or a combination'
Grooves	Microgrooves or microthreads

The diameter of the platform is also important. Platform size is essentially the maximum diameter of the implant head, which is often described by manufacturers by the use of a sliding scale, for example small, medium and large. Generally speaking larger diameter implants are used for molars, medium diameter implants are used for all teeth bar molars, and small diameter implants are used for upper and lower lateral incisors, and lower central incisors. These general principles of size selection are modified by the need for at least 3 mm of bone between adjacent implants and 2 mm of bone between implants and adjacent natural teeth to ensure retention of bone and therefore soft tissue support.

Abutments

Abutments can be classified as follows.

- Healing abutments – Attached to the implant body at implant placement (first stage or non-submerged surgery) or at abutment connection (second stage) surgery to allow healing and maturation of gingival margin before the placement of temporary or definitive prosthesis.
- Temporary abutments – Used to allow a temporary prosthesis to be attached to help further refine the gingival emergence contour and establish occlusal and aesthetic parameters prior to the placement of definitive abutment and prosthesis.
- Definitive abutments – These can be pre-manufactured ('stock' abutments, including precision attachments), modifiable or custom made. They can allow the emergence trajectory of the prosthesis to be significantly different to that of the implant itself.

Abutments are generally secured to the implant by a screw. Following on from this the temporary or definitive prosthesis can be secured to the abutment either by a further screw or by cement. The selection of cement versus screw for securing the prosthesis depends on a number of factors, including the need for easy retrievability and position of any screw access hole, etc.

Treatment planning for implants

History and examination

The history and examination of the patient should follow exactly the same principles as described in Chapter 1. An overview of some of the additional considerations in the history and examination are outlined in Table 11.2.

The history and examination are key to determining:

- If an implant borne prosthesis is appropriate for, or desired by, the patient.
- What hard and soft tissue considerations there might be for any implant borne prosthesis provided.
- Whether the patient will be able to tolerate the procedures involved in surgical placement and restoration of implants.

Table 11.2 Some of the additional considerations in the history and examination for treatment planning an implant patient. Please note that the list below is not exhaustive

History	History of presenting complaint	Looking to identify reason for loss of teeth as will give information on a number of potential factors affecting the treatment plan including: likely loss of bone through periodontal disease or trauma Looking to identify why patient doesn't tolerate existing prosthesis and what they expect of implant-based treatment to check they have realistic and achievable expectations
	Medical history[1]	Looking for contraindications or confounders to providing implant-based treatment. Examples may include impaired host response or healing potential, etc. Also looking to identify any factors that may impair the patient's ability to maintain oral hygiene around complex crown and bridge work, e.g. decreased manual dexterity. This may mandate a simpler implant borne prosthesis
	Social and past dental history	Looking for contraindications or potential confounders to implant-based treatment for example: smoking, inability to comply with oral hygiene regimens
Examination	Extraoral	A natural smile will give you opportunity to see the smile line Assess facial symmetry and occlusal vertical dimension Muscular hypertrophy may indicate parafunctional habit Temporomandibular disorders' signs Active functioning of existing prosthesis
	Intraoral	Survey of existing dentition to ascertain long-term prognosis and any bruxist facets to help with treatment planning and location of implants Hard and soft tissue inspection and palpation. Looking for deficiencies, severe undercuts, mucosal thickness and quality Ascertain vertical and horizontal space availability for implant borne prosthesis Examination of existing prosthesis gives a lot of important information for example: amount of pink acrylic gives an idea of amount of tissue lost; positioning of teeth in relation to ridge to see if position reproducible with implant borne prosthesis etc

[1] A good summary of relative and absolute contraindications can be found in Zitzmann *et al.* (2008).

It is *imperative* to base the final treatment plan on the desired prosthetic result, as this should, except for a few situations that demand pragmatism, determine the number, positions and characteristics of the implants. Careful surgical planning and technique remain important, but a fully osseointegrated implant that is malpositioned such that it emerges outwith the prosthetic envelope or is totally unrestorable due to its poor trajectory is no use to anyone. Even apparently quite subtle implant malpositioning can result in significant aesthetic compromise, which though not precluding a mechanically stable end result, may not be regarded as satisfactory by the patient.

Both restorative and surgical aspects of treatment planning are crucial. Guidance for the appropriately trained practitioner has been specifically produced to help classify cases as simple, advanced or complex from both restorative and surgical perspectives (FGDP Training standards in implants; SAC classification). Simple cases are clearly those that could be accomplished by an individual alone, the other classifications may merit a team approach dependent on the individuals involved, their experience and the boundaries of their competence.

Treatment planning adjuncts and special investigations

The choice of treatment planning adjuncts and special investigations for implants will depend on the complexity of the case. Table 11.3 gives some of the main adjuncts and special investigations.

Discussions about the final treatment plan and alternative non-implant options must be recorded. There must be explicit notes made regarding risks, procedures, timings, responsibilities and costings.

Overview of surgical procedures in implant placement

Placement of two piece implant

Surgical placement of implants demands all the same principles of surgery as described in Chapter 7. In fact, as the end product is the placement of a foreign body in the patient's jaw(s), it is of the utmost importance to ensure these principles are upheld. The surgical process is shown in Figure 11.8.

For a two-piece implant system, the surgery commonly involves the following two procedures.

First stage surgery

A mucoperiosteal flap may be lifted, depending on the system used. If it is lifted, great care must be exercised to ensure the periosteum is cleanly reflected from the alveolus. If a flap is not lifted, either a tissue punch is used to remove a circumscribed area of mucosa and then the osteotomies are performed, or the osteotomies are performed through the gingiva. 'Flapless' placement is only

Table 11.3 Treatment planning adjuncts and special investigations

	Function
Adjunct	
Diagnostic wax-up on study models	Allows: – assessment of occlusion – visualisation of potential result – temporisation via use of putty matrix over wax-up – creation of radiographic guide to enable visualisation of the prosthetic envelope on radiographic images – creation of surgical guide to assist in accurate implant positioning
Trial denture (complete or partial)	Allows a trial of the final prosthetic result Assessment of tolerance, for example to the palatal coverage that might be produced by an overdenture
Ridge mapping	Once anaesthetised the depth of soft tissue and the width of the bone can progressively be mapped using a graduated sharp probe. This information can then be transferred to a study model
Special investigation	
Panoramic tomography (DPT, OPG)	Gives an approximation of the position of the nearby anatomical structures such as maxillary sinus, floor of nose, inferior alveolar nerve and mental foramen Gives an overview of the condition of the dentition as a whole, such as alveolar bone levels around teeth
Long cone periapical radiograph	Gives accurate information of the immediate area for potential implantation
Cone beam volumetric tomogram or conventional computed tomographic (CT) scan	Gives an accurate three-dimensional image of the jaws Through the use of a radiographic guide and commercially available software, allows virtual placement of implants and construction of machine made surgical guides. Especially useful when bone volume or height is in question

used when the surgeon is certain that a good height and volume of bone exists and no vital structures are likely to be damaged.

Irrespective of whether a flap is raised, a series of progressively larger osteotomies are performed in the alveolar bone using a series of gradated drills running with copious irrigation at low speed, high torque. The osteotomies are developed in a predetermined sequence dependent on a number of factors including: osteotomy site; quality and density of bone; size and length of implant.

If the implant system and features of the bone site require the bone to be thread tapped, a thread-tapping tool is used at very slow speed (~15 rpm) with copious irrigation to create a thread in the final osteotomy site prior to placing the implant.

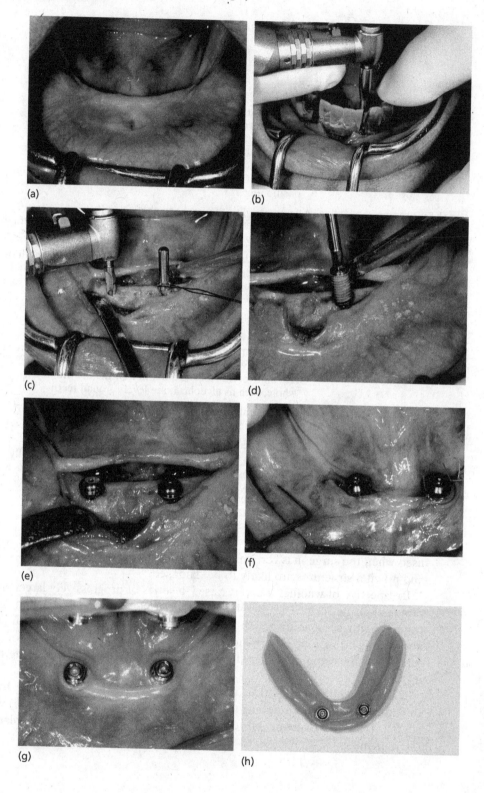

Figure 11.8   Implant placement. Surgical process. (a) Preoperative clinical examination showing good width of keratinised attached gingival and reasonable ridge morphology. (b) Pilot osteotomy prepared with the use of custom-made stent to guide placement of osteotomy site. (c) Left-sided osteotomy occupied by direction indicator to help guide angulation and direction of osteotomy being conducted on right side. (d) Implant insertion. (e) Cover screws placed onto both implants. Wound ready for closure. (f) Implants covered by mucoperiostium during period of osseointegration. Exposure of implants performed and healing abutments placed. Healing abutments left permucosal. (g) After period of healing and maturation of gingival margin the healing abutments are replaced by the definitive Locator (ZestAnchors, Escondido, CA) abutments. (h) Fitting surface of lower denture adjusted and Locator (ZestAnchors, Escondido, CA) male denture caps now included.

Once the osteotomy is complete, the implant is carefully seated at slow speed (~15 rpm). The aim is to achieve a tight fit to the osteotomy, so-called good 'primary stability'. Machine-driven or hand-held devices enable the extent of this tightness (degree of torque in Newton centimetres) to be measured.

The achievement of good primary stability is considered to be one of the critical requirements to allow the possibility of immediate restoration of the implant with a temporary or even definitive prosthesis in carefully selected cases.

If the intention is to allow a period of completely undisturbed healing once the implant is seated, a cover screw is used to close off the implant platform to prevent ingress of debris or bone. The wound is toileted and debrided and the flap repositioned with sutures.

Second stage surgery

This is undertaken after a period of osseointegration; classically this was 3 months for the mandible, 6 months for the maxilla. However, osseointegration is now achieved sooner with evolving implant surface technologies. The surgery involves exposing the cover screw, removing it and placing either a healing abutment or a temporary abutment with a temporary prosthesis. The exposure of the cover screw can be accomplished by a number of methods; the choice between these methods is largely dependent on the state of the soft tissue around the head of the submerged implant. The aim is to achieve a healthy band of attached mucosa around the emerging abutment. The second stage surgery also gives the opportunity of manipulating tissues to achieve this goal.

Dealing with inadequate hard tissue height and volume

Ultimately the surgeon should always try to preserve alveolar bone using the techniques outlined previously. Unfortunately it is not uncommon for there to be less than the ideal amount of bone, caused by hypodontia, traumatic avulsion of teeth and alveolus, traumatic extractions by another practitioner or the late effects of progressive alveolar resorption.

Circumventing inadequate bone height or width may be possible through the use of shorter or angled implants, although these techniques may lead to compromises in the final prosthetic result. Further advancement in implant technology may produce comparable stability from shorter implants.

If bone at the site of the planned implantation requires augmentation, this is possible by a variety of methods:

- guided bone regeneration
- ridge splitting and ridge dilation techniques
- bone grafting using autogenous bone blocks: onlay bone grafting; interpositional bone grafting
- procedures to augment the thickness of the floor of the maxillary sinus: 'sinus lift procedure'; closed or open procedure.

Guided bone regeneration (GBR)

The primary principle behind this technique is that epithelial cells and fibroblasts migrate into an extraction socket or bone defect clot quicker than osteoblasts. Preventing these non-bone cells reaching the clot will positively discriminate towards the slower-migrating bone-forming cells. The osteoblasts migrate into the clot from the walls of the socket or defect and thus one of the requirements for this technique is a walled defect over which a resorbable or non-resorbable membrane is placed to protect the clot. One of the most common uses of GBR is around exposed threads of an implant to encourage new bone to form.

Autogenous, allogenous, xenogenous bone or alloplastic material can also be placed below the membrane and therefore used in combination with GBR.

Ridge splitting/dilation techniques

This technique is only useful to enhance residual alveolar ridge width. Indications for this technique include (Misch, 2004):

- residual alveolar residual ridge thickness >3 mm
- more than single tooth site
- good bone quality – preferably in the maxilla rather than the mandible due to thinner cortex, although splitting in the posterior mandible is possible as long as there is >12 mm bone above the inferior alveolar nerve canal
- no concavity to buccal plate
- no vertical deficiency.

The technique is performed through a minimal mucoperiosteal flap to help maintain blood supply to the bone that is split. The two cortical plates, buccal and palatal/lingual, are initially separated with a scalpel. A series of progressively wider tapered osteotomes are then used to separate the two plates sufficiently to accommodate the desired width of implant. The implant osteotomy is then prepared in the usual manner and the fixture placed. Primary wound closure over the implant fixture is achieved through releasing the periosteum and the implant is left for the usual period of undisturbed healing.

It is also possible to dilate an osteotomy site using round profile tapered instruments to avoid losing critical bone wall.

Box 11.1 Donor sites for grafts	
Extra-oral	Intra-oral
Iliac crest	Tori
Tibia	Ramus or symphysis of mandible
Rib	Tuberosity of maxilla
Calvarium	Palatal bone

Bone grafting

All autogenous block bone grafting has the disadvantage of a second surgical site (the donor site) for the harvesting of bone, which increases the morbidity of the procedure.

Donor sites that have been used to provide grafts for the oral cavity include intra- and extraoral sites (Box 11.1).

Three of the main uses of bone grafts in implant surgery are:

1 as an onlay (or veneer) to the alveolus thereby increasing width of the ridge
2 as an interpositional graft to the ridge thereby increasing height of the ridge
3 as an onlay to the crest of the ridge to increase height.

In onlay bone grafting, carefully shaped autogenous bone is laid onto the prepared recipient alveolar surface underneath the mucoperiosteum. The graft can be secured using titanium bone screws. Implants may be placed at the time of grafting or more usually after the graft has stabilised at around 4 months.

Interpositional bone grafting involves a horizontal osteotomy in the alveolar ridge to allow the placement of a block of bone between the basal bone and the alveolus.

Distraction osteogenesis

A modification of interpositional bone grafting is distraction osteogenesis where the horizontal osteotomy is performed and a small mechanical device fitted to the two halves of the osteotomy. After a healing period of about 10–14 days the distracting device can be activated. The patient then uses the screw in this mechanical device to gradually increase the gap between the two halves of the osteotomy by 0.25–0.5 mm/day over the course of a number of weeks. This creates the formation of new bone and soft tissue height. Once the desired height is achieved the distraction device is left *in situ* for a consolidation period of a number of months to allow mineralisation of the new bone formed before implants are placed (Iizuka *et al.*, 2005). Theoretically this approach removes the need for a graft between the two halves as the slow expansion allows the body to lay down new bone between the two halves of the osteotomy. This is of course wholly dependent on the vascularity of the segment that is being moved away from the basal bone, which makes the procedure very technique sensitive.

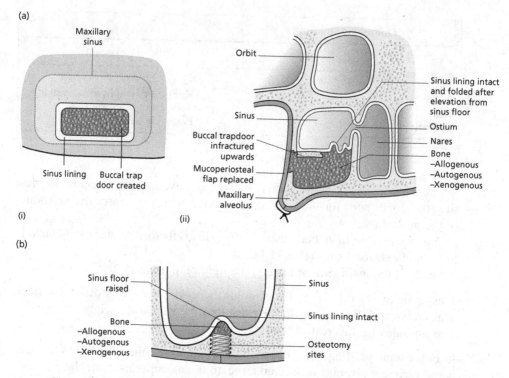

Figure 11.9 (a) Left: a buccal view of the maxillary alveolus overlying the maxillary sinus. An ellipsoid-shaped trapdoor is created in the maxillary alveolus overlying the lateral wall of the sinus using either a rotary bur or ultrasonic cutting instrument. Right: a coronal view of the 'lifted' ellipsoid trapdoor increasing the height of bone available to place implants by the placement of autogenous, allogenous, or xenogenous bone underneath the trapdoor. (b) 'Tenting' up of the lining of the maxillary sinus by the use of osteotomes through the osteotomy site. The height of bone available for implant placement is then increased by placing autogenous, allogenous, or xenogenous bone through the osteotomy in to the space created by this tenting.

Sinus lift procedure

This procedure is performed to increase bone height in the posterior maxilla. It can be performed in an open (Tatum sinus lift procedure or lateral open sinus lift procedure (Figure 11.9ai and ii)) or a closed (Summer's sinus lift (Figure 11.9b)) manner.

In the open procedure a mucoperiosteal flap is reflected and the sinus lining is exposed by either a modified Caldwell-Luc approach or by the creation of a bony trapdoor in the lateral wall of the sinus. A bur or a piezoelectric cutting instrument can be used to create the access into the sinus. The exposed sinus lining is carefully dissected from the underlying bone and positioned more superiorly than its original position. Autogenous, allogenous or xenogenous bone or artificial bone substitute materials are then placed under the sinus lining and or bony trapdoor thereby increasing the depth of bone for placement of implants. Despite autogenous bone being traditionally accepted as the gold standard because of its osteogenic properties, a recent review has shown no clear reason for the clinician to select autogenous bone over any of the alternatives for the sinus lift (Nkenke and Stelzle, 2009).

If the pre-existent bony anatomy is favourable (5 mm residual ridge present below sinus floor; >6 mm residual ridge width; Jensen *et al.*, 1998), implants can be placed at the same time as the sinus lift, otherwise they can be placed after a period of healing of around 4–6 months. The remaining orifice in the lateral wall of the sinus can then be covered with a resorbable membrane dependent on the material placed in the sinus, using the principles of GBR. The flap is then repositioned and sutured, and any dentures should be left out for 1–2 weeks, dependent on resolution of postoperative oedema.

The closed sinus lift procedure involves the use of specialised osteotomes through an under-prepared implant osteotomy in the maxilla to gently push up the sinus floor and lining. Autogenous, allogenous or xenogenous bone can be placed into the extra space created by the osteotomes and the implant can then be seated. The sinus floor can be raised some 2–4 mm using this technique.

Dealing with unfavourable soft tissue configurations and relationships

The surgical procedures outlined earlier in relation to preparing the mouth for tissue-borne prostheses can equally be applied for implant borne prostheses.

There are a number of advanced perioplastic procedures that can be undertaken in relation to implants, including procedures to try to recreate papilla(e), improve papilla(e) appearance, increase the amount of attached (keratinised) gingiva around implants and provide mucosal coverage of exposed implant threads. These are outwith the remit of this chapter and a suggestion for further reading on this subject is at the end of the chapter.

References and further reading

Dawson A, Chen S (2009) *The SAC Classification in Implant Dentistry.* Quintessence, London.

Esposito M *et al.* (2002) Interventions for replacing missing teeth: different types of dental implants. *Cochrane Database Syst Rev*, CD003815.

Faculty of General Dental Practitioners RCS Eng (2008) Training standards in implants. Available at: http://www.fgdp.org.uk/pdf/training_stds_imp_dent_guide_2008.pdf (accessed 25 May 2010).

Froum SJ (ed.) (2010) *Dental Implant Complications: etiology, prevention, and treatment.* Wiley-Blackwell, Oxford.

Iizuka T *et al.* (2005) Bi-directional distraction osteogenesis of the alveolar bone using an extraosseous device. *Clinical Oral Implants Research* **16**: 700–7.

Jensen OT *et al.* (1998) Report of the Sinus Consensus Conference of 1996. *International Journal of Oral and Maxillofacial Implants* **13**(Suppl): 11–45.

Laney WR (ed.) (2008) *Glossary of Oral and Maxillofacial Implants.* Quintessence, London.

Misch CM (2004) Implant site development using ridge splitting techniques. *Oral Maxillofacial Surgery Clinics of North America* **16**, 65–74, vi.

Nkenke E, Stelzle F (2009) Clinical outcomes of sinus floor augmentation for implant placement using autogenous bone or bone substitutes: a systematic review. *Clinical Oral Implants Research* **20** (Suppl 4): 124–33.

Sclar A (2003) *Soft Tissue and Esthetic Considerations in Implant Therapy*. Quintessence, London.

Stanford, C.M. (2008) Surface modifications of dental implants. *Australian Dental Journal* **53**(Suppl 1): S26–33.

Zitzmann N, Margolin M, Filippi A, Weiger R (2008) Patient assessment and diagnosis in implant treatment. *Australian Dental Journal* **53**: 3–10.

Chapter 12
Treatment of Surgical Infections in the Orofacial Region

- Acute infections
- Diagnosis
- Bacterial investigations
- Principles of treatment of acute infections
- Infections of the face, head and neck
- Chronic infections of the jaws

Acute infections

Acute infections of the orofacial region are due to the pathogenic activities of micro-organisms, including viruses, fungi and bacteria. Surgical infection is mainly due to bacterial infection. The progress of any infection is governed by the host response to the invading organisms. Factors related to the organism that are important include their number and virulence. Organisms vary in their virulence and can be divided into:

- commensals
- potential pathogens
- pathogens.

Commensals

These may become pathogenic by a change of site or host resistance. Host factors that are important concerning the establishment of an infection include:

- age (resistance is decreased at the extremes of age)
- concurrent disease
- drugs (immunosuppressants)
- therapeutic irradiation (this decreases the local blood supply).

Principles of Oral and Maxillofacial Surgery, 6th Edition. Edited by U. J. Moore
© 2011 Blackwell Publishing Ltd

Spread of infection

Once established, infection may spread and this is governed by host and pathogen factors. Local anatomy is an important host factor in the direction of spread. There are three serious sequelae of spread of infection in the orofacial region:

- airway obstruction
- intracranial spread
- septicaemia.

Infection may spread by one of three routes:

- tissue planes and spaces
- the lymphatics
- the blood.

The prompt treatment of oral infection requires an understanding of both systemic and local factors.

Diagnosis

The diagnosis is made from the history and examination of the patient supported by additional special investigations. The five classical signs of acute inflammation are diagnostic:

- swelling
- redness
- pain or tenderness
- heat
- loss of function.

In addition, there may be a discharge of pus and regional lymphadenopathy. The systemic signs include:

- raised temperature
- rapid pulse
- general malaise.

The typical picture of the acute phase may be altered where antibacterial drugs have been ineffectively used. They may not have overcome the infection but have produced a state of balance between the invading bacteria and the patient's defences.

The formation of pus in a superficial abscess causes softening with fluctuation, redness and marked tenderness at the centre of the inflamed area. In a deep abscess affecting the neck, pus may spread widely and fluctuance may be masked by tense, oedematous swelling in the overlying tissue, which can be indistinguishable from cellulitis. The patient's temperature continues to rise with a swinging temperature suggesting the presence of suppuration.

A clear and concise medical history is recorded with special regard to metabolic or blood disorders. In very acute, recurrent or persistent infections, special investigations should be performed such as:

- urinalysis
- haemoglobin
- full blood count and differential white cell count – leucocytosis
- fasting blood sugar
- blood cultures
- C-reactive protein (CRP).

Radiographs may be uninformative in early acute infections of the jaw, unless there has been a previous chronic condition. Initially, a dental abscess may appear as a diffuse radiolucency associated with the apex of a non-vital tooth (Figure 12.1) After a period of approximately 10 days, bone changes may be seen as either localised periapical areas (Figure 12.2) or more diffuse changes in the case of osteomyelitis.

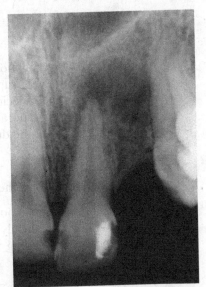

Figure 12.1   Acute periapical infection associated with a non-vital upper lateral incisor. The radiological appearance is often less marked than the history would suggest.

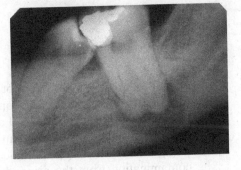

Figure 12.2   An established infection in a lower molar. The margins are more defined due to a long-standing chronic reaction. An acute episode may cause the patient to seek care.

The underlying cause, such as a non-vital tooth, should be sought, although treatment should not be delayed until the cause is found.

From the history the clinician should record:

- duration of infection
- changes in signs and symptoms
- sequence of events
- treatments sought, including antibiotics prescribed.

From the examination the clinician should record:

- swelling, diffuse or localised (fluctuant)
- lymphadenopathy
- trismus
- presence of sinus
- changes in the jaws and teeth
- presence of pyrexia (raised body temperature).

Bacterial investigations

Microbiological investigation can play an important role in the management of a patient with orofacial suppurative infection. All efforts should be made to obtain an appropriate specimen for any patient suspected of having a bacterial infection. Within the laboratory the organisms will be cultured, identified and an indication given of the drugs to which the bacteria will be sensitive.

Culture and sensitivity

This is imperative where there is:

- rapidly spreading infection
- infection in the medically compromised patient
- infection not responding to antibiotic therapy
- recurrent infection
- osteomyelitis
- postoperative infection.

Methods of sampling

Aspiration

Where collections of pus have not discharged, aspiration is preferred to prevent loss of oxygen-sensitive strict anaerobes prior to processing. The overlying tissue is first thoroughly cleaned and dried. An 18-gauge needle in a syringe is inserted into the most dependent part of the swelling and a sample aspirated (Figure 12.3). The sample should be immediately sealed to avoid drying and contamination from the air, and sent to the laboratory accompanied by the

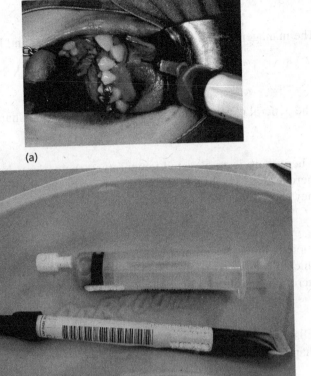

Figure 12.3 (a) Aspiration of a buccal swelling in the maxilla. (b) The aspirate is sealed into the syringe to allow anaerobic culture to proceed. An oral swab is also sent in a culture medium.

appropriate microbiology form with the date and time of collection, nature and site of the sample, method of collection, current and previous antibiotic therapy, together with any relevant clinical information. Culture and sensitivity results should be available within 36 to 48 hours, although anaerobic cultures can take longer.

Swabs

A bacteriological swab may be used for taking pus either from an extraoral sinus or from an abscess drained through an extraoral incision, providing that the skin and surrounding area have been thoroughly cleansed beforehand. However, swabs taken inside the mouth are liable to contamination from the saliva so that growths obtained are often reported as mixed oral flora. Swabbing is the least reliable method for obtaining a specimen for culture and sensitivity, but may be required when aspiration is unsuccessful.

Principles of treatment of acute infections

The management of an infection relies on general and local measures.

General measures

The general care of patients has been discussed in Chapter 2.

Rest

Where there is an elevated temperature, the patient should rest in bed. When there is gross swelling of the neck or floor of the mouth, or the patient is toxic, they should be admitted to hospital.

Nutritional support

Copious fluids are administered, often intravenously, to combat dehydration, which is a complication of high fever. Circulating toxins are diluted and their excretion encouraged by an increased turnover of water.

Diet

A balanced diet of easily digested proteins and carbohydrates is required (see Chapter 2).

Analgesia

Orofacial infections are painful and an important part of management is good pain control. Non-steroidal analgesics are the drugs of choice, many of which have the benefit of being anti-pyretic. In the case of airway problems, any drugs with a respiratory depressant effect, such as opioids, should be avoided.

Control of infection

Antibacterial drugs are not always necessary in the treatment of infections. Drainage, removal of the cause and applications of heat may be enough to enable the patient to overcome the condition, and antibiotics must not be prescribed to replace or delay these local measures.

Indications for antibiotic therapy

- Where culture and sensitivity has been obtained
- Continuing unresponsive infection
- Systemic spread
- Chronic infections
- Postsurgical infections in medically compromised or debilitated patients
- Postoperative infections at the operative site.

Unfortunately in many of these situations it is not feasible to await the result of a culture and thus antibiotics are often prescribed blind. Amoxycillin, which is a broad spectrum penicillin, is often the preferred drug. A loading dose of 3 g amoxycillin orally rapidly achieves bactericidal concentrations in the blood, and may be followed by 250 mg or 500 mg 8-hourly. Metronidazole (200–400 mg 8-hourly) targets anaerobic bacteria, which are often the causative organisms in many dental infections. A combination of amoxycillin with metronidazole may be appropriate in more severe infections and it may be necessary to admit the patient to provide antimicrobial therapy intravenously, together with surgical drainage. Once an antibiotic has been prescribed it should not be changed within the first 48 hours unless there is bacteriological evidence of resistance. If clinical improvement is occurring despite laboratory evidence of resistance it is not essential to change the regimen. There is no set duration of administration of antibiotics and no rationale in 'completing the course'. Antibiotic therapy should not be maintained after clinical resolution has occurred. Hyperbaric oxygen therapy is useful in promoting bone healing. It increases the effectiveness of antibiotics and the vascularity of tissues that have been subjected to radiation therapy.

Local measures

Local measures include:

- removal of the cause
- institution of drainage
- prevention of spread
- restoration of function.

Removal of the cause

This is the most important principle in the management of infection. In well-localised minor infections it may cure the condition immediately. In other cases it may initially be simpler to institute drainage and prevent spread. However, if the cause is not removed, infection will recur. Causes of orofacial bacterial infections include:

- necrotic pulps, periapical pathology (see Figure 12.4)
- periodontal disease
- avascular bony remnants (sequestrae)
- foreign bodies
- salivary calculi.

Once the cause has been identified it should be effectively removed, e.g. extraction of the tooth, extirpation of necrotic pulp, removal of salivary calculus, etc.

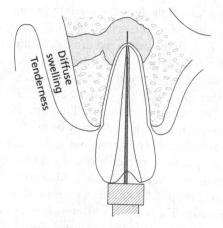

Figure 12.4   A necrotic pulp may be treated by opening the tooth and removing the dead pulp. The tooth can be left open to allow drainage of the collection of pus.

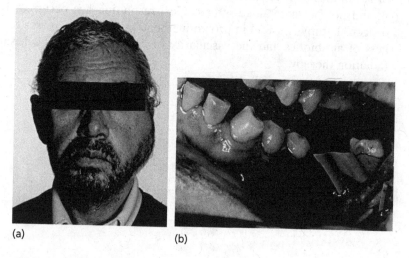

(a)

(b)

Figure 12.5   Acute infection. (a) Acute painful buccal and submasseteric swelling associated with grossly carious lower molar; (b) intraoral drainage following tooth removal.

Institution of drainage

Reddening of the skin, fluctuance and a point of maximum tenderness indicate localisation of pus (pointing). When this occurs the pus must be drained and a surgical incision leaves much less scarring than if pus bursts through the skin spontaneously. To be effective, drainage must be provided at the lowest point of the abscess. A drain (see Figure 12.5) should always be inserted to keep the opening patent for as long as the discharge continues. In cellulites, drainage is not established until the condition has localised, usually after 3 or 4 days. However, where a brawny, spreading swelling of the floor of the mouth and neck might involve the larynx and jeopardise the airway, surgery will reduce the tension in the tissue spaces and should not be withheld.

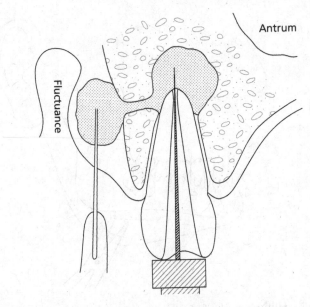

Figure 12.6   A localised swelling may be treated by opening the tooth and removing the dead pulp, together with an incision in the sulcus.

Intraoral incisions

In the mucous membrane incisions are made parallel to the occlusal surface of the teeth, 1 to 2 cm in length, with due regard for underlying structures such as the mental nerve. Smaller incisions are ineffective. This may be performed in conjunction with pulp extirpation or extraction (Figure 12.6).

Extraoral incisions

Incisions through skin should avoid the branches of the facial nerve. Where the abscess is deep and a free discharge is not obtained through a simple skin incision, Hilton's method of blunt dissection is performed (Figure 12.7). This involves inserting closed sinus forceps into the wound, and then opening them slowly but firmly to separate the soft tissue planes; the forceps are then withdrawn open to avoid damaging nerves or vessels by closing them blind. This procedure is repeated until the abscess is reached and pus discharges. In dental infections, an area of rough cortical bone can be felt on the mandible or maxilla where the periosteum has been raised. A drain is placed to allow drainage to continue for the required duration (Figure 12.8).

Prevention of spread

This is achieved by rest, drainage and the use of antimicrobial drugs. Rest of the affected part may be difficult when dealing with the orofacial region. However, trismus, when present, achieves this naturally.

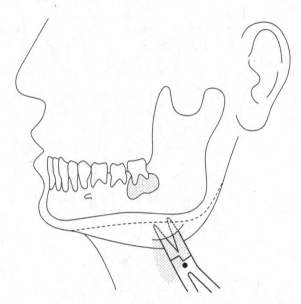

Figure 12.7   Hilton's method of drainage using sharp dissection through skin followed by blunt dissection through the tissues to open the abscess cavity.

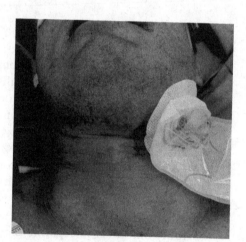

Figure 12.8   The drainage pathway is maintained by insertion of a suitable drain and the discharge collected – here in a stoma bag – until the abscess settles.

Restoration of function

The patient should be reviewed following the acute phase to ensure that function is restored. Trismus may persist and require treatment to improve mouth opening (see Chapter 17), and dental units may require restoration or replacement. Other causes such as periodontal disease or sialadenitis should be treated to prevent recurrence.

Timing

The decision when to perform various procedures is of great importance and requires considerable experience.

- In acute infection with a high temperature, immediate treatment with intravenous antibacterial drugs should be commenced.
- If pus has localised this must be drained without delay and culture and sensitivity tests performed.
- Antibacterial drugs can be commenced blind and continued until the results of the sensitivity tests are available.
- If not possible before, the cause should be removed as soon as the acute phase has passed.

Maintenance of the airway

Infections in the neck may cause oedema of the glottis with acute respiratory embarrassment. In all acute swellings where swallowing is difficult, patients should be watched for signs of difficulty in breathing and everything necessary for emergency tracheotomy should be at hand. To maintain control of the airway an awake bronchoscopic intubation may be necessary as a general anaesthetic may precipitate respiratory arrest when the accessory muscles of respiration stop functioning. Anaesthesia may be induced after control of the airway has been achieved.

Common infections in the mouth

Pericoronitis

Pericoronitis commonly presents as inflammation around the crown of a partly erupted, or impacted, tooth. In adults it is common in the mandible, particularly associated with the lower third molar tooth. The causes of the inflammation are:

- infection
- trauma from an opposing tooth
- foreign body reaction due to food packing.

An acute attack may be precipitated by the upper third molar traumatising the operculum of the lower third molar (Figure 12.9), which then becomes infected. The patient complains of pain and tenderness in the operculum and a foul taste. When severe, there is swelling of the floor of mouth and face, with trismus. There may be difficulty in swallowing and a raised temperature. The condition is rare in the maxilla.

Diagnosis

Diagnosis is made after confirming the presence of the impacted tooth with radiographs, and eliminating apical or periodontal disease in neighbouring teeth.

Treatment

Treatment is in two stages, directed first to the infection and second to the impacted tooth. For the acute inflammation hourly hot salt water mouth baths

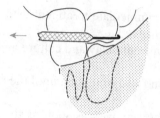

Figure 12.9   As it is often difficult to see if the upper third molar is biting on the inflamed gingival flap over a partly erupted lower third molar, a dental probe may be placed distal to the upper third molar and drawn forward over its occlusal surface with the teeth in occlusion. This will not be possible where the upper cusps are in contact with the swollen gum flap.

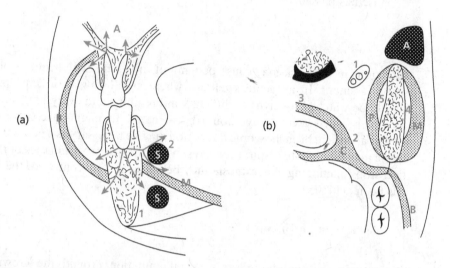

Figure 12.10   Spread of infection. (a) Coronal section through the tissue spaces of the face and neck. Note *A* the maxillary sinus, *B* the buccinator muscle, *M* the mylohyoid muscle, *S* the submandibular salivary gland. Spaces shown are (1) the submandibular and (2) the sublingual. (b) Transverse section through the tissue spaces of the face and neck. Note *A* the parotid salivary gland, *B* the buccinator muscle, *C* the superior constrictor muscle, *M* the masseter muscle, *P* the medial pterygoid muscle and (1) the carotid sheath. Spaces shown are (2) the lateral pharnygeal, (3) the retropharyngeal, (4) the submasseteric, (5) the pterygomandibular.

held over the affected operculum should be carried out. It is essential to eliminate any trauma from the opposing tooth. Where the upper tooth is nonfunctional it can be extracted at once under local anaesthesia, providing access is satisfactory, but where the tooth is functional the cusps may be ground clear of the operculum. If the temperature is raised or trismus is present, antibacterial drugs are prescribed. Spread of the infection from this site can quickly involve tissue spaces close to the airway (Figure 12.10), and prompt and effective treatment is essential. The surgical treatment of the impacted tooth may have to be delayed until the acute phase, particularly the trismus, has resolved, which may take some 2–3 weeks, but consideration should be given to immediate removal of the tooth as this will institute drainage and remove the cause.

Operculectomy has been practised but the results are unsatisfactory and it is of little value except where the tooth will erupt into a functional occlusion.

Acute periapical abscess without soft tissue involvement

Periapical infection from non-vital teeth or periodontal disease may either be contained and present as a low-grade chronic condition or apical granuloma with mild symptoms, or may suppurate to form an acute periapical abscess.

Diagnosis

The patient with an acute periapical abscess will complain of severe pain and the affected tooth feels raised in its socket. At first the pain may be eased by biting on the tooth but later it becomes exquisitely tender to touch. Examination at an early stage shows no involvement of the oral mucosa or soft tissue and systemic symptoms are usually absent.

Treatment

Where it is hoped to retain the tooth, the root canal is opened through the crown to provide drainage and access for root canal therapy. Otherwise the tooth may be extracted.

Subperiosteal abscess and spread into the soft tissues

Pus from an acute periapical abscess takes the track of least resistance through the medullary bone and points on the nearest epithelial surface. This is usually the buccal aspect of the maxilla or mandible where the alveolar bone is thinnest. Pus breaks through the bone above or below the attachment of buccinator. This determines whether the discharge occurs intraorally or through the soft tissues onto the skin of the face (Figure 12.10).

In the maxilla, the lateral incisor and palatal roots of the molar teeth commonly present as palatal abscesses. Anterior teeth may discharge into the nose and posterior teeth into the maxillary sinus. In the mandible, the relationship of the roots to the insertion of mylohyoid determines where lingual discharge will occur. The apices of the lower third molar and on occasions the second molar lie below the insertion of mylohyoid and thus pointing on the skin can occur. The remaining apices lying above mylohyoid cause discharge into the floor of the mouth. Periapical abscesses can discharge through the root canal or periodontal membrane.

Presentation and diagnosis

The cardinal signs of acute inflammation with mild systemic symptoms are present. Initially there is a tense very painful subperiosteal swelling near to the tooth with some facial oedema. Pain reduction usually occurs once pus is released through the mucoperiosteum into the mouth or through the periosteum into the soft tissues of the face and neck.

Treatment

If there is inflammatory oedema present the treatment is as for an acute peri-apical abscess. Pus below the mucoperiosteum is unlikely to drain through an extraction socket and must be incised and drained. Systemic symptoms require antibiotic therapy.

Infections of the face, head and neck

Spread of infection via tissue spaces, the lymphatics and blood may lead to the serious consequences of airway obstruction, intracranial spread and septicaemia.

Spread through muscle and fascial planes

Spread of infection takes place through potential spaces, normally filled with loose areolar tissue. These spaces lie between muscles, bones and viscera that are covered by condensations of fascia which form strong fibrous sheaths. The fascial planes of importance are:

- deep cervical
- pretracheal
- prevertebral
- carotid sheath.

Deep cervical fascia

The superficial layer encloses the neck and prevents deep infections pointing easily onto the skin. Arising from the scapula, clavicle and manubrium sterni it sweeps up the neck as a continuous tube, attached posteriorly to the ligamentum nuchae and anteriorly to the hyoid bone. It divides at the lower border of the mandible to form the submandibular space and is then attached lingually to the mylohyoid line and buccally to the outer aspect of the mandible. Buccally the fascia is then reflected up onto the zygomatic arch where posteriorly it ensheaths the parotid gland and is inserted into the mastoid process and the superior nuchal line on the skull. Invaginations are formed in the neck; the pretracheal fascia, a continuation of the deep surface, which invests the trachea and thyroid gland; the prevertebral fascia, lying anterior to the prevertebral muscles; and the carotid sheath, which surrounds the great vessels of the neck. All these extend down into the thorax and can provide a pathway for spread of infection to the mediastinum.

A number of potential tissue spaces exist in the neck and orofacial region through which infection may spread. They include the following superficial spaces:

- sublingual
- submental

- submandibular,
- submasseteric

and the following deeper spaces:

- infratemporal
- pterygomandibular,
- lateral pharyngeal
- retropharyngeal.

Sublingual space

There are two spaces on the medial aspect of the mandible lying above mylohyoid, both continuous across the midline and bounded by the insertion of the suprahyoid muscles into the hyoid bone. The superficial space lies between the mylohyoid and geniohyoid, and a deep space lies between the geniohyoid and genioglossus.

Infection can track laterally across the floor of the mouth or posteriorly to cause inflammatory oedema of the larynx and respiratory embarrassment.

The deep part of the submandibular gland lies in the sublingual space and curves round and down below the mylohyoid muscle to allow communication between the sublingual and submandibular spaces (Figure 12.10a).

Submental space

The submental space below the chin drains to the submandibular spaces.

Submandibular spaces

This is continuous across the midline and bounded by the deep cervical fascia laterally and the mylohyoid muscle superiorly. The superficial part of the submandibular gland lies in this space.

Infection can track from the lower molars and contralateral space, which communicates with the fascial planes of the pharynx and neck (Figure 12.11).

Submasseteric space

This is a potential space between the masseter and the lateral aspect of the mandible. Postoperative infection in this space can contribute to trismus.

Infratemporal space

This is bounded anteriorly by the maxillary tuberosity, medially by the lateral pterygoid plate and inferior belly of the lateral pterygoid muscle and laterally by the tendon of temporalis and the coronoid process.

Pterygomandibular space

This lies between the medial aspect of the ascending ramus and the medial pterygoid muscle and is limited superiorly by the lateral pterygoid muscle. It

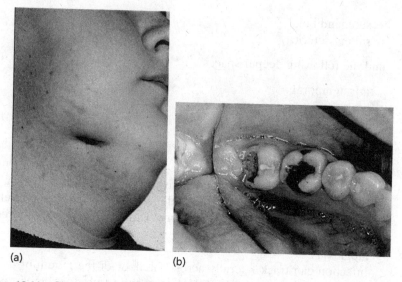

(a)   (b)

Figure 12.11   Chronic infection. (a) Extraoral submandibular sinus associated with; (b) grossly carious lower molar. Infection has tracked lingually, passing below mylohyoid to emerge in the submandibular space (see Figure 12.9).

communicates with the lateral pharyngeal and infratemporal spaces (Figure 12.10b).

Lateral pharygeal space

The boundaries of this space are: medially the superior pharyngeal constrictor muscle, laterally the medial pterygoid muscle and anteriorly the pterygomandibular raphe where the fascia covering superior constrictor is reflected onto the medial pterygoid muscle. Posteriorly lies the styloid process and stylohyoid and stylopharyngeous muscles, along which infection can spread to the larynx.

It is close to the carotid sheath and communicates with the submandibular and sublingual spaces round the submandibular salivary gland, the posterior part of which protrudes into the lateral pharyngeal space. The submandibular gland can play an important part in the spread of infection as it links the submandibular, sublingual and lateral pharyngeal spaces (Figure 12.10).

Retropharyngeal space

This lies between the constrictor muscles of the pharynx and prevertebral muscles and connects the right and left lateral pharyngeal spaces (Figure 12.10b).

Spread via lymphatics

- Scalp and facial skin drains into the superficial group of nodes in a circle around the head. These are the occipital, posterior auricular, parotid and facial nodes. Efferent vessels from these pass down to the superior lymph glands of the deep cervical chain.

- The lower lip and incisor region of the mandible drain to the submental lymph nodes lying between the anterior bellies of the two digastric muscles.
- Anterior tongue and floor of mouth lymph then passes to the submandibular nodes or direct to the deep cervical chain.
- Submandibular lymph nodes lie in the submandibular triangle and drain the remaining ipsilateral lymph vessels of the lips, cheeks, tongue and jaws, and thence to the deep cervical nodes accompanying the internal jugular vein.
- Anterior mouth drains to the lower group of nodes in this chain while the posterior mouth drains to the upper group of nodes.
- Pathological conditions of the tonsil and mouth may result in early enlarge- ment of the jugulodigastric node (superior nodes) at the level of the posterior belly of the digastric.

The response of the lymphatic system varies with the severity of the infection. Acute infections lead to lymphangitis – inflammation of lymph vessels. Organisms and their toxins in the node lead to lymphadenitis (or lymphaden- opathy) – enlargement due to inflammation. Virulent infections may lead to suppuration and abcess formation in the node. It is important to exclude other possible causes of lymph node enlargement.

Spread via the bloodstream

Entry of infected material into the bloodstream can lead to septicaemia or toxaemia. These are potentially life-threatening conditions. The intravenous route is also a means of intracranial entry.

Intracranial spread of infection

From an intraoral source this may lead to:

- cavernous sinus thrombosis
- brain abscess.

Cavernous sinus thrombosis

This is a rare but serious condition. The sinus may be infected by general spread in the blood either via the angular veins of the orbit (following infection from a maxillary anterior tooth) or by a short venous connection from the pterygoid plexus (from posterior maxillary teeth). Among the structures that pass through this sinus are the nerves which supply the muscles of the orbit, branches of the trigeminal nerve and the internal carotid artery. The presenting eye signs are:

- opthalmoplegia (inability to move the eye)
- ptosis (drooping upper eyelid)
- proptosis (extrusion of the eye).

Brain abscess

Direct entry of infected material may occur via tissue planes, access to the brain being achieved along the carotid sheath. Another route is via the nasal sinuses following infection of an upper molar tooth gaining access to the maxillary sinus. Once here, spread to other nasal sinuses may occur and breach of a sinus wall in contact with the brain can result in intracranial spread.

Mediastinal spread of infection – mediastinitis

This is a very severe infection that may spread through orofacial fascial spaces via the deep cervical spaces to affect the mediastinum. It presents as fever, chest pain, general malaise and a raised temperature. Management is tailored to remove the source. Incision and drainage of cervical spaces and mediastinal drainage with long-term high doses of antibiotics are necessary. There is a high level of morbidity and mortality with the possible sequelae of damage to large vessels and cardiac failure.

Spread of maxillary infections

(See Figure 12.12)

Where pus points buccally above the buccinator it will form an abscess in the cheek and may spread over a wide area as there is nothing to contain it. An abscess from the anterior teeth leads to an infraorbital abscess, which is serious because thrombosis of the facial vein may follow. This vessel anastomoses with orbital veins that drain into the cavernous sinus. In this way infection may pass from the face into the cavernous sinus.

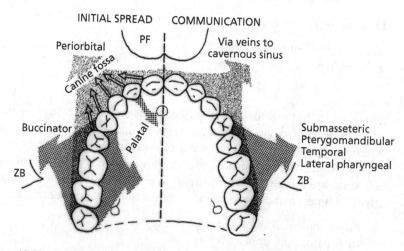

Figure 12.12   Possible routes of spread of infection in the maxilla (PF – pyriform fossa; ZB – zygomatic buttress).

Abscesses in the cheek may point anywhere on the face, and when drained the incision is made parallel to the branches of the facial nerve. Infection of the infratemporal space may be caused by posterior superior dental nerve injections given behind the tuberosity of the maxilla or by spread from the maxillary third molar tooth. This space may be drained intraorally through the buccal sulcus lateral and posterior to the tuberosity.

Spread of mandibular infections

(See Figure 12.13)

Spread of infection buccally, below the attachment of the buccinator, causes a swelling in the cheek over the lateral aspect of the mandible, but the inferior border of the bone remains palpable if the submandibular space is not involved. Incision for drainage may have to be made over the lateral aspect of the mandible.

An infection in the submandibular space gives rise to swelling over the lower border of the mandible and into the neck. It is drained by an incision parallel with the lower border of the mandible and about 2 cm below it to avoid the mandibular branch of the facial nerve and the facial vessels.

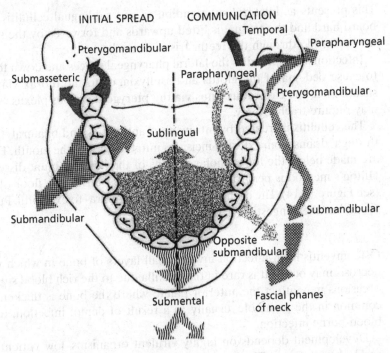

Figure 12.13 Routes of spread in the mandible. The intial spread of infection may continue to encroach on more distant spaces.

The sublingual spaces are involved when spread takes place above the mylo-hyoid into the floor of the mouth, which becomes swollen and is raised with difficulty in swallowing. These spaces may be drained by an incision in the floor of the mouth, but if the submandibular space is also involved an extraoral approach is more satisfactory.

Infection of the pterygomandibular space, with symptoms of trismus and pain on swallowing, may follow an inferior dental nerve injection or spread of infection from the lower third molar tooth. This space and the submandibular space communicate with the lateral pharyngeal space, which, if involved, gives rise to swelling in the lateral wall of the oropharynx and mesial and posterior to the angle of the mandible, accompanied by trismus and difficulty in swallowing.

The lateral pharyngeal, and through it the pterygomandibular space, may be drained by an incision made 2 cm below the angle of the mandible. In those rare cases where only the pterygomandibular space is affected it may be opened by incising down the anterior border of the ascending ramus intraorally.

Infection from the lower third molar tooth may also occasionally track buc-cally either under the skin superficial to the masseter or less often into the submassetric space (Figure 12.10).

Persistent and spreading infection

Ludwig's angina

This presents as bilateral submandibular and sublingual cellulitis. Swelling is board hard and the tongue is lifted upwards and forwards by the swelling and may protrude through the teeth. Trismus may be severe.

Infection may spread to the lateral pharyngeal spaces and down to the larynx, to cause oedema of the glottis and asphyxia, or to the thorax via the carotid sheath or to the cavernous sinus via the pterygoid venous plexus. Severe cases may require tracheotomy.

The cellulitis is treated by intravenous antibiotics and bilateral 'through and through' drains from external incisions into the floor of the mouth. The incisions are made below the lower molar regions of the jaw, and blunt dissection using Hilton's method is performed up to second incisions in the floor of the mouth (see Figure 12.14). The drains are brought from intra- to extraoral. Pus is seldom found but the congestion is usually relieved.

Osteomyelitis

Osteomyelitis is an infection involving all layers of bone in which widespread necrosis may occur. It is rare in the maxilla due to the rich blood supply, but on occasions may affect the anterior palate where the bone is thicker. It is more common in the mandible, usually as a result of dental infection, trauma or a blood-borne infection.

Development depends on highly virulent organisms, low patient resistance and lack of drainage. The incidence has been reduced by antibiotic therapy. The

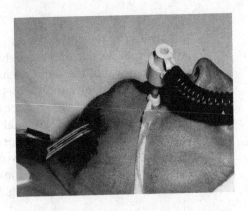

Figure 12.14 Ludwig's angina. The swelling is described as brawny and is often hard without discernible fluctuance. Drainage may decrease the pressure and reduce the rate of spread.

presentation of chronic inflammatory swellings complicated by subacute episodes is more common, which may be settled by a long period of antibiotic therapy. Short courses of antibiotics may suppress but not cure, contributing to extensive destruction of bone.

Presentation

Pus tracks through the medulla of bone (rather than through a narrow track into the soft tissue). It reaches the cortical plate at several points to lift the periosteum and deprive large areas of the blood supply. Pus may then discharge through a sinus and the situation enters a chronic phase.

Limitation of the infection is achieved by osteoclasts separating away the dead bone (sequestrum), which is walled off by granulation tissue. Osteoblasts initiate repair and support of the weakened bone by laying down a new layer of bone (involucrum). Discharge continues until the sequestrum is removed. If drainage is inadequate, slow spread with formation of new sequestra may continue indefinitely.

Diagnosis

Symptoms can include those of acute infection, severe pain, pyrexia, teeth tender to percussion and loose, intermittent mental sensory loss in the mandible. Facial swelling soon follows, followed by discharge of pus and sinus formation. Bare rough bone is palpable at the base of the sinus.

Radiographs are initially negative but after 10 days irregular radiolucent areas are seen. Later, sequestra appear as radiopacities surrounded by a radiolucent zone. Bone destruction may lead to pathological fracture visible on radiographs.

Treatment

Immediate admission to hospital is advisable. High-dose antibiotics and the establishment of drainage via an extraoral incision are the priorities. Only very loose or non-vital teeth should be removed while the application of heat should be avoided as it may lead to spread of infection. Hyperbaric oxygen may be useful and antibiotics are continued for at least 14 days after disease has settled.

Sequestrectomy

Removal of sequestra under antibiotic cover is an essential part of treatment. A clear radiolucent line around the sequestra on radiograph should suggest simple removal of the sequestrum. Sequestra above the inferior alveolar canal may be removed intraorally with the resultant defect packed open. ower border sequestra require a lower border incision; where a sinus is present incorporate this in the incision line. Non-vital bone is excised and the area gently curetted to expose healthy bleeding bone; a drain is placed.

Mowlem's decorticectomy involves removal of the thick poorly vascularised buccal plate over the diseased area, which promotes ingrowth of granulation tissue and speeds wound healing.

Acute necrotising fasciitis

This rapidly spreading and aggressive infection of fascia and muscles presents following trauma or post-surgery in debilitated patients. The skin is mottled and dusky with sloughing. Both aerobic and anaerobic organisms are involved and management consists of drainage, debridement of necrotic tissue and high dose intravenous antibiotics.

Acute maxillary infection in children

A rare, acute staphylococcal infection affects the maxilla, usually in infants a few weeks old.

Aetiology

The infection follows birth trauma, mouth abrasions or blood-borne infection.

Presentation and diagnosis

The disease is of rapid onset with all the signs of acute infection. The child is very ill with a high temperature, swelling of the cheek with eye closure, pus discharge from the nostrils and/or intraoral sinuses. Partially calcified teeth may be devitalised and sequestrate. Occasionally, thicker bony margins such as the infraorbital margin may sequestrate. Radiographs are not helpful as the maxilla, at this age, consists of thin bone around a 'bag of teeth'.

Treatment

The patient should be admitted under the care of a paediatrician for antibiotics and drainage. Later any sequestra (bone, teeth) may require removal to avoid a chronic phase.

Osteomyelitis in children

This may occur acutely in the mandible following exanthematous fevers, tonsillitis, sinusitis or middle ear disease. Symptoms are similar to those of the adult.

Unerupted teeth may be exfoliated and complications include involvement of growth centres and subsequent deformity or ankylosis of the joint. Treatment is as for an adult.

Chronic infections of the jaws

Chronic periapical abscess

An acute periapical abscess can become chronic if the cause is not removed and it drains through a sinus. Sinus blockage may contribute to acute exacerbations. Treatment includes extraction or root canal therapy with or without subsequent apicectomy. On rare occasions extraoral sinuses may occur, which if unsightly may require excision (see Figure 12.11).

Tuberculosis

Tuberculosis is now more common, particularly in immigrant populations. It may spread to the mouth in infected sputum or by the haematogenous route, usually secondary to lung infection. The causal organism is mycobacterium tuberculosis. Cervical tuberculous adenitis may be a primary infection, presenting as enlarged non-tender lymph nodes.

Presentation and diagnosis

The tongue is often affected with deep ragged painful ulcers. Smears from mouth ulcers should be cultured and the chest radiographed for other foci of infection. Osteomyelitis of the jaw can occur, characterised by long-standing localised tender swellings, which may discharge at the lower border of the mandible. Sequestra may be present and secondary infection may occur.

Treatment

This is first directed to the general care of the patient. Local measures include antibiotics, drainage and sequestrectomy where appropriate. Drugs such as isoniazid, rifampicin and pyrazinamide are administered and routine sputum and wound cultures are carried out.

Actinomycosis

This is a chronic infection caused by *Actinomyces israelii* which may affect the face and neck, the lungs or abdomen.

Diagnosis

The patient complains of a 'board' hard, lumpy swelling usually over the angle of the mandible (see Fig 12.15). It is sometimes bluish in colour and tends to

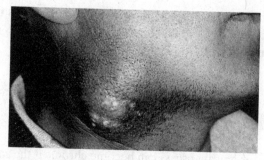

Figure 12.15 Actinomycosis. The classic presentation is in the neck with a localised board hard swelling. Sulphur granules can be seen in the discharge.

form multiple sinuses which discharge pus containing 'sulphur granules'. These, if examined microscopically, show the organisms.

Sometimes the disease occurs as a mixed infection and presents as a typical acute abscess that fails to clear up normally. In these cases frequent anaerobic cultures should be made as there is often difficulty in isolating the organisms and the diagnosis cannot be definitely established without a positive culture. Rarely the bone is also involved.

Treatment

Antibacterial drugs are prescribed, for a period of 4–6 weeks. Penetration of antibiotics may be limited by the fibrous nature of the lesions.

Surgery is limited to draining superficial lesions, which may on occasions necessitate repeated episodes of draining, but if bone is involved the affected area may be curetted and packed open and the teeth involved extracted.

Further reading

Bagg J, MacFarlane TW, Poxton IR, Smith AJ (2006) *Essentials of Microbiology for Dental Students*, 2nd edn. Oxford University Press, Oxford.

Ingham HR, Kalbag RM, Tharagonnet D, High AS, Sengupta RP, Selkon JB (1978) Abscesses of the frontal lobe of the brain secondary to convert dental sepsis. *Lancet* **2** (8088): 497–9.

Iwu GO (1990) Ludwig's angina: report of seven cases and review of current concepts on management. *British Journal Oral and Maxillofacial Surgery* **28**: 189.

Lewis MAO, MacFarlane TW, McGowan DA (1990) A microbiological and clinical review of the acute dentoalveolar abscess. *British Journal Oral Maxillofacial Surgery* **28**: 359.

Rud J (1970) Removal of impacted lower third molars with acute pericoronitis and necrotising gingivitis. *British Journal of Oral Surgery* **7**(3): 153–60.

Ward Booth P, Schendel S, Hausamen J (2006) *Maxillofacial Surgery*, 2nd edn. Churchill Livingstone, Elsevier.

Chapter 13
Treatment of Cysts of the Jaw

- Diagnosis
- Treatment
- Developmental cysts of non-dental origin
- Non-epithelial lined cysts
- Soft tissue cysts

A cyst may be defined as a radiolucency that is usually fluid filled and has a lining. The lining is frequently epithelium and in the mouth is either of dental or non-dental origin. A cyst must be differentiated from other pathology that might mimic it, particularly neoplasia.

The common cysts of the jaw arising from epithelium of dental origin are:

- dental (radicular) or periodontal cysts
- residual cysts
- dentigerous cysts
- eruption cysts
- keratocysts.

Dental (radicular) or periodontal cysts

These form from the epithelial cells or rests of Malassez, which are the remnants of Hertwig's sheath. They remain throughout life, scattered in clusters, in the periodontal membrane. Chronic infection may stimulate them to proliferate and form epithelial lined cysts in the jaws. These occur chiefly over the apex of a dead tooth, but may occasionally be found on its lateral aspect, when they are called lateral periodontal cysts.

Residual cysts

These occur in edentulous areas of the jaws and are dental cysts believed to have been present before the dead tooth was extracted and which continue to grow.

Principles of Oral and Maxillofacial Surgery, 6th Edition. Edited by U. J. Moore
© 2011 Blackwell Publishing Ltd

Dentigerous cysts

These form between the reduced enamel epithelium of the follicle around a developing tooth and its crown. The cyst lining is therefore attached to the tooth at the amelocemental junction.

Eruption cysts

These are cysts forming over erupting teeth and they have a dentigerous relationship also. Those over deciduous or permanent teeth with no deciduous predecessor are believed to originate from the cells of the enamel organ. Where there has been a deciduous predecessor, the epithelial rests of Malassez from this tooth could give rise to one of these cysts.

Cyst growth

Osmotic growth

The above cysts of dental origin are believed to increase in size either from continual liquefaction of their shed cells (which forms the cholesterol that gives the contents a characteristic golden appearance) or as a result of the positive osmotic pressure of the hypertonic contents that draws water in from the tissues.

Mural growth

Direct growth of the epithelium lining the cyst wall from which keratin squames are shed is a characteristic of keratocysts (see below). This ability to grow means that if any lining remains recurrence is more likely.

Keratocysts (primordial cysts)

These are said to arise from the dental lamina or from the enamel organ of a tooth germ. Their lining is of well-differentiated epithelium which may show ortho- or parakeratosis. They are believed to increase in size by mural division. Beneath the epithelium is thin fibrous tissue, which is easily torn, and satellite cysts lying outside the main body of the lesion are often found. For these reasons keratocysts are well known to be difficult to eradicate and likely to recur after treatment. The recurrence rate has been reported to be anything between 5 and 60%. The complete removal of all the lining of these cysts to avoid recurrence is of great importance. Their contents have less soluble protein (below 5 g/100 ml) than dental cysts.

Diagnosis

Diagnosis on clinical grounds alone should be treated with caution. Histological confirmation of any diagnosis should be vigorously pursued (Figure 13.1).

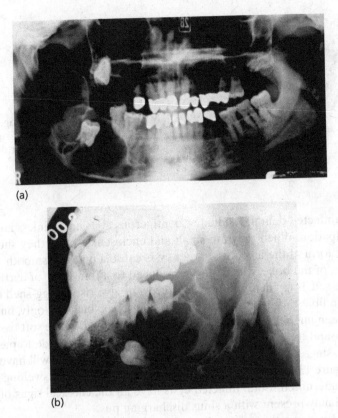

(a)

(b)

Figure 13.1   Diagnostic difficulties. (a) Histologically this lesion was a dental cyst; (b) this lesion was an ameloblastoma.

Presentation

In many cases the presentation is on routine radiograph. The process of diagnosis follows established routines.

History

The patient often gives no history, as many cysts may escape attention until they become infected. Larger cysts may cause swelling of the jaw or face, which in the edentulous may be associated with difficulty in wearing dentures. In the mandible, pressure on the inferior dental nerve almost never gives rise to mental anaesthesia or paraesthesia, an important point in differentiation from tumours. Occasionally cysts reach such proportions that excessive resorption of bone leads to pathological fracture. Eventually the majority of cysts become infected, with acute symptoms and, in those that have expanded into the soft tissues, an increase in the swelling.

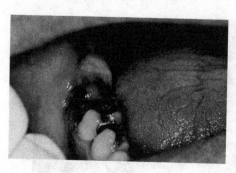

Figure 13.2 A dentigerous cyst around the unerupted lower right third molar. Note the blue colour due to the fluid content of the cyst.

Examination

Uninfected dental, residual or dentigerous cysts are painless and non-tender on palpation. When they are small and enclosed in bone they show no change in the form of the alveolus. Larger cysts cause a marked, smooth, rounded expansion of the bone, which may be reduced to a thin layer of cortical plate. This, if pressed, is resilient but may fracture and give rise to egg-shell crackling. In the mandible this expansion is said to take place buccally only, but occasionally it is seen lingually as well. Where the cyst has invaded the soft tissues the swelling is found to be fluctuant and a definite thrill can be made to pass through it. At this stage, if the mucous membrane covering is thin, it will have a bluish colour (Figure 13.2). An eruption cyst presents as a small blue swelling in the gum over an unerupted tooth. Infected cysts have all the classical signs of acute infection and may present with a sinus discharging pus.

Missing teeth must be charted and the standing teeth carefully examined for caries, periodontal disease and mobility. A dentigerous cyst may be suspected where a tooth is missing from the arch without any history of previous extraction. Dead and root-filled teeth are associated with dental cysts. The vitality of all teeth near the lesion must be tested with an electric pulp tester and the results compared with similar teeth on the unaffected side. If there is any delay between diagnosis and operation these tests should be repeated immediately before operation, for cysts not only arise from dead teeth but their expansion may also devitalise adjacent teeth.

Keratocysts may present like dental cysts but occur most commonly in the lower third molar region or distal to it and invade the ascending ramus extensively. They tend to expand anteroposteriorly in the medullary bone of the mandible and reach some size with minimal expansion of the cortical plate. Diagnosis may result from an infective episode or as a result of discovery on a scanning radiograph (Figure 13.3).

Gorlin–Goltz syndrome

Multiple recurrent keratocysts are associated with basal cell carcinomas and some skeletal abnormalities in this syndrome. These patients require careful management and appropriate referral when necessary. Recurrence of the cystic

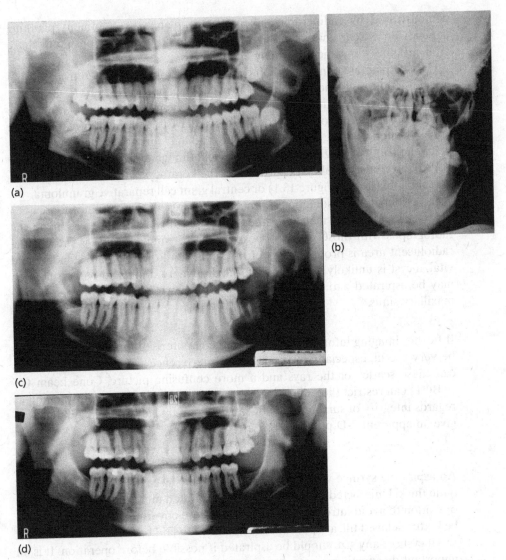

Figure 13.3   Keratocyst. (a, b) At presentation; note resorption of apex of first molar; (c) immediate postoperative appearance; (d) appearance at 6 months showing bone healing. Inferior alveolar nerve function was not affected.

lesions in this syndrome requires regular reviews and radiography to identify lesions early and reduce morbidity.

Radiography

Intraoral apical films usually suffice for small dental cysts. Larger ones may need extraoral and occlusal views of the jaws to show their full extent. This is demonstrated by radiographs taken in two planes, as treatment planning depends on a clear understanding of their size and their relationship to those vital structures on which they may encroach.

Cysts appear as rounded, radiolucent areas sharply demarcated from normal bone by a thin, radiopaque, limiting line of compact or cortical bone (Figures 13.1 and 13.3). This line is not usually present on radiographs of apical granulomas and is often absent or hazy round infected cysts. Apical periodontal cysts are associated with the roots of dead teeth and may throw a shadow over or displace the roots of neighbouring teeth, which, though apparently involved, may yet still be vital. Dental cysts, particularly the keratocyst, if loculated may simulate ameloblastoma (Figure 13.1) or central giant cell reparative granuloma.

In the maxilla it is sometimes difficult to tell whether a radiolucent area is a cyst or a locule of the maxillary sinus. Therefore it is necessary to compare the radiographs with those of the opposite side; if a similar locule is present the radiolucent area is probably part of the sinus. If all the teeth are standing and vital, a cyst is unlikely to be present. Finally, where doubts still exist, the area may be aspirated and if air, not fluid, is withdrawn it is certainly part of the maxillary sinus.

CT scan and cone beam CT (CBCT)

If further imaging information is required computerised tomography (CT) can be very useful, especially in the maxilla. Interference with metal restorations can cause scatter of the rays and a more confusing picture. Cone beam CT (CBCT) can restrict the radiation dose and give very clear local information as regards integrity of surrounding bone. The digital image can be manipulated to give an apparent 3-D picture.

Aspiration

An aspirating syringe with a broad-bore needle is used, as the contents can be quite thick. Uninfected cysts should not be aspirated more than 24 hours before operation to avoid introducing infection. In those covered by thick bone it may be better delayed till, at operation, a flap has been laid back and bone removed.

All cysts of any size should be aspirated if possible before operation. It is an important diagnostic measure that can save the surgeon much embarrassment from accidentally opening a solid tumour, or worse a central haemangioma. Microscopic examination of the aspirate may show the presence of cholesterol.

Further, only in this way may a keratocyst be differentiated from other odontogenic cysts before operation. This is done by electrophoresis of the aspirate, which for keratocysts will show less than 5 g in 100 ml of soluble protein, whereas other dental cysts will have quantities similar to that in the patient's serum.

Differential diagnosis

These lesions may all mimic cysts in their radiographic appearance:

- solitary bone cyst
- Stafne's bone cavity

- aneurysmal bone cyst
- central giant cell granuloma
- ameloblastoma
- myeloma.

Where doubt exists, blood chemistry, aspiration and biopsy should be performed.

Assessment

This includes an estimation of the size of the cyst and, particularly in the mandible, the extent of bone resorption. Should there be a risk of a pathological fracture, the means to reduce and internally fix the mandible should be available (see Chapter 14). Many cysts, however, which on lateral radiographs occupy the whole of the depth of the mandible, usually have a sturdy lingual plate that adequately maintains the continuity of the bone through the operation.

The relationship of the cyst to adjacent structures is more important. Vital teeth that have a satisfactory periodontal condition and are functional, should be preserved. Consideration should be given to retaining dead teeth in well-cared-for mouths. This may be done by root-filling and apicectomy providing that at the very least the whole of the coronal half of the root is firmly held in sound alveolar bone. Dead teeth should be extracted where they are non-functional, mobile, the periodontal condition is poor and the patient already wears denture. Where a diagnosis of keratocyst has been confirmed, extraction of involved teeth may be wise to ensure removal of all the lining in view of the high reported recurrence rate.

Dentigerous cysts surround the crowns of teeth and, in the young where these are reasonably well placed, treatment may be directed at saving the tooth and allowing it to erupt into the arch.

Cysts may be closely related to the maxillary sinus, floor of nose or to the inferior dental canal, which are important structures not to be damaged and may modify the treatment plan. The maxillary antrum can be partially or even completely obliterated by a large cyst. In the mandible the inferior dental nerve may be grossly displaced in a similar way.

Treatment

Acutely infected cysts are treated with antibacterial drugs and by drainage; further surgery is delayed until the acute phase has settled. There are two methods for treating cysts: enucleation and marsupialisation.

Enucleation

In this operation the whole of the cyst lining is removed. For this reason, and because healing proceeds more rapidly after this has been done, it is the best treatment, particularly for keratocysts, and should be used whenever possible.

Though applicable to all types of cyst it is seldom necessary in treating cysts of eruption and is contraindicated in dentigerous cysts if the enclosed tooth is to be preserved.

Small apical cysts where the tooth is to be retained (apicectomy)

These often resolve or remain static following adequate orthograde root canal treatment. If there is evidence of an enlarging radiolucency, or root canal treatment is mechanically impossible, then removal of the cyst together with the apical third of the root may be indicated. A full thickness mucoperiosteal flap should be raised. A number of different designs have been used that preserve the gingival margin around crowned teeth and these may be preferred, but only if these designs do not compromise the surgical access. A two- or three-sided flap may be required in the anterior region. The incision is made round the neck of the affected tooth with one or two vertical incisions diverging into the buccal sulcus. The flap is then reflected to expose the bone over the apex (Figure 13.4).

The position of the root in the alveolar bone is estimated and the apical third exposed. This may be done with a medium-sized rosehead bur. Bone is then removed to expose the cystic area, taking care to avoid damaging, or even exposing, the roots of neighbouring teeth. The apical third of the root is divided using a No. 5 fissure bur. The anterior part of the root should be cut flush with the alveolar bone but bevelled to allow retrograde access to the root canal (Figure 13.4).

The use of loupes at this stage can facilitate vision and make both removal of the cyst and other aspects of apical surgery more accurate. The cyst lining is then enucleated. This does not mean curettage, but implies a careful, methodical separation of the cyst from bone to remove the lining intact without tearing if possible (Figure 13.4). Curettes (Mitchell trimmer) can be used, if kept well against bone, to dissect out the cyst gently (Figure 13.5). Where the lining is firmly attached, 1.5 cm ribbon gauze soaked in saline or in diluted hydrogen peroxide may be packed carefully into the cavity to separate the two tissues (Figure 13.5). The lining is sent for histological examination. The cavity is examined for any remnants of granulations or cyst lining. These are frequently far back behind the root of the tooth and are removed by scraping the bony walls; none must be left if a recurrence is to be avoided. Where the tooth has been root filled the apical seal is checked. Should this be inadequate a retrograde filling is placed in the apex. The cavity is thoroughly washed out and the flap replaced and sutured.

Where a prosthetic crown is present it is unwise to incise around the gingival margin and a semi-lunar incision is made within the unattached gingivae, leaving an adequate margin for suturing. Care must be taken when removing bone to ensure that at the end of the operation the flap margin is adequately supported on bone.

Enucleation of the larger odontogenic cysts

The chief problems in the treatment of large cysts by enucleation are to provide a flap which will give adequate closure and to establish the maximum

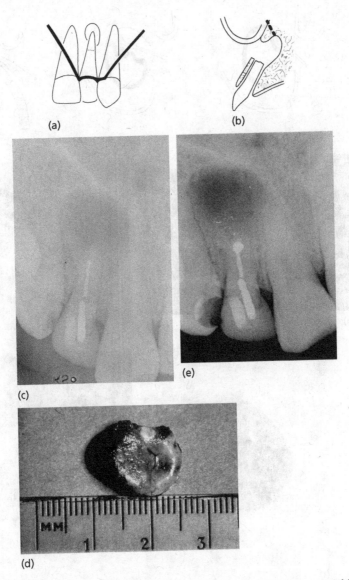

Figure 13.4   Apicectomy. (a) Apicetomy flap – dotted line shows proposed level of section of root; (b) after root section. Note root cut level with bone margin. Saucerisation may be completed by removing buccal plate to level of dotted line; (c) radiograph shows cyst associated with apex of incisor; (d) enucleated cyst – note apex contained within cyst; (e) postoperative radiograph showing retrograde root filling sealing apex. Note amalgam has been used in this image; a calcium hydroxide based material is in more common current usage.

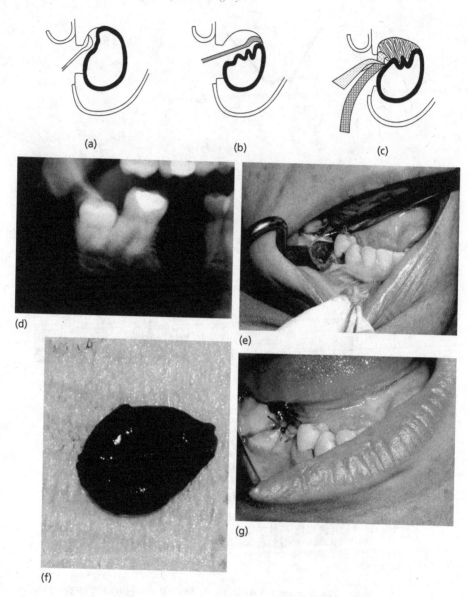

Figure 13.5 Enucleation of cyst. (a) Curette used to enucleate cyst with the back of the spoon turned towards cyst lining; (b) at greatest diameter of cyst the curette is reversed to present concavity of spoon to the cyst lining; (c) packing wet ribbon gauze between cyst lining and bone to separate them; (d) radiograph of residual cyst; (e) cyst exposed via two-sided flap; (f) enucleated cyst; (g) closure.

amount of clot that will organise without liquefying or becoming infected. When these objects are achieved the cyst will heal by first intention with minimal deformity.

Flap

The incision is made at the cervical margin of the teeth or along the alveolar crest in edentulous patients. The design should ensure that at closure the margins are on sound bone and thus it should be adequately extended to allow for the extraction of teeth that might become necessary during the procedure. An envelope flap or three-sided design is suitable for most situations (see Chapter 8). Where the bone resorption has brought cyst lining and mucoperiosteum into apposition the two should be separated without tearing either, and the flap reflected beyond the cyst lining on to bone. This is usually the most difficult part of the operation.

Bone removal

It may be possible to peel thin layers of bone from the cyst lining if this is sufficiently thin, but some bone must usually be removed with burs to allow full access to the cavity. The alveolar ridge should be spared as much as possible to facilitate the wearing of dentures. Any tooth with a poor prognosis should be removed. If it is in close relation to the lining it should accompany the rest of the specimen for histological examination.

Enucleation

The whole of the cyst lining must be enucleated. After its removal it is carefully examined for any tears or deficiencies. Only where it is intact can the surgeon be sure no lining has been left behind. The cavity is systematically searched and any soft tissue remnants curetted out. This is particularly important where a keratocyst is suspected. The bone edges are saucerised to provide a smooth transition from cyst cavity to the surface of the bone (Figures 13.6, 13.7 and 13.8). Saucerisation can be extensive providing that the alveolar crest is preserved to leave a satisfactory ridge for dentures and that vital structures are not damaged. Anteriorly the bony support to the ala of the nose must not be undermined as an ugly deformity can occur.

Closure

This needs to be done with care to achieve the elimination of as much dead space as possible. In addition there should a good seal around the margin of the cyst cavity. Postoperative bleeding will cause bulging of the flap and may contribute to breakdown of the wound. A small quantity of a haemostatic agent such as oxidised cellulose may be used to prevent this. The flap should be encouraged to lie in close apposition to the cyst cavity and mattress sutures may help. Added support may be given by an external pressure dressing, particularly in the lower anterior region. This can be removed after 48 hours or

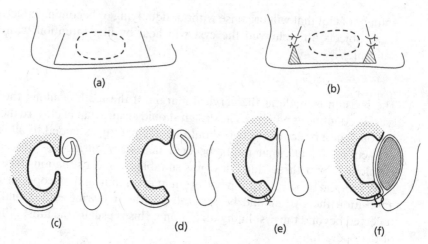

Figure 13.6 Enucleation of large dental cysts. (a) Design of flap with more vertical incisions to allow mucosa to line cavity; (b) flap replaced, some areas of bone are exposed (shaded areas); (c) section of cyst cavity before saucerisation; (d) after saucerisation; (e) flap replaced.

when postoperative haemorrhage has ceased. Alternatively, the clot may be reduced by adequate drainage. For cysts in the mandible a drain can be placed from the cavity through the lingual wall below the floor of the mouth and brought out onto the skin of the neck. The drain is removed after 48 hours.

Various substances have been packed into the cyst cavity to obliterate the dead space. Fibrin foam and gelatine sponge only form a matrix for a large clot, which may still become infected. The use of bone is more rational and chips have been successfully employed, but also carry a risk of infection. Rarely, in very large cysts of the mandible, the bone can be so weakened at operation that it may be necessary to place an immediate bone graft in the cavity. Osteoconductive substances can also be placed at the time of operation to promote bone production and save a further operative site (see Chapter 11).

Pathological fracture

Before, during or after operation pathological fracture may occur in cysts that have caused large amounts of bone loss. If this occurs, the fracture should be managed as outlined in Chapter 14. At operation a plate may be adapted to the bone before enucleation to allow rapid fixation if fracture should occur. If bone loss is excessive reconstruction plates (bicortical) may be required.

Wound breakdown

If the wound should break down the cavity will become contaminated with saliva and food debris. In this event the cavity should be gently packed with half-inch ribbon gauze soaked in bismuth iodoform paraffin paste (BIPP) (or Whitehead's varnish, also an iodoform preparation, if available) to maintain an antiseptic occlusion of the space for up to 3 weeks. After this time the pack should be changed at intervals until epithelialisation of the wound has occurred.

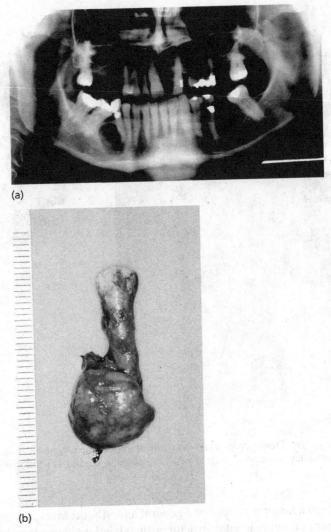

(a)

(b)

Figure 13.7 Dental or radicular cyst. (a) Radiographic appearance; (b) following removal; note association with apex of premolar.

The patient may then be furnished with a syringe to keep the cavity clean. Healing even under these circumstances is remarkably rapid.

Marsupialisation

An opening into the cyst is made so that the contents drain out and the lining epithelium is exposed to the mouth. The advantages of marsupialisation are simplicity, speed of operation, minimal trauma and that no bone is exposed to contamination from the mouth. This makes it ideal for ill patients unable to

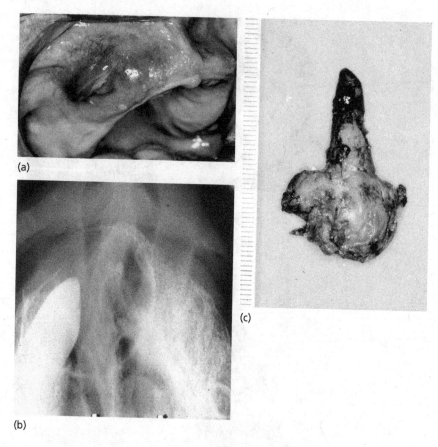

Figure 13.8 Dentigerous cyst. (a) Clinical appearance; denture trauma; (b) large radiolucency associated with crown of unerupted canine; (c) following removal.

undergo a long procedure or a general anaesthetic. Marsupialisation lessens the danger of damaging vital structures, the alveolar ridge is preserved and indeed, if properly planned, the operation may improve the depth of the buccal sulcus and the retention of dentures, particularly in the lower jaw. It has two major disadvantages: pathological tissues are left and healing is slow. It should be the treatment of choice only for eruption cysts and dentigerous cysts where the tooth is to be preserved and expected to erupt. In large cysts where the jaw may fracture or vital structures, particularly teeth, could be damaged by enucleation, marsupialisation may be used as a first procedure. Once bone has reformed the remaining lining is enucleated at a second operation. This technique has also been successfully used for large keratocysts of the ascending ramus where, because the lining is in contact with periosteum over a wide area and dissection is difficult, there is a danger of seeding into the soft tissues. Even in this group of cysts new bone appears to reform and make later enucleation safe.

Operation

A buccal incision is made along the occlusal margin of the cyst and curved at each end to follow its contour in the bone. The flap should be large. Some operators make a small hole, which tends to close and requires packing over a long period because a satisfactory obturator cannot be fitted. It must be accepted that where many natural teeth are present only a small opening can be made.

The flap is then reflected and the bone removed as widely as possible over the cyst. A window that closely follows the bone margins is cut in the lining with scissors. This tissue should be sent for histological examination. The mucosal flap is now excised so that cyst lining and mucosa can be sewn together round the edges of the window (Figure 13.9). The cavity is washed out and temporarily dressed with BIPP or Whitehead's varnish on ribbon gauze. With a large window in an edentulous area the pack and sutures may be removed after 10 days and an obturator constructed on a denture. The patient is given a water syringe to keep the cavity clean. As the cavity obliterates the obturator will require reduction. Where the aperture is small and an obturator cannot be worn, packing must continue until healing is complete. In dentigerous cysts containing an erupting tooth the same procedure is followed, care being taken not to disturb the tooth (Figure 13.10).

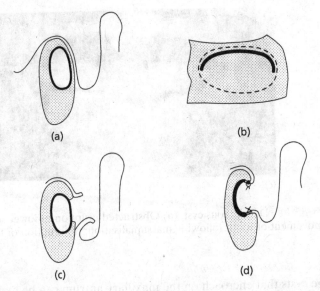

(a)   (b)

(c)   (d)

Figure 13.9   Marsupialisation. (a) The preoperative outline of cyst in mandible; (b) black line shows line of incision in buccal mucoperiosteum and following the outline of the cyst (dotted line); (c) removal of buccal bone to expose cyst but preserve the alveolar ridge; (d) cyst opened, drained and lining sutured to mucous membrane.

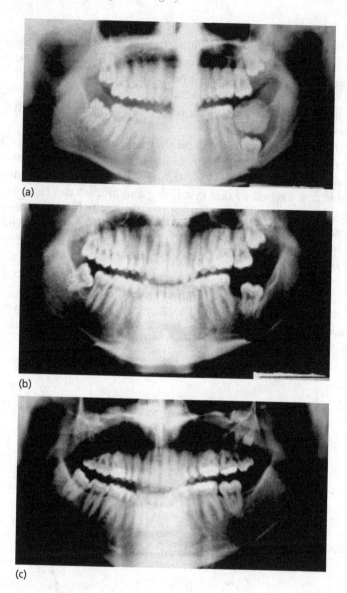

Figure 13.10   Dentigerous cyst. (a) Obstructed eruption of lower second molar; (b) movement of tooth following marsupialisation; (c) eruption of tooth into function.

Marsupialisation into the antrum

Large cysts that encroach on the maxillary antrum can be marsupialised into it. This avoids a gross deformity in the buccal sulcus, which may take a long time to heal. The cyst is exposed as for enucleation and a window cut in the lining. Through this a direct opening into the antrum is made where cyst and antrum lining are in apposition. This should be as large as possible and never less than 2.5 cm across. This technique may be combined with enucleation of cysts that are adherent only to the antrum lining. The operation can also be performed through a Caldwell–Luc approach into the antrum when a hole is cut from the antrum into the cyst.

Combined enucleation and open packing

Large cysts can be enucleated, but instead of an immediate closure the mucosal flap is turned into the cavity to cover some of the raw bone and a pack is inserted to protect the rest. This technique overcomes the risk of breakdown of the blood clot present in immediate closure. As the pathological lining has all been removed, healing is far faster than when the cavity is marsupialised.

Follow-up

Long-term follow-up of all cysts is advisable lest retained epithelial fragments cause a recurrence. Satisfactory healing can be assessed by clinical examination, and by radiopaque lamina around the periphery of the cyst and new bone formation filling the radiolucent area.

Keratocysts may recur a long time after operation; follow-up of these lesions must continue over a long period of years (at least five).

Developmental cysts of non-dental origin

Inclusion or fissural cysts of the jaws

These arise from the inclusion of epithelial remnants at the site of fusion of the various processes that form the mouth and face. They are epithelial lined and usually contain mucoid fluid. As they do not arise from the teeth, vitality testing is essential in the differential diagnosis.

Nasolabial cysts

These occur at the junction of the globular, lateral and median nasal processes, under the ala of the nose. They are diagnosed by their position as they lie in a depression on the maxilla, and not in the bone.

Median cysts

These very rare cysts are found in the midline where fusion of the two halves of the palate and mandible takes place.

Incisive canal cysts

These develop from epithelial remnants in the incisive canal. They present as a swelling under the incisive papilla, which, on an anterior occlusal radiograph, shows as an expansion of the incisive foramen. The latter is normally under 7 mm in diameter. Occasionally the presenting symptom is a complaint of a salty taste.

Globulomaxillary cysts

These occur at the junction of the globular and maxillary processes. They arise between the maxillary lateral incisor and canine, characteristically separating the roots of these teeth, which are not concerned with the formation of the cyst and should be vital.

Diagnosis and assessment

This is approached in the same way as for cysts of dental origin and the differential diagnosis is made by their special features. These are their site, fluid contents and the fact that adjacent teeth are vital because the cysts are of non-dental origin.

Treatment

They are treated like other cysts of the jaws by enucleation, or by marsupialisation followed by enucleation where there is risk of damaging adjacent teeth.

Non-epithelial lined cysts

Solitary bone cyst

These so-called traumatic bone cysts occur in the jaws, usually in the tooth-bearing area. However, they are not associated with dental pathology and are discovered purely on routine radiography. On opening the cyst cavity, little or no lining or contents are found. Any lining present is connective tissue rather than epithelium. They heal spontaneously following light curettage (Figure 13.11).

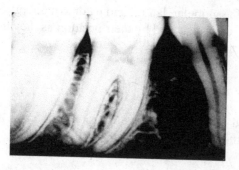

Figure 13.11   Solitary (traumatic) bone cyst.

Soft tissue cysts

Dermoid cysts

These arise from inclusion of ectoderm at lines of fusion anywhere in the body. In the mouth they may be found in the floor, the palate or the tongue. They are teratomas lined by stratified squamous epithelium and may contain hair, nails, teeth, etc.

Diagnosis

Those in the floor of the mouth may occur in the midline or laterally. They do not become obvious until adolescence or later. The patient complains of a slowly enlarging swelling under the tongue, occasionally affecting speech, and which is visible in the neck. Examination reveals a fluctuant or soft swelling in the floor of the mouth either above or below the mylohyoid. It does not move up or down on swallowing, which is important in distinguishing it from a thyroglossal cyst. Aspiration produces a thick sebaceous material, where this can be withdrawn. Dermoid cysts at other sites are similarly diagnosed.

Treatment

Sublingual dermoids may be enucleated through an external approach below the mandible or intraorally though an incision in the floor of the mouth, just at the reflection of the lingual mucosa from the mandible. The latter flap is reflected lingually and will contain the ducts of the submandibular glands, which must not be damaged. The cyst is then exposed but may have to be emptied to remove it, as otherwise it may be too large to pass out of the incision. Its thick lining makes it easy to enucleate. Satisfactory drainage must be provided for a few days for the large sublingual deficiency.

Salivary cysts (mucocele)

There are discussed under diseases of the salivary glands (Chapter 16).

Further reading

Chapelle K, Stoelinga P, Wilde P, Brouns J, *et al.* (2004) Rational approach to diagnosis and treatment of ameloblastomas and odontogenic keratocysts. *British Journal Oral and Maxillofacial Surgery* **42**: 381–90.

Cawson RA, Langdon JD, Eveson JW (1996) *Surgical Pathology of the Mouth and Jaws.* Wright, Oxford.

Meechan JG (2006) *Minor Oral Surgery in Dental Practice.* Quintessence, London.

Soames JV, Southam JC (2005) *Oral Pathology,* 4th edn. Oxford University Press, Oxford.

Chapter 14
Management of Maxillofacial Trauma

- Initial assessment
- Applied anatomy
- Diagnosis
- Treatment planning
- Principles of treatment
- Definitive treatment
- Complications of fractures

The commonest causes of fractured jaws are fights, road accidents, falls and sport. They occur chiefly in males between 15 and 35 years of age and twice as frequently in the mandible as in the maxilla. Fractures may be direct, following a blow at the point where the break occurs, or may be indirect as a result of a blow on the bone at some distance from where the lesion occurs. They may be single, linear or comminuted, that is fragmented into two or more small pieces, and are said to be compound when they communicate with a wound in the skin or mucous membrane of the mouth, nose or air sinuses. Where there is a tooth in the line of the fracture the latter is almost certainly compound into the mouth through the periodontal membrane. In the young, incomplete or greenstick fractures of the mandible can occur. Diseases of the bone predispose to spontaneous pathological fractures. All traumatised patients need to be fully assessed.

Initial assessment

The American College of Surgeons has established a pattern of assessment of the traumatised patient that has been adopted as the gold standard in many countries around the world. This is disseminated through advanced trauma life support courses (ATLS). The initial assessment should not concentrate on the most obvious injury but involve a rapid survey of the vital functions to allow management priorities to be established. The primary survey involves:

Principles of Oral and Maxillofacial Surgery, 6th Edition. Edited by U. J. Moore
© 2011 Blackwell Publishing Ltd

- A – airway maintenance with cervical spine control
- B – breathing and ventilation
- C – circulation with haemorrhage control
- D – disability: neurological status
- E – exposure: complete examination of the patient.

During the primary survey, resuscitation is performed and afterwards shock management is initiated with fluid replacement while the vital signs are monitored for any deterioration in the status of the patient.

Once the patient is stabilised a secondary survey is carried out to ensure that all traumatic injuries are evaluated, after which definitive care can be prioritised.

Airway and cervical spine

In unconscious patients respiratory obstruction may be caused by blood clot, or a foreign body in the oropharynx or larynx. In bilateral fractures of the mandible through the canine region the tongue may fall back to occlude the airway. In maxillary injuries the palate can be displaced down and back to occlude the oropharynx. Cervical spine injury should be suspected in any blunt trauma above the clavicle and excluded by appropriate radiographs. Until then a hard cervical collar should be worn.

Control of the airway is an absolute priority. The tongue or palate is drawn forward and the mouth and pharynx sucked or wiped clear of debris to re-establish the airway. To keep the tongue forward, a suture may be passed through it, or the patient turned on their side, with control of the cervical spine, to allow saliva and blood to drain out of the mouth. Where these measures are ineffective, intubation may be necessary and consideration given to a tracheostomy. Before giving an anaesthetic to the unconscious patient soon after the accident, the stomach must be emptied of swallowed blood using an orogastric tube.

Haemorrhage

Acute bleeding can be life threatening if major vessels are involved and should be controlled as described in Chapter 7.

Surgical shock

This condition is as a result of excessive blood loss, leading to circulatory collapse. In closed wounds, blood and plasma may bleed from the vessels into the tissue spaces. The abdomen is a common reservoir following major trauma. If the initial loss is over one litre this cannot be compensated for by general vasoconstriction. Where fluid is not replaced, the falling blood pressure and vasoconstriction cause oxygen lack in the tissues and an increased permeability of the capillaries with still further loss of fluid into the tissues.

Signs and symptoms

The patient is typically cold, sweating and pale or cyanosed. In the limbs the degree of swelling in closed injuries gives some indication of the fluid loss into the tissues, but this is of little use in facial injuries. Increased respiratory rate, rapid pulse and falling blood pressure are strong indications of deterioration.

Treatment

Prompt and energetic measures are necessary. Immediate replacement of fluid is lifesaving whilst arrest of haemorrhage must be undertaken to prevent further loss. Blood pressure and pulse must be continually monitored to gauge the effectiveness of replacement therapy until the patient stabilises. A patient with a pulse rate persistently over 100, and systolic blood pressure of under 100 mmHg (13.3 kPa), requires transfusion of whole blood. Grouping and cross matching should be done early, and intravenous access to allow a saline or plasma substitute drip should be established immediately.

Haemoglobin estimations are of little use in the acute phase owing to the haemoconcentration which usually occurs, but should be checked after haemodilution has taken place.

The circulation to the head is improved by raising the foot of the bed, and oxygen should be administered. Warmth should be applied with blankets to keep the patient in an environmental temperature of 32°C.

Head injury

Many patients who sustain facial injuries may also have lost consciousness. All these patients, however short the time they were unconscious, must be fully assessed using the Glasgow Coma Scale (GCS) and referred to a neurosurgeon. The Glasgow Coma Scale consists of ranking of behavioural responses (Table 14.1). Motor responses, verbal responses and eye opening are independently assessed and scored numerically out of a total of 15. The patient's condition must be carefully observed and recorded for change in GCS status. In addition pulse, blood pressure and pupil reaction to light are monitored, as these reflect changes in intracranial pressure. A rise in intracranial pressure is denoted by a slow reaction to light of the pupil on the affected side and as the pressure increases the pupil becomes fixed and dilated. As the condition of the patient worsens the opposite pupil also dilates. In the initial stages of assessment and resuscitation following acute trauma, monitoring may be virtually continuous but should be maintained even in the apparently stable patient at intervals up to one hourly for 24 hours after the initial trauma.

Table 14.1   Glasgow coma scale (GCS). Take the best score from each category to give a total coma score

Eye opening		Motor		Verbal	
Spontaneous	4	Moves to command	6	Converses	5
To speech	3	Localises to pain	5	Confused	4
To pain	2	Withdraws from pain	4	Gibberish	3
None	1	Flexes	3	Grunts	2
		Extends	2	None	1
		None	1		

Prevention of infection

External wounds are kept covered with dressings and a prophylactic course of antibacterial drug is administered. The wounds should be closed as soon as possible, under local anaesthesia if necessary.

Pain

This can be severe, particularly with comminuted and grossly displaced fractures, but can sometimes be less than anticipated. Morphine or its derivatives must not be given because they may mask the signs of increasing intracranial pressure or depress the patient with a compromised airway. Non-steroidal anti-inflammatory drugs (NSAIDs) may be prescribed to reduce both peripheral and intracranial pressure.

Temporary immobilisation or fixation

This has mainly fallen into disuse as early reduction and fixation is to be preferred. However, the use of a barrel bandage to support the comminuted mandible may be advocated. Careful consideration must be given to the effect this may have on the fragments, as an ill-applied bandage may increase the displacement. A bridle wire between teeth either side of the fracture line can be useful to stabilise a mobile fracture.

Supportive treatment

This has been discussed in Chapters 2 and 4.

The management of maxillofacial injuries will now be considered.

Applied anatomy

For describing injuries the face is divided into three parts. The lower third is the mandible and the soft tissues covering it. The middle third is bounded below by the occlusal line of the maxillary teeth and above by a line drawn through the pupils. The upper third lies above this.

The mandible

The commonest sites of fracture in the mandible are the condyle neck, the angle and the canine region. The condyle may fracture through its thin neck, either within the capsule or below it, and may be bilateral as a result of blows to the chin, particularly if the mouth is open, or unilateral following blows to the body of the mandible on the opposite side. Fractures of the coronoid process are uncommon.

The angle of the mandible is a weak point because there is a change in the direction of the grain of the bone, which occurs where the vertical ascending ramus and horizontal body meet. Further, the shape of the mandible in cross-section changes as the thick lower border of the body becomes thin at the angle, so that the lower third molar sits in bone with little basal support lingually. Finally, the third molar, particularly if it is unerupted, may occupy up to two-thirds of the depth of the bone.

The body is the strongest part of the lower jaw but is weakened by the presence of the tooth sockets. The canine has a long broad root and its socket is a common site of fracture. The symphysis may also be involved as a result of blows on the chin. Alveolar fractures occur chiefly in the incisor region.

Displacement

Displacement depends on three factors: the force of the blow, gravity and the pull of the muscles inserted into the bone. The muscles concerned are the suprahyoid group attached to the lingual aspect of the anterior part of the mandible, which depress the lower jaw, and the muscles of mastication (masseter, temporalis and medial pterygoid) inserted into the ascending ramus, which elevate the mandible and move it laterally. The lateral pterygoid muscle, inserted into the condyle and meniscus of the temporomandibular joint, draws the condyle forward and therefore assists in opening the mouth.

Condylar fractures

In these cases the lateral pterygoid muscle draws the fractured head forward medially and, in certain cases, over the eminentia articularis and out of the glenoid fossa to produce a fracture dislocation. The other muscles of mastication raise the ramus of the affected side to produce an anterior open bite between the incisors and canines on the opposite side. On opening the mouth the body of the mandible is displaced towards the affected side with marked deviation of the midline. In bilateral condylar fractures both ascending rami are drawn up and back equally so that gagging occurs on the posterior teeth causing an anterior open bite on both sides.

Fractures of the angle or body

In these the suprahyoid group of muscles depresses the anterior part of the mandible. Posteriorly the pull of the muscles of mastication attached to the ascending ramus draws it upwards. The posterior fragment is also drawn inwards as the pull of the medial pterygoid muscle is stronger than that of the masseter (Figure 14.1). Displacement is resisted by the periosteum, if it is intact, by the occlusion of the teeth and by the impaction of the fractured bone ends against each other. This last depends on the angle of the line of fracture which is said to be *unfavourable* if it would allow the posterior fragment to displace or *favourable* if it prevents it doing so.

As displacement can take place in two planes, upwards and inwards, fractures are described as favourable or unfavourable when viewed from the side or horizontally, and from above or vertically. Thus a horizontally unfavourable fracture displaces upwards, a vertically unfavourable fracture inwards (Figure 14.1).

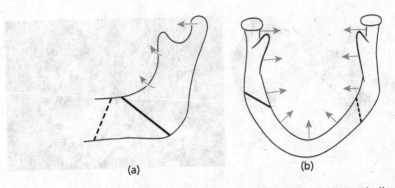

(a)   (b)

Figure 14.1   Effects of muscle pull on mandibular fractures. Arrows indicate the direction of muscle pull. (a) Horizontal view of mandible showing horizontally favourable fracture (dotted line) and horizontally unfavourable fracture (continuous line); (b) vertical view showing vertically favourable (dotted line) and unfavourable (continuous line) fractures.

Where a bilateral fracture occurs in the anterior region through the canine sockets it is possible for the geniohyoid, genioglossus and mylohyoid muscles to displace the loose anterior portion downwards and backwards, with loss of control of the tongue, which may fall back into the pharynx and obstruct the airway.

Midline fracture

In oblique fractures through the symphysis of the mandible, one half may be displaced lingually by the mylohyoid muscle to cause over-riding in the midline.

Age

In children, facial trauma more often involves the upper and mid third of the face as the relative size of the face is smaller (Figure 14.2a). With developing facial structure trauma is seen more evenly distributed and with an adult dentition the trauma seen fits the same pattern as adult patients regardless of chronological age. The mandible of a child is greatly weakened by the numerous crypts of the developing teeth, but the greater elasticity of the bone compensates for this (Figure 14.2b). In older patients the bones become more brittle and tend to break more easily and the mandible is weakened by resorption of the alveolar bone after the teeth are lost. The periosteum does, however, form a complete envelope round the edentulous mandible which, if not torn in the accident, holds the fractured ends in apposition. With advancing years the mandible becomes more dependent for its blood supply on the periosteum than on the inferior dental artery. For this reason methods of reduction or fixation that involve stripping of the periosteum must be avoided in the elderly. Classical plate fixation is compromised in these extremes of age.

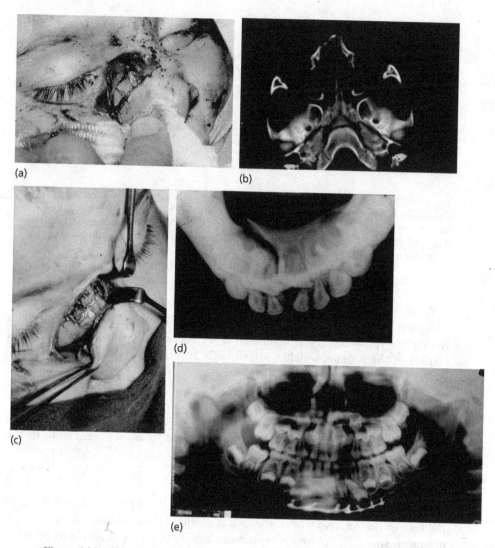

Figure 14.2　Trauma in children. (a) Nasal bone fracture in a 3-year-old child; (b) CT shows displacement; (c) ORIF via existing laceration to give good anatomical reduction of comminuted fragments; (d) displaced symphyseal fracture in a 6-year-old; lower occlusal radiograph giving clear view of fracture; (e) displaced symphyseal fracture in a 6-year-old; OPG shows ORIF applied at lower border via extraoral approach as very limited bone for classic sites of plate fixation due to developing dentition.

Middle third of the face

Fractures of the middle third of the face involve a complex of bones, which include the paired bones, the maxilla, palatine, zygomatic, nasal, lachrymal and inferior conchae, together with the single vomer and ethmoid bones. The structure of the maxillary complex consists of a grid system of buttresses

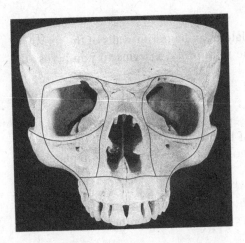

Figure 14.3   Grid structure of face: these are the principal lines of reconstruction.

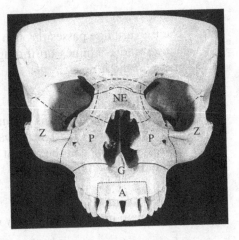

Figure 14.4   Fractures of the mid-third of the face: A – alveolar; G – Guérin's (Le Fort I); P – pyramidal (Le Fort II); Z – zygomatic (malar); NE – naso-ethmoidal; Le Fort III is shown by the upper dotted line.

(Figure 14.3). Strong vertical buttresses are formed by the frontal process of the maxilla, the zygomatic process of the maxilla and the zygomatic bone, and the pterygoid plates of the sphenoid with the tuberosity of the maxilla. Horizontal buttresses are formed by the supraorbital margin, the infraorbital margin and the palatine bones in continuity with the alveolar process. The spaces between are closed with thin bone plates, which enclose several large cavities, the maxillary air sinuses, the nasal cavity and the orbits. The vertical buttresses are more functionally challenged through the forces of mastication, particularly in the first permanent molar and canine regions, and the middle third is thus more resistant to upward forces but less to shearing stress from a horizontal blow.

Fractures of the middle third of the face fall into six categories (Figure 14.4):

- alveolar
- Guérin's/Le Fort I
- pyramidal/Le Fort II
- high transverse/Le Fort III
- naso-ethmoidal complex
- malar/zygomatic.

Alveolar fractures

Alveolar fractures occur in the tooth-bearing areas of the jaw.

Guérin's/Le Fort I

These occur where the palate and alveolus are separated from the maxillary complex by a transverse fracture just above the floor of the nose and the antrum.

Pyramidal/Le Fort II

The fracture line passes through the lateral and anterior walls of the maxillary sinuses and continues up through the infraorbital margins to join across the bridge of the nose.

High transverse/Le Fort III

The maxillary complex is virtually separated from the cranium by a fracture that traverses the lateral walls of both orbits and both orbital floors and crosses the midline at the root of the nose to involve the cribriform plate of the ethmoid.

The nasal bones and naso-ethmoidal complex

This may be involved separately or in combination with other fractures.

The malar bone (zygoma)

This can be fractured by a direct blow which may drive in the prominence of the cheek. The fracture line passes through the infraorbital margin, the anterior wall of the antrum, the malar buttress, the zygomatic arch and the frontal process of the zygoma.

It is important to understand that facial fractures rarely fall into such neat classifications. There is often a combination of injuries of the midface depending on the direction of the trauma. This can make exact classification difficult with fracture distribution being different on either side of the face. The clinical importance of this classification is that the Le Fort I involves only the alveolar process, the palate, nasal floor and maxillary antrum. The Le Fort II involves in addition the antrum, floor of the orbit and the nasal bones. The Le Fort III includes the structures affected by the Le Fort II and also the zygomas and anterior cranial fossa. It is emphasised that all Le Fort III fractures are head injuries and should be monitored as such. Further, as the anterior cranial fossa communicates with the nose through the fractured cribriform plate there is a grave danger of an ascending infection. The patient must be protected from a meningeal infection by the prescription of appropriate antibiotics. A cerebrospinal fluid (CSF) leak may require an intracranial dural repair by neurosurgeons, which may be effected at the same time as fracture fixation. Thus the management of such injuries calls for a team approach.

Displacement

In maxillary fractures the displacement is caused by the force of the blow and not by muscle pull as none of the muscles attached to the maxilla are strong enough to move the fragments. The most usual displacement is backwards and downwards, causing a typical concavity of the face (dish face) with anterior open bite due to gagging on the posterior teeth. This open bite is particularly marked in the Guérin's type fracture.

Diagnosis

The oral surgeon should proceed to make a diagnosis in the usual way unless some urgent condition identified in the primary survey requires immediate attention.

History

In the unconscious patient the history may have to be taken from those who witnessed or attended the initial scene of trauma. The time of the accident is important in assessing the urgency of treatment, and the degree of infection in compound fractures. Soft tissue lacerations should be closed as soon as possible and certainly within 24 hours. The difficulty of reducing misplaced fractures increases as healing progresses. A history of any previous facial injury is important as old injuries can cause confusion in the diagnosis. The patient's general condition and any tenderness or bruising of the head, chest or abdomen is noted. Shock is unusual in facial injuries and, unless the blood loss has been excessive, the cause should be sought elsewhere.

The patient should be asked if there was any loss of consciousness. In unconscious or confused patients, causes other than concussion, such as alcohol, recreational drugs, insulin or diabetic coma, or a cardiovascular catastrophe, should be considered. Any drug administered previously, especially sedatives, analgesics or antibacterials, should be recorded.

Examination

The surgeon must consider all the possible tissues that might be involved in the trauma – skin, connective tissue, blood vessels, nerves (both sensory and motor), muscles, underlying bones – together with special structures such as the eyes and salivary glands. The following signs of a fracture must be looked for. Swelling and bruising are usual at the point where the patient was struck, but may not coincide with the site of an indirect fracture. Deformity of the bone contour can be masked by swelling, but examination may reveal a break in the continuity of the bone or displacement. Intraorally, derangement of the occlusion may localise the fracture. Abnormal movement in the bone is diagnostic and when it occurs may be accompanied by pain and crepitus or grating as the rough bone ends rub against each other. Loss of function in the jaws is common as a result of trismus or pain.

The facial bones can be conveniently examined in the dental chair, but should the patient be too ill to get out of bed the headboard may be removed to allow the patient to be examined from above and behind.

Extraoral

The patient is first looked at full face for obvious signs of injury. Lacerations should not be probed or touched but are immediately covered with a dressing. Clots present in the nose and ears should not be disturbed but a discharge of CSF from these orifices is an important finding, indicating a fracture of the cranial base. To distinguish it from nasal secretion it should be tested for glucose, a constituent of CSF. CSF in contradistinction to blood does not clot and this can usefully differentiate them.

Facial skeleton

The surgeon should then move behind the patient and, looking down from above, use the tips of their fingers to palpate and compare the right and left sides, and to determine points of tenderness or breaks in the continuity of the facial bones. This starts with the superior, lateral and inferior margins of the orbit and then proceeds to the bridge of the nose, where any deviation from the midline or depression is noted. The malar prominences are compared to detect loss of contour. Where there is marked oedema if may be very difficult to do this with certainty, but firm steady pressure on the swelling for a few moments will push it away and allow the bone to be felt.

The fingers then move over the zygomatic arch, to the temporomandibular joints. The patient is asked to open and close the mouth and perform lateral movements. The range of opening and of lateral movement is assessed. Fractures of the zygomatic arch may prevent opening as the coronoid process may jam against the displaced zygomatic process. In fractures of the condyle or ascending ramus there is little movement of the condyle head on the affected side or the mandible towards the opposite side. When the joint is difficult to palpate the little finger may be put into the external auditory meatus and the condyle felt through the anterior wall. Palpation is then continued to compare the ascending ramus, the angles and the lower border of the body of the mandible.

Eye

The surgeon then moves to face the patient and examines the eyes for damage, particularly depression, proptosis or a difference in level. The intercanthal distance should be measured from the midline. Any difference in the values on either side or a marked increase from the normal range suggests a traumatic detachment of the medial canthal ligaments. Subconjunctival haemorrhage without posterior limit in the upper half of the eye suggests bleeding from a fracture of the roof of the orbit, and in the lower part of the conjunctiva a fracture of the orbital floor, but in severe injuries the whole of the conjunctiva may be involved. Each eye is checked individually for vision and then both together for movement vertically and horizontally and for double vision (diplopia) in all fields. This can be done by moving a finger up, down and across where it can be clearly seen by both eyes at once. Abnormalities of movement and diplopia may be due to paralysis of the extrinsic muscles of the eye as a result of cranial injury. Diplopia alone may be caused by detachment of the suspensory ligament in malar or maxillary fractures, herniation of orbital fat through defects in the orbital floor, or by oedema, all of which may alter the position of the globe. Oedema can also mask diplopia by compensating for a fall in level that may only become apparent when the swelling recedes. Visual acuity should also be tested in the conscious patient.

An ophthalmic opinion should be sought in cases where visual acuity or diplopia is encountered. Assessment of these injuries preoperatively is vital to ensure correct treatment planning.

Sensory and motor acuity

The examination concludes with tests for loss of sensation in the branches of the trigeminal nerve, particularly the infraorbital, which is affected in malar and maxillary fractures, and the mental nerve involved in mandibular injuries. Function of the facial nerve is checked by asking the patient to move their forehead, eyelids and lips. This nerve is most frequently involved in lacerations of the face.

Intraoral

The lips are gently parted and the mucosa, floor of the mouth and tongue examined for lacerations or haematoma. A haematoma of the floor of the mouth is a sign of a fracture of the mandible. The teeth are charted and those that are lost, grossly carious or fractured are noted, together with any disturbance of the occlusion. The patient's opinion is valuable as to whether this is normal or not. Where teeth (or denture fragments) are missing and cannot be accounted for, particularly if the patient has lost consciousness, the chest should be radiographed. Percussion of the teeth may give a 'cracked teacup' note suggestive of a broken tooth or a fractured jaw, particularly in the maxilla. The upper buccal sulcus is palpated for any sharp edges of bone or bruising diagnostic of a fracture through the malar buttress.

Fractures of the maxillary alveolus or a midline split of the palate are detected by grasping the alveolar segments and trying gently at first to move them by grasping the alveolus and the teeth in one hand and trying to elicit movement, while the other hand palpates extraorally to determine the level at which the fracture has occurred. The fingers are placed in turn over the root of the nose, at the infraorbital margins and in the canine fossa.

Similarly the mandible is grasped in both hands, with the fingers over the occlusal surface of the teeth and the thumbs under the lower border, and tested in segments for mobility. The clinical findings should be written down and a provisional diagnosis made before radiographs are ordered.

A summary of the diagnostic features of various fractures is shown in Table 14.2.

Radiographs

Radiographs (Table 14.3) are taken to establish the presence of fractures, the direction in which they run and the amount by which they are displaced,

Table 14.2 Diagnostic features of fractures. All these signs and symptoms are not found in every case. Radiographs will show a lack of continuity in the bone at the site of the fracture

Site	Signs and symptoms
Unilateral condyle	Affected side: Pain in joint, worse on moving
	Tenderness and swelling
	Absence (or abnormality) of movements of condyle head
	Deviation of mandible towards this side
	Gagging on molar teeth
	Opposite side: Open bite
	Limitation of lateral excursion to that side
Bilateral condyle	Pain, tenderness and swelling over both joints
	Gagging on the posterior teeth and an anterior open bite
	Restricted lateral movements
	Absence of movement of condyle heads
Body of the mandible	Pain on moving jaw
	Trismus
	Movement and crepitus at site of fracture
	Step deformity of lower border of mandible
	Derangement of the occlusion
	Mental anaesthesia
	Haematoma in the floor of mouth and buccal mucosa
Malar	Depression of the prominence of the cheek
	Step deformity in the infraorbital ridge
	Subconjunctival haemorrhage and diplopia
	Infraorbital nerve anaesthesia
	Haematoma intraorally over the malar buttress
	Blood in the antrum
	Trismus due to the coronoid process impacting against the displaced malar or zygomatic arch
	Circumorbital ecchymosis
Guérin's (Le Fort I)	Floating palate
	Blood in the antrum
	Bilateral haematoma in buccal sulcus
	Deranged occlusion with anterior open bite

Table 14.2 (Continued)

Site	Signs and symptoms
Low pyramidal (Le Fort II)	Gross swelling and, after oedema subsides, dish-faced deformity
	Subconjunctival haemorrhage and diplopia
	Bilateral infraorbital nerve anaesthesia
	Bilateral haematoma intraorally over malar buttresses
	Retroposed upper dental arch with anterior open bite
High transverse (Le Fort III)	Gross swelling and, after oedema subsides, dish-faced deformity
	Subconjunctival haemorrhage and sometimes diplopia
	Retroposed upper dental arch with anterior open bite
	Cerebrospinal fluid leak from nose
	Signs of head injury

Table 14.3 Facial radiographs in maxillofacial trauma

Site of injury	Radiographic views	Area visualised
Mandible	DPT, OPT	All areas except lower anterior
	Lateral oblique	Good for angle, body, and condyle
	PA mandible	Shows horizontal displacement at angle and condyles
	Lower occlusal	Anterior region
Zygoma	Occipitomental (OM) 10°–30°	Orbital margins, malar buttress, antrum
	Submentovertex	Zygomatic arch, supraorbital margin
	Computerised tomography (CT)	Orbital blowouts
Maxilla	As for zygoma	As above
	Lateral face	Shows backward displacement, pterygoid plates anterior open bite
	Computerised tomography (CT)	Orbital contour, optic nerve, naso-ethmoidal complex
Naso-ethmoidal complex	Computerised tomography (CT)	Good detail, can get reconstructions from CT

and to identify radiopaque foreign bodies such as glass in the soft tissues. Medicolegally they are considered a diagnostic measure of the first importance. They also provide a visual record of the patient's progress.

Radiographs of all fractures must be taken in two planes. The following views usually give a satisfactory survey of the facial bones and wherever there is doubt about the extent of the injuries all should be taken. They are a dental panoramic tomograph (DPT or OPT), or if the patient is non-ambulatory lateral oblique views of the mandible can be used instead, a postero-anterior view of the mandible, occipitomental views of the sinuses (10, 15 or 20 degrees), a submentovertex and a true lateral of the facial bones. Note that the midline of the mandible is difficult to see except on an occlusal film. Fractures involving the nasoethmoidal complex should always be visualised using computerised axial tomography (CT). It is common practice now for all mid-third fractures involving the orbital floor to have CT.

Examination of the radiographs is first made to identify all the normal structures and the bony margins of the facial bones. Both sides of the jaws are compared for differences in outline. It is important to recognise shadows thrown by such normal structures as the oropharyngeal airway, hyoid bone or intervertebral spaces, which may simulate fractures in certain projections.

The dental panoramic tomograph (DPT)

This tomographic radiograph of the jaws has largely replaced the lateral oblique views. However, it is unsuitable for any patient who is unable to stand or sit while the radiograph is being taken and in this case lateral oblique views should be considered. The mandible from condyle to condyle is seen, but due to superimposition of the cervical spine the canine and incisor regions may not be well visualised. As the rotation of the X-ray tube changes direction in the premolar region, caution is needed in interpretation in this area. The principal indication for this view is in the diagnosis of fractured mandibles, but some information about the lower part of the middle third can also be gleaned (Figure 14.5).

The postero-anterior view of the mandible

The whole of the mandible from the condyle neck to the midline on both sides is shown. As the rays pass through the angle of the mandible from the lower border to the occlusal surface they give a vertical view of this area and allow vertically favourable and unfavourable fractures to be assessed (Figure 14.6). The midface is also visualised but there is a great deal of superimposition.

The occipitomental view

This is examined in a series of transverse sweeps following the bony contours at the levels of the supraorbital ridges, the infraorbital margins and the zygomatic arch, of the antral wall, nasal wall and vomer, and finally the level of the mandibular/maxillary occlusion and the lower border of the mandible. It demonstrates fractures of the maxillary complex and radiopacity of the maxillary sinus, which may be the result of bleeding into the antrum from a fracture of one of its walls (Figure 14.7). Fifteen- or thirty-degree occipitomental and stereoscopic occipitomental views are both of assistance in detecting displacement not shown on the standard views.

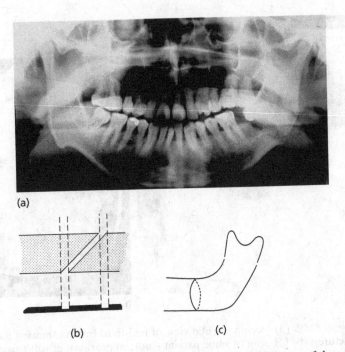

(a)

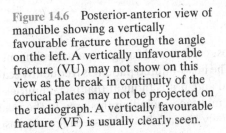

(b)   (c)

Figure 14.5   (a) An orthopantomogram showing a displaced fracture of the mandible. Drawing (b) shows how one oblique fracture passing through inner and outer cortical plates may give a false appearance of a double fracture on radiograph. (c) In such a case the fracture lines are always seen to meet at the upper and lower border of the bone.

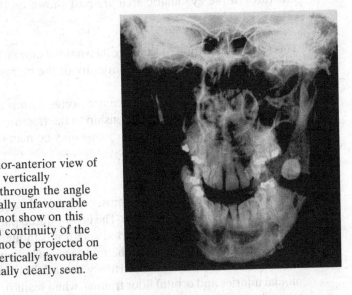

Figure 14.6   Posterior-anterior view of mandible showing a vertically favourable fracture through the angle on the left. A vertically unfavourable fracture (VU) may not show on this view as the break in continuity of the cortical plates may not be projected on the radiograph. A vertically favourable fracture (VF) is usually clearly seen.

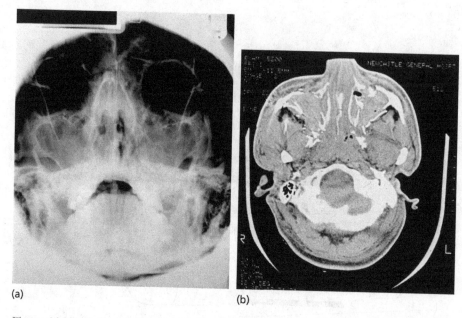

(a)   (b)

Figure 14.7   (a) Occipitomental view of mid-third trauma showing pan-facial fractures; (b) CT scan of same patient – note appearance of soft tissue. This patient is seen in Figure 14.13.

Submentovertex view

Fractures of the zygomatic arch are best shown on this film.

True lateral of facial bones

This shows separation of the maxilla from the cranial base, or of the palate from the maxilla, as well as any discontinuity of the pterygoid plates.

Other radiographs of importance are occlusal films and intraoral apical views of the teeth showing their relationship to the fracture line of their roots. Special views of the temporomandibular joints may be necessary to show the condyles and the condyle neck.

Computerised axial tomography (CT)

This is now readily available in most centres and can give valuable information when plain films cannot be taken. The head-injured patient is frequently scanned during the initial assessment period and, if it is thought that facial injuries have been sustained, particularly in the mid-face, including this area in the scan can save time in diagnosis. CT is virtually essential in the assessment of nasoethmoidal injuries and orbital floor trauma, when scans in all planes (coronal, sagittal and transverse) give a comprehensive picture of the injury. Computed reconstructions of these areas can be particularly useful to give a virtual 3-D image.

Study models

Frequently the patient is unable to bring their teeth into occlusion or the fractures are badly comminuted so that the normal relationship of the teeth can only be seen on study models. These are also useful for the construction of custom arch bars where these are indicated.

Treatment planning

The aims of treatment are to restore function and to achieve a good aesthetic result, but treatment must be modified according to the patient's general condition. The only immediate local measures required are attention to the airway, arrest of haemorrhage and control of infection. Where multiple injuries are present the surgeon is responsible for explaining the degree of urgency for treatment of the jaws to achieve a satisfactory result. Thereafter, planning is done jointly with the other specialists involved. It is generally agreed that bony injuries heal better the earlier they are treated, but in the presence of gross oedema or large haematomas they may be left a few days for these to settle.

Natural repair of bone

The healing of fractures takes place entirely by the natural process of bone repair. Treatment is directed to providing ideal conditions for this to take place.

Between the fractured ends of the bone a blood clot forms. Within 4 days capillaries, fibroblasts and inflammatory cells invade this and begin replacing it with granulation tissue. Along the bony margins of the fracture osteoclasts appear which resorb the bone; this is seen on radiographs as a widening of the fracture line. Osteoblasts from the periosteum and cancellous bone invade the granulations and lay down a collagenous matrix called osteoid. The acidity of the tissues caused by the initial inflammatory reaction subsides after 10 days and this allows calcification to proceed. Bony union takes place in 4–6 weeks.

The pattern of the new bone or callus is at first irregular but later, over a period of about 6 months in the mandible, reorganisation to normal bone structure takes place. In long bones an excess of callus is formed round the bone ends, and its presence on radiographs is accepted as a sign that satisfactory union is proceeding. This does not happen in the mandible, where formation of callus is usually limited to the space between the bone ends and therefore shows little on radiographs. Maxillary fractures may heal by fibrous union only.

Principles of treatment

Control of infection

Repair, particularly new bone formation, cannot take place in the presence of infection. To prevent this occurring all foreign bodies, dead bone and tissue are removed from the wound, which is then closed to cover the exposed bone. Any movement of bone fractures may predispose to infection and fracture treatment should aim to eliminate this. Antibacterial drugs are administered prophylactically until the inflammatory reaction has resolved and the soft tissue wounds have healed satisfactorily. Drainage is provided if suppuration occurs and causes of infection should be sought and treated as appropriate.

Tooth in the line of fracture

In the jaws, the fracture line often passes through a tooth socket, leaving one side of the root exposed in the wound. The fracture is then compound into the mouth as tearing of the gingival attachment provides a portal of entry for oral micro-organisms. Exposed cementum on the surface of the root rapidly dies and repair may not take place between this inert cementum and new bone, so that healing is delayed. As a result of the accident the pulp may become non-vital and a focus of infection. It is wise, therefore, to extract teeth in the line of fracture where there is gross displacement, unless they are to be retained temporarily to establish the occlusion. Where there is little displacement of the fracture the teeth may be kept unless they delay union. The vitality must be checked and non-vital teeth treated as appropriate. In the maxilla, vital teeth may be kept, as experience has shown that teeth in the fracture line seldom affect union in the upper jaw.

Reduction of fractures

In reducing fractures the object is to reappose the bone ends as accurately as possible. Although the surgeon should attempt to get perfect reduction, the aim is to treat not a radiograph, but a patient, and where displacement is acceptable and function is not impaired the patient should not be subjected to unnecessary surgery.

Perfect reduction may be impossible where there has been gross comminution or tissue loss, and healing will not take place between the fractured ends if the gap is too wide (more than 6 mm). In comminuted fractures all fragments attached to periosteum must be kept.

The best guide to accurate reduction is the occlusion of the teeth, because of the precise way in which the teeth interdigitate. Further, if the occlusion is restored, masticatory function should be satisfactory. In edentulous patients the dentures are the only sound guide. Where they are lost, the site of the accident should be searched or a spare set may be available. The fractured jaw is reduced to the sound jaw, but where many teeth are missing or both jaws badly comminuted, the problem is more difficult. The surgeon must then rely more on anatomical reduction of the bony margins, appearance of the patient and the results shown on postoperative radiographs.

Reduction should be done as soon as possible, but where delay is unavoidable it should be remembered that greater difficulty will be experienced in reducing maxillary fractures after 10 days and mandibular fractures after 3 weeks.

Immobilisation of the fragments

Any movement in the fracture line after reduction may disturb or tear the granulations or osteoid tissue. It may also cause the bone to heal with a deformity. Immobilisation should therefore be complete, and continued until union has taken place, which in the mandible is about 4–6 weeks, and in the maxilla, fibrous union is accepted as 3–4 weeks.

Open reduction and rigid internal fixation (ORIF)

This technique relies on open reduction and rigid fixation of the bone with plates and screws to eliminate movement of the fragments and thus can make further immobilisation unnecessary. It allows uneventful bone healing to occur even under function.

Anaesthesia

Fractures with appreciable displacement are usually reduced under a general anaesthetic. In mandibular fractures a cuffed intranasal endotracheal tube can be passed quite easily despite some preoperative trismus, but in maxillary fractures involving the cranial base there is often some degree of difficulty and danger in passing a tube through the nose as it may pass into the anterior cranial fossa with disastrous consequences. In this situation an oral tube may suffice if it does not interfere with the occlusion. In the fully dentate patient a submental approach allows an oral tube to be passed through a small submental incision into the floor of the mouth and thus into the larynx. If it is anticipated that more than one surgical intervention is likely, then the need for a tracheostomy to provide a safe and efficient anaesthetic must be considered. This may be chosen in the polytraumatised patient in order to maintain respiratory function in those slow to regain consciousness.

Where the jaws are to be fixed together under an anaesthetic, a tongue suture may be employed. This is placed well back to enable the tongue to be drawn forwards out of the pharynx during the recovery period and can be removed once the patient has full control of their airway. The throat pack must be removed prior to the jaws being fixed together. This may best be achieved with elastics, which are easily cut with scissors in an emergency, but if wires are to be used then the ends should be left long to enable them to be easily identified.

Definitive treatment

Soft tissue repair

All wounds are first carefully explored and foreign bodies and dirt removed. Glass is not easy to find and road or coal dust is difficult to get out, but if left gives rise to a tattooed scar. To clear wounds or skin abrasions they are scrubbed with water, soap and a soft brush, and thoroughly irrigated.

All tissues about the face are precious and, fortunately, because of their rich blood supply are very viable. Excision is not practised except on tags of loose, dead skin or mucous membrane, or around the edges of wounds that are several days old and may have started to epithelialise. Lacerations are then closed in layers by primary suture, with drains inserted where necessary.

Where there has been loss of skin, the edges must not be drawn together under tension as this leads to deformity and scar formation. Full thickness loss in cheek or lips may be temporarily repaired by sewing skin to mucous membrane. This prevents scarring, protects the deeper tissues and provides a satisfactory base for reconstruction.

Tears in the mucosa must be closed to cover exposed bone. Mucous membrane is easier to manipulate than skin so that by undermining edges and rotating flaps, deficiencies can usually be made up.

Where bone and soft tissue surgery are being done at the same operation, soft tissue repair is completed after the fractures have been reduced and fixed.

Management of fractures

Open reduction and rigid internal fixation (ORIF)

This concept has been accepted as the standard treatment for the vast majority of facial fractures. The technique relies on exposing the fractures through intra- or extraoral incisions and accurate reduction of the bony fractures, which are then held rigidly in place by the application of malleable metal plates. This method was originally developed for use in the mandible but is now routinely used to treat all facial fractures. The application of rigid fixation enables bone healing to take place without immobilisation of the bone. Long periods of intermaxillary fixation (IMF) are thus not necessary and return to function is much more rapid. A well-designed plating toolkit integrated with a selection of plate sizes graded by screw diameter (from 2mm down to 1mm) provides a flexible system of fixation for all the facial bones (Figure 14.8).

Intermaxillary fixation (IMF)

The mandible is immobilised by fixing it to the maxilla. This establishes the occlusion and is an accepted part of the treatment of maxillary fractures. It may be employed in mandibular fractures, particularly when one or both condyles are involved. IMF may be achieved in a number of ways.

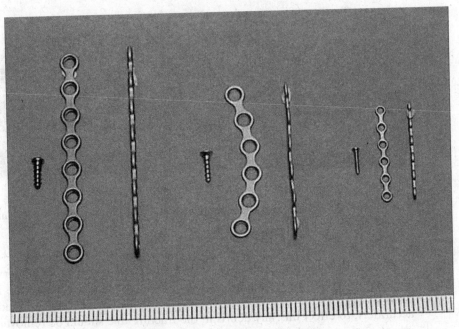

Figure 14.8 Titanium plates for facial fractures from left: 2 mm used in mandibular fractures, 1.7 mm (low profile) and 1 mm used in mid-third fractures.

IMF (bone) screws (temporary)

Monocortical bone screws placed between the roots of the canines and pre-molars in each quadrant can allow IMF to be established during the operative procedure but will not withstand long periods of immobilisation.

Arch bars

Close fitting cast arch bars may be constructed from study models if time allows, but preformed bars are also available for immediate use (Figure 14.9). These are bent to fix closely to the teeth in the upper and lower arches while the fractures are held in their reduced position. Wires are passed around the teeth to hold the bar in place. Once the arch bar has been tied across the fracture line further adjustment to the reduction is difficult.

Mandibular fractures

ORIF of mandibular fractures

Plating of the mandible has the advantage that postoperative intermaxillary fixation is not essential but may be applied while the plate is being placed.

Monocortical miniplates

Titanium miniplates are inserted across the fracture line via an intraoral approach. The incision is made through the mucoperiosteum below the attached

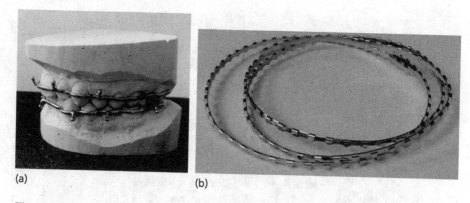

(a)   (b)

Figure 14.9   Arch bars. (a) Custom-made arch bars; (b) preformed arch bars can be cut to length from a roll.

gingivae with due consideration of vital structures such as the mental nerve. To expose the symphysis region the incision should be flared out into the lip to reduce the chance of wound breakdown. The fracture is identified and reduced accurately; to effect this, any debris in the fracture line should be removed and irrigation performed to allow good visualisation. The occlusion is established and may be maintained by an assistant or by the application of temporary IMF.

Titanium miniplates of 2 mm are used as standard in the fixation of mandibular fractures. It is crucial that the plate is accurately adapted to the contour of the bone and the operator should strive to achieve this. Holes are then drilled through the outer cortical bone to enable monocortical self-tapping titanium screws to be placed. The holes are drilled with burs slightly smaller than the screw diameter to ensure firm screw fixation. The screw should be inserted at the same angle as the drill and advanced slowly through the bone. After each forward turn a reverse half-turn should be made until the self-tapped hole is established. The screw is then tightened, but care should be taken not to strip the threads in the bone. Emergency screws of a greater diameter are available should this arise. Care should be taken to avoid damaging the teeth and suitable screw lengths should be chosen; screws of between 6 and 8 mm length are used as standard in the mandible. The plate should be selected to allow at least two screws to be placed either side of the fracture. In comminuted fractures longer plates may have to be used to achieve this, but four or five hole plates suffice in most situations. In the anterior region of the mandible two plates are placed across the fracture to counteract increased torsional forces, while in the body and angle one plate only may be needed (Figure 14.10). The plates counteract lines of tension at the upper border of the mandible. Titanium is a bio-inert material and thus plates do not have to be removed unless they become exposed or the patient becomes aware of them. If rigid fixation is achieved bone healing will take place even in the presence of infection.

Bioresorbable plates

Research and development into resorbable plates continues in order to eliminate the long-term sequelae of plate retention, such as infection.

Bicortical plates

More rigid plates in conjunction with screws that engage both cortices of the bone are available; these must be placed at the lower border of the mandible to avoid traumatising the teeth. As this often requires an extraoral approach these plates are most frequently used when loss of bone from the fracture site has occurred.

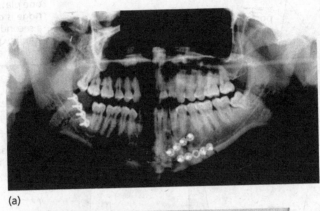

(a)

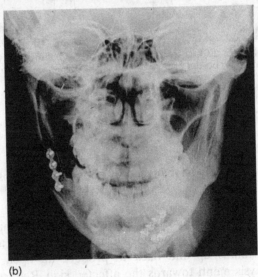

(b)

Figure 14.10 Plating of mandibular fractures – note two plates at parasymphysis and one at angle: (a) orthopantomogram; (b) posterior-anterior view of same patient; (c) diagrams to show tension and compression and placement of plates.

Tension and compression in mandibular body fractures

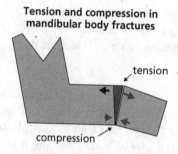

tension

compression

Mandibular body fractures

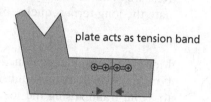

plate acts as tension band

Mandibular angle fractures

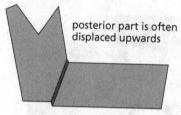

posterior part is often displaced upwards

Mandibular angle fractures

one plate at external oblique ridge is often sufficient but a second plate may be used if stability problems are encountered

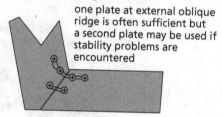

Parasymphyseal fractures

Tension at upper border remains

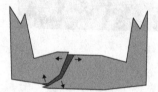

Rotational forces distract fracture at lower border

Parasymphyseal fractures

Two plates are necessary to stabilize the rotational forces

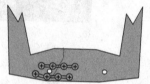

Care must be taken to safeguard the mental nerve

Figure 14.10   (Continued).

Condylar fractures

These fractures may be managed by either open or closed methods.

Closed method (IMF)

The fractured condyle head is usually displaced forward and medially by the lateral pterygoid muscle, while the muscles of mastication tend to draw the ascending ramus up and back to produce an open bite, with rotation of the symphysis menti towards the affected side. Reduction is directed to correcting the displacement of the mandible only. Many patients can be taught to do this, using their hands at first to assist in re-educating the muscles of mastication. The patient should be told to stay on a soft diet and analgesics should be prescribed. Where swelling and pain make this difficult, IMF may be applied for 1–2 weeks using arch bars and elastics to encourage the re-establishment of the occlusion. In fracture dislocations the same treatment is adequate, as it has been shown that, though union occurs in an abnormal position, the head of the condyle remodels to make a functional joint. Where other mandibular fractures are present these should be treated as indicated and the need for IMF assessed following this.

Open method (ORIF)

The close proximity of the facial nerve makes the surgical approach to the condylar neck more exacting. A retromandibular approach is most often used, although intraoral approaches have been described. Once exposed, fixation of the fracture with monocortical plates is completed using principles as outlined above. The application of IMF may still be needed.

Bilateral condylar fractures

The management of bilateral condylar fractures is complicated due to an increased incidence of anterior open bite and this does not always respond to a period of IMF. Open reduction and internal fixation of at least one of the fractured condyles may be indicated if these fractures lie outside the joint capsule. This particularly applies in panfacial fractures where the spacial geometry of the face may be difficult to reconstruct without this important dimension.

Mid-third fractures

The advent of miniaturised plating systems has allowed the technique of open reduction and internal fixation to be applied to these areas. The same general rules of ORIF apply, but as fewer displacing forces are applied to the mid-face, smaller plate sizes (1.7–1 mm) can be used to allow reconstruction of delicate areas such as the infraorbital margins (Figure 14.11). The concept of reconstruction of the main buttresses of the face is crucial to re-establish the facial geometry. Study models and custom arch bars can be of great value to establish the occlusion pre- and peroperatively and the use of intraoperative IMF is advocated.

Reduction of malar bones and zygomatic arch

This may be achieved either extraorally or via an intraoral approach. ORIF of the zygoma is complicated as approaches to the zygomaticofrontal suture and the infraorbital margin require a skin incision with consequent scarring. An intraoral approach avoids this and gives access to the malar buttress for ORIF to fix an unstable fracture.

Gillies approach

The external approach devised by Gillies is made through an incision in the skin above the hairline and over the temporal fossa. It is made at an angle to

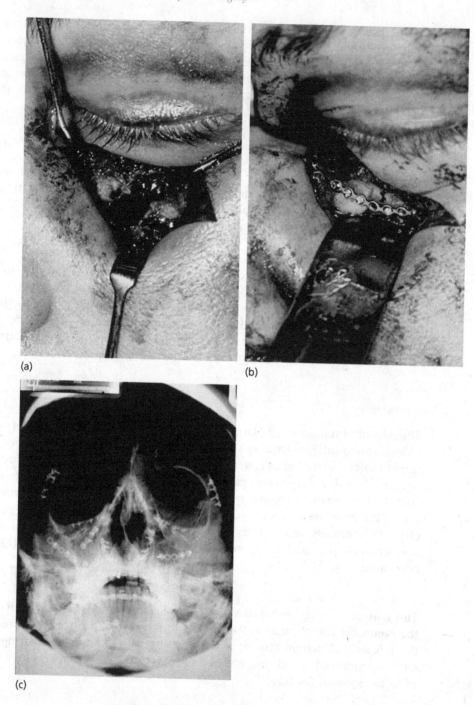

Figure 14.11   Plating of infraorbital margin fracture. (a) Fracture exposed showing displacement; (b) 1 mm plate across reduced fracture; (c) postoperative radiograph of same patient showing plated panfacial fractures. Note the reconstruction of the vertical and horizontal buttresses as seen in Figure 14.3.

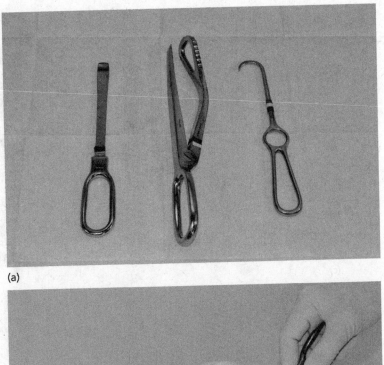

(a)

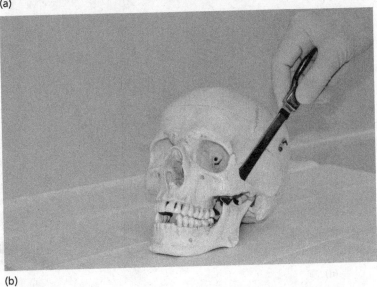

(b)

Figure 14.12 Elevation of left malar. (a) Elevators: l–r Bristow, Rowe, malar hook. Position of elevators deep to the malar and zygomatic arch; (b) Bristow, note the index finger used to protect the temporal bone; (c) Rowe; (d) malar hook.

avoid the terminal branches of the superficial temporal artery. The temporal fascia is exposed and divided to give access to an elevator (Figure 14.12). This is passed deep to the fascia and to the zygomatic arch. It is used to lift the depressed malar forwards, upwards and outwards. Considerable force is often necessary and the fulcrum must never be the temporal bone, lest the thin lateral wall of the skull be fractured. The assistant keeps the head stabilised while the

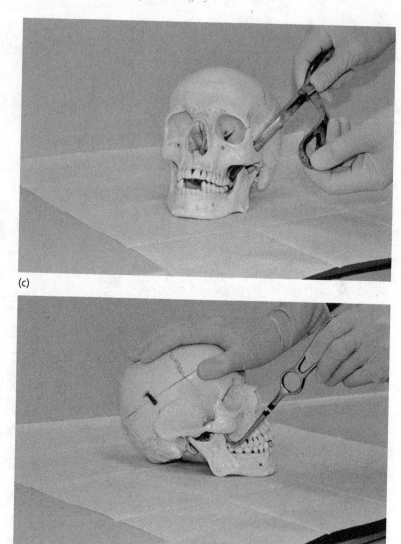

(c)

(d)

Figure 14.12   (Continued).

operator applies the force and checks to ensure that reduction is satisfactory. The malar often clicks into place and is stable without fixation, but if not it may be held by a bone plate at the zygomaticofrontal suture, the infraorbital margin or intraorally at the malar buttress.

Malar hook

The zygoma may also be reduced using a malar hook inserted through a stab incision in line with the lateral canthus at the level of the alar of the nose, although this is not suitable if the zygomatic arch is also depressed (Figure 14.12). Alternatively an elevator may be passed under the zygoma through a buccal sulcus incision, which may be combined with an intraoral approach to bone plate fixation at the malar buttress.

External fixation

An intraosseous pin in the body of the malar may be employed, attached by a vertical bar to a pin placed in the supraorbital rim.

Orbital exploration

The orbital floor may require exploration if there is clinical or radiographic evidence of a defect with loss of orbital contents into the maxillary sinus (orbital blowout). Enophthalmos may be masked initially by swelling. Exploration may be combined with reconstruction of the infraorbital margin. Exposure is achieved via infraorbital, blepharoplasty or transconjunctival incisions. Defects may be repaired with bone graft, silastic sheets or titanium mesh (Figure 14.13). The orbital roof and both walls may also require exploration. CT scans in three planes can give very exact information as to the extent and site of injury.

Retrobulbar haemorrhage

This is a severe though rare hazard following orbital trauma, reduction of zygomatic fractures or any intervention involving the orbit. Bleeding behind the globe during or after the operation can cause proptosis, pain and decreasing visual

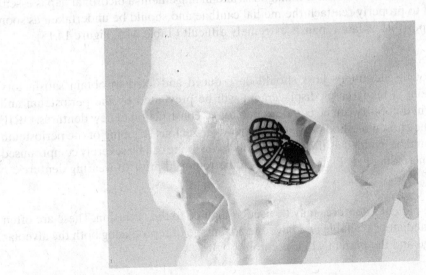

Figure 14.13 Preformed titanium orbital floor reconstruction plate. The plate can be trimmed to fit the size of the defect. Note that the medial wall and floor can be reconstructed as required. Image by permission from Synthes (Ltd).

acuity, which, if the pressure is not relieved, may result in blindness. The blood may be drained via an infraorbital or lateral canthal incision; however, medical management, in the form of steroids, acetazolamide and mannitol, can also be successful in reducing the pressure on the optic nerve (Table 14.4). Postoperative eye observations every 15 minutes for 2 hours, then every 30 minutes for 2 hours will aid in the early diagnosis and treatment of this condition.

Le Fort I and II fractures

These can usually be exposed from an intraoral 'horseshoe' incision and the vertical buttress system accurately reduced and fixed at the malar buttress and canine fossa regions. The infraorbital margins may need to be exposed from an extraoral approach and this can allow exploration of the orbital floor if this is involved in the trauma.

Le Fort III fractures

These may require fixation in the same areas, depending on the degree of comminution, and will require further exposure to allow their fixation to solid bone at the zygomaticofrontal suture and at the nasal bridge. The use of a bicoronal scalp flap gives excellent exposure for the reduction of the fractures in this area. The objective is to rebuild the vertical and horizontal buttress system to re-establish the facial geometry as accurately as possible (Figure 14.14).

Nasoethmoidal complex fractures

These fractures, in which the intercanthal distance has been traumatically increased, demand careful diagnosis and management; a bicoronal flap is essential to properly reattach the medial canthae and should be undertaken as soon as possible as late repair is extremely difficult (Table 14.5, Figure 14.15).

Edentulous jaws

Though edentulous jaws should be reduced and fixed to obtain satisfactory union, in many cases displacement will be prevented by the periosteum and slight deformity can be compensated for by construction of new dentures. ORIF is the chosen method of treatment but over-zealous stripping of the periosteum should be avoided as the blood supply to the bone can be severely compromised in increasing age. Plates may have to be removed prior to wearing dentures.

Dentures

The patient's dentures may be used as a guide to the occlusion. These are often immediately available and have the advantage of reproducing both the alveolar ridge and the patient's bite accurately.

Other techniques

The following techniques have been used historically but are now used infrequently and not described in detail. They may be useful in certain circumstances.

Table 14.4 Retrobulbar haemorrhage

Signs and symptoms	Time of onset	Treatment	
		Surgical	Medical
Decreasing visual acuity Tunnel vision Eye pain Proptosis	After mid-third trauma, during treatment of zygomatic or Le Fort II/III fractures, after treatment (up to 4 hours)	Drainage of blood from behind eye via infraorbital or lateral canthal incisions	Dexamethasone 20mg, acetazolamide 1g, mannitol 10%, all given IV at onset of symptoms can be repeated
Eye observations Quarter-hourly for 2 hours Half-hourly for 2 hours Hourly for 2 hours		Observe for: visual acuity, reaction to light, pain	

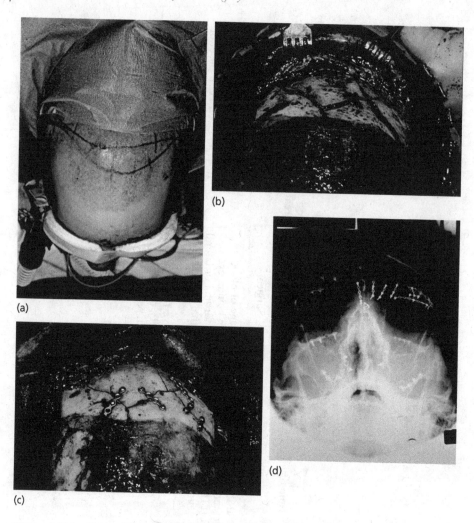

Figure 14.14   Craniofacial fractures. (a) Bicoronal flap approach; (b) fractures of frontal bone exposed; (c) reconstruction of frontal bone and supraorbital margin; (d) postoperative occipitomental radiograph showing reconstruction of whole of facial skeleton.

Eyelet wiring

Eyelet wiring is a simple method of IMF using wires passed around the teeth. Loops in the wire allow the upper and lower jaws to be wired together.

Gunning splints

These are the standard splint for immobilising edentulous jaws. They are an upper and lower bite block made in acrylic. They have a shallow periphery, a hole anteriorly for feeding and cleats for intermaxillary fixation. They are

Table 14.5 Surgical approaches to the facial bones (see accompanying Figure 14.15)

	Intraoral		Extraoral	
	Area	Approach	Area	Approach
Mandible	Angle Body Parasymphysis Symphysis Condyle	Ramus	Condyle Lower border	Retro- mandibular Preauricular Submandibular
Zygoma	Malar buttress	Incision below attached gingivae	Zygomatico-frontal suture Infraorbital margin Zygomatic arch	Brow, upper blepharoplasty Blepharoplasty Infraorbital Transconjunctival Preauricular Bicoronal
Maxilla	Malar buttress Canine fossa	Incision below attached gingivae – extending to 'horseshoe'	As for zygoma + supraorbital	As above Bicoronal
Naso-ethmoidal			Nasal bridge Medial canthae	Bicoronal

constructed from casts of the patient's dentures, which are also used to register the bite, or by direct impressions of the patient's jaws.

Gunning splints or dentures may be wired to the jaws (see below) to reduce the bone fragments, following which IMF may be applied.

Circumferential and transalveolar wiring

These may be used to secure splints to the jaws. In the lower jaw three wires are passed around the mandible to emerge intraorally, one on each side in the first molar region and one anteriorly. The upper splint may be attached to underlying bone with titanium mini-plate screws or held in position by transalveolar wires, one on each side in the molar region and one anteriorly.

External fixation

Craniomaxillary fixation

The maxilla may be fixed to the skull to hold it firmly in place. This is done by attaching metal rods to locking plates on arch bars or Gunning splints. These rods come out of the mouth and are connected by means of universal joints (Clouston-Walker joints) and rods to a metal halo frame or supraorbital intraosseous pins joined by a connecting bar (Levant frame) (Figure 14.16).

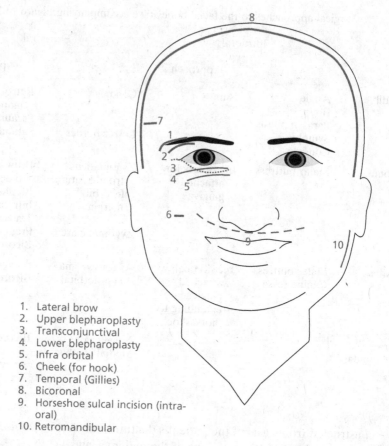

1. Lateral brow
2. Upper blepharoplasty
3. Transconjunctival
4. Lower blepharoplasty
5. Infra orbital
6. Cheek (for hook)
7. Temporal (Gillies)
8. Bicoronal
9. Horseshoe sulcal incision (intra-oral)
10. Retromandibular

Figure 14.15 Surgical approaches to facial bones. The diagram shows the common approaches. There are more choices around the infraorbital margins where scarring is a greater aesthetic issue.

Halo head frame

This is screwed to the head by means of pins that penetrate the skin and engage the outer bony cortical plate of the skull. Two pairs of opposing pins in the occipital and frontal regions are placed above the hairline to avoid unsightly scars. The temporal vessels should be identified to avoid damage to these when placing the frontal pins. Once in position rods from arch bars will provide rigid fixation of the maxilla.

Complications of fractures

Removal of bone plates

Infrequently, titanium bone plates will have to be removed. This is due to patient request, plate exposure or, rarely, involvement of the plate in infection. The most

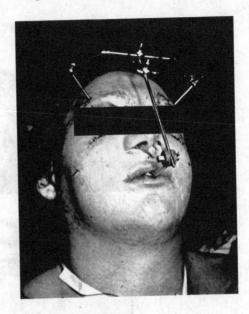

Figure 14.16 Levant frame attached to upper metal cap splint by bars and universal joints. Note facial laceration extended for open reduction.

frequent area from which plates are removed in the mandible is the parasymphyseal region and in the maxilla at the zygomaticofrontal suture region. The plates should ideally remain until bone healing is complete before removal, unless rigid fixation is lost due to loosening of the screws or breakage of the plate.

Delayed union

Normally fractures unite in about 4–8 weeks, but take longer in elderly patients. This time may be greatly increased in comminuted, compound or infected fractures. Rigid internal fixation will allow these fractures to heal but some may take several months, during which time they must be carefully observed. Radiographs may be taken at intervals if movement of the fracture is evident clinically, to determine whether non-union has occurred (Figure 14.17).

Malunion

This is union with the bone ends still misplaced or badly reduced. It may be slight and cause the patient little disability or it may be such as to interfere with function or appearance. Slight deformity affecting the occlusion can be treated by grinding or extracting teeth, and the provision of dentures. More severe deformities may require re-fracture and reapposition of the bone ends by an osteotomy operation.

Non-union

This term refers to the failure to obtain bony union, where healing has occurred by fibrous union only. In facial trauma it is significant only in the mandible. Clinically, movement is found across the fracture line. On radiographs a smoothing over of the bone ends is seen, which is later followed by a deposition of cortical bone (eburnation). The chief causes of non-union are a failure to achieve

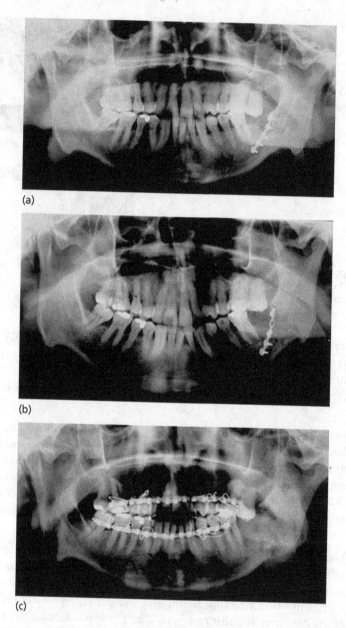

Figure 14.17   Loss of fixation. (a) Good reduction of fracture at left angle; (b) 3 weeks postoperatively, note loss of screws and movement of fracture; (c) IMF applied with arch bars following removal of fixation. The patient may have been involved in further trauma.

satisfactory apposition, bone loss, and movement or infection in the fracture line. Treatment of non-union is necessary in the body of the mandible but may be acceptable in the ascending ramus and the condyle, if function is unimpaired.

Bone loss

In severe injuries, particularly in gunshot wounds, there may be bone loss. In the mandible, if this is slight, a satisfactory result can be achieved by approximating the bone ends. Otherwise, the gap is accepted and the fragments are reduced into their normal position and held there by bicortical bone plates or external pin fixation. When soft tissue healing has taken place and the inflammatory reaction has settled, the defect is repaired with bone grafts. This may be delayed several weeks, or even months. Monocortical plates are not rigid enough to bridge large bone defects effectively.

Infection

This may reach the fracture from wounds in the skin or more commonly from the mouth. The mandible is more susceptible to infection than the maxilla. In the latter, drainage is downwards into the mouth and the thin plates of bone with a good blood supply make it more resistant to infection. Infection from the mouth may enter the fracture through a tear in the mucous membrane, from dead teeth, particularly those in the line of fracture, or by direct or lymphatic spread from other infected teeth in the jaw. If rigid fixation has been achieved with a bio-inert material, such as titanium, fracture healing should continue if energetic treatment with antibacterial drugs and drainage, together with the removal of infected teeth, is instituted. On rare occasions the fixation may have to be removed and IMF applied.

Residual trismus

In mandibular fractures residual trismus may be due to scarring in the traumatised muscles or rarely due to ankylosis in intracapsular condylar fractures. In poorly reduced zygomatic arch fractures bony interference may occur with the coronoid process. The cause must be carefully ascertained and treated either surgically or with exercises and physiotherapy.

Further reading

Advanced Trauma Life Support Student Manual, 8th edn. American College of Surgeons. Chicago, IL.

Champy M, Lodde JP, Jaegar JH, Wilk A, Gerber JC (1978) Mandibular osteo-synthesis by miniature screwed plates via a buccal approach. *Journal of Maxillofacial Surgery* **6**: 14.

Symposium on management of the bilateral fractured condyle (1998) *Journal of Oral Surgery* **27**: 244–67.

Ward Booth P, Schendel S, Hausamen J (2006) *Maxillofacial Surgery*, 2nd edn. Churchill Livingstone, Elsevier.

Williams JL (ed.) (1994) *Rowe and Williams Maxillofacial Injuries*, 2nd edn. Churchill Livingstone, Edinburgh.

Chapter 15
Tumours of the Mouth and the Management of Oral Cancer

- Oral precancer
- Oral cancer
- Aetiology and risk factors
- Clinical presentation
- Spread of oral cancer
- Principles of management
- Surgery
- Radiotherapy
- Chemotherapy
- Recent advances

A tumour is a swelling or mass caused by excessive, continued growth of cells within a tissue; growth is unco-ordinated with that of normal tissue and persists in the same excessive manner after cessation of the stimulus that evoked it, in distinction to developmental abnormalities such as haemangiomas which are termed hamartomas. Tumours may be either benign or malignant (Table 15.1).

Oncology is the study and science of new growths, while a neoplasm refers to any new, diseased form of tissue growth. Cancer is the overall name applied to malignant growths, more than 90% of which are derived from epithelial tissues, and is essentially a genetic disease caused by somatic mutation. The multistage theory of carcinogenesis believes that individual cancers arise from several sequential mutations in cellular DNA. There is a close correlation between cancer incidence and increased age, reflecting the time required to accumulate the critical number of genetic abnormalities needed for malignant change.

The two most significant characteristics of malignant growths are: local invasion, in which malignant cells either singularly or as cords or sheets infiltrate and destroy adjacent normal tissue, and metastasis, in which secondary tumours, by dissemination of tumour emboli through lymphatic and vascular channels, are formed at sites discontinuous from the primary. Death from cancer usually

Principles of Oral and Maxillofacial Surgery, 6th Edition. Edited by U. J. Moore
© 2011 Blackwell Publishing Ltd

Table 15.1 Benign tumours of the mouth

Pathological characteristics	Clinical features	Common oral tumours	Treatment
Slow growing Expansile Localised Encapsulated Well differentiated	Mucosal or submucosal swelling Local pressure or displacement effects	Squamous cell papilloma Adenoma Fibroma Neurofibroma Lipoma Osteoma	Local excision

Table 15.2 Oral precancer

Classification	Definition (WHO 1978)	Clinical examples
Precancerous lesions	Morphologically altered tissue in which cancer is more likely to occur than in its apparently normal counterpart	Leukoplakia Erythroplakia Speckled leukoplakia
Precancerous conditions	Generalised states associated with a significantly increased risk of cancer	Immunosuppression Submucous fibrosis Sideropaenic dysphagia Discoid lupus erythematosus Actinic keratosis Lichen planus Syphilis

results from tumour deposition within vital organs such as the liver, lungs or brain, from a generalised carcinomatosis, or from uncontrolled disease at the primary site causing airway obstruction or haemorrhage from large blood vessels.

Oral precancer

Fundamental to reducing cancer morbidity and mortality is the ability to recognise the earliest possible neoplastic changes in oral tissues. Dental practitioners have a unique opportunity during routine oral examination to detect malignant neoplasms while they are asymptomatic and often precancerous. In 1978 the World Health Organization (WHO) divided oral precancer into: precancerous lesions, altered tissues in which oral cancer is more likely to occur, and precancerous conditions, which are generalised states associated with a significantly increased risk of cancer (Table 15.2).

While this remains a useful distinction, WHO terminology changed in 2005 to combine lesions and conditions into a unified category of potentially malignant disorders. This reflects the clinical reality that patients often present with widespread mucosal disease rather than isolated single lesions.

Epithelial dysplasia is defined as a collection of epithelial changes seen by light microscopy (primarily disordered tissue maturation and disturbed cellular proliferation) and is the most important determinant of the risk of malignant transformation of precancerous lesions. Pathologists qualitatively divide dysplasia into mild, moderate, severe or carcinoma-in-situ, depending on the extent of dysplastic features and the resultant risk of malignant change.

Epithelial dysplasia does not mean that a lesion will inevitably proceed to an invasive cancer, but an increased risk exists which worsens as the epithelium becomes increasingly dysplastic. Erythroplakic lesions generally contain more severely dysplastic epithelium than leukoplakia, and carry a higher risk of malignant change, as do speckled (red and white) lesions, while rough or nodular leukoplakias carry more risk than smooth (homogeneous) leukoplakias. Lesions arising in the floor of mouth and ventral tongue display higher rates of malignant transformation than other oral sites.

Box 15.1 outlines a pragmatic management protocol for patients with oral precancer. Laser surgery, a technique involving high-temperature tissue vaporisation and coagulative necrosis, allows accurate dissection and excision of premalignant lesions with reduced morbidity; minimal blood loss, reduction in postoperative pain, reduced scarring and rapid healing without skin grafting facilitate an acceptable strategy in patients for whom multiple or recurrent oral lesions are not uncommon.

Field change

An important complicating factor is that following surgical removal of individual precancerous lesions the rest of the patient's upper aerodigestive tract mucosa may display widespread precancerous change, rendering patients susceptible to other primary cancers of larynx, oesophagus and lungs.

Box 15.1   Management protocol for oral precancer

1 Eliminate risk factors – tobacco, alcohol
2 Clinical photographic record
3 Baseline haematology – full blood count, serum ferritin, B_{12}, folate
4 Candidal swab
5 Incisional biopsy and dysplasia characterisation
6 Careful clinical follow-up and consider repeat biopsy for mild dysplasias
7 Laser excision for moderate/severe dysplasias
8 Long-term clinical follow-up
9 Monitor oral mucosa for field change

Table 15.3   Malignancies of the oral cavity

Primary tumours	Secondary tumours (metastases)
Squamous cell carcinoma (>90%) Minor salivary gland carcinomas Lymphoma Malignant melanoma Sarcoma	Adenocarcinomas primarily from breast, renal and gastrointestinal tract primaries

Oral cancer

While the term oral cancer encompasses a range of malignant tumours arising within the lip, oral cavity and oropharynx (Table 15.3), more than 90% of oral cancers are primary squamous cell carcinomas arising from the oral mucous membrane.

Worldwide, the incidence of oral cancer varies, with India and parts of Asia having the highest rates (40% of all cancers), while in Western countries the incidence is about 3% of all new cancers. However, this incidence is rising, particularly in younger patients and women, and oral cancer is a particularly lethal disease. Approximately 3400 new cases of oral cancer occur each year in the UK and there are about 1600 deaths.

Overall, the 5-year survival rate for patients with oral cancer is only 50%, although small, slow-growing lesions, tumours detected early and those presenting at the front of the mouth tend to do better. Posteriorly sited, rapidly growing tumours invading bone and with demonstrable lymph node metastases at presentation have the worst prognosis.

Aetiology and risk factors

The principal aetiological factors involve the use of tobacco and alcohol, which are known mucosal irritants and mutagenic agents. There is an important synergistic relationship between the two, which significantly increases the risk of cancer for those who both smoke and drink.

Patients who have had oral cancer previously, or those who have had lung, throat or oesophageal tumours, are also at high risk of developing new oral tumours or recurrence of their original cancers. Immunocompromised patients, such as those with AIDS or post-transplant patients on long-term immunosuppressive agents, are also at risk. Other postulated aetiological agents include viruses, chronic candidal infections, anaemias, nutritional and vitamin deficiencies, and for lip cancer, exposure to ultra-violet radiation.

Clinical presentation

The most frequent clinical presentation is an indurated area of ulceration, often surrounded by leukoplakic or erythroplakic patches, while the commonest sites involved are the floor of the mouth, ventrolateral tongue and the soft palate complex (soft palate, retromolar trigone and anterior tonsillar pillar).

Oral cancer is usually asymptomatic in the early stages. Late presentation is common, although patients report non-specific symptoms over several months prior to their seeking attention. (Table 15.4 summarises the salient signs and symptoms suspicious of oral malignancy.)

Spread of oral cancer

The most significant behavioural feature of oral cancers is their ability to invade and destroy local structures and to spread via lymphatics into the neck (Table 15.5). An appreciation of the pattern of spread is essential for effective treatment in order to control the disease within the mouth and neck.

Local invasion

Cancers can infiltrate widely into adjacent connective tissue, within muscle bundles, perineural spaces or local blood vessels. Direct extension via periodontal membrane or cortical deficiencies in edentulous ridges allows invasion of alveolar bone.

Table 15.4   Clinical presentation of oral cancers

Early lesions symptoms	Late lesions symptoms	Signs
Asymptomatic Irritation Discomfort	Pain and swelling Paraesthesia Dysarthia Dysphagia	Non-healing ulcer Induration and fixation of tissues Exophytic growth White/red mucosal patches Unexplained localised tooth mobility Non-healing tooth socket

Table 15.5   Spread of oral cancer

(1) Local invasion	(2) Regional lymph node metastasis	(3) Distant spread
Soft tissues and muscles Perineural spaces Blood vessels Bone		Lungs Liver Bones

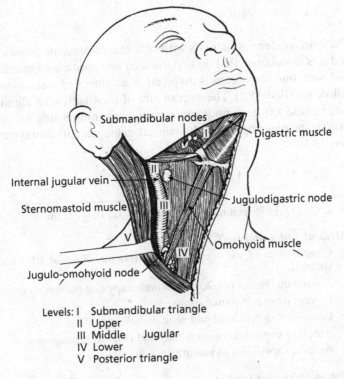

Levels: I   Submandibular triangle
        II Upper
        III Middle   Jugular
        IV Lower
        V   Posterior triangle

Figure 15.1   Surgical anatomy of cervical lymph node groups. Levels: I, submandibular triangle; II, upper; III, middle jugular; IV, lower; V, posterior triangle.

Lymph node metastasis

The likelihood of lymphatic spread increases with the size of the primary tumour. While the precise group of cervical lymph nodes affected depends on the location of the primary, intraoral cancers tend to spread initially to ipsilateral submandibular, upper, middle and lower deep cervical nodes (Levels I to IV in Figure 15.1). Tumours of the tongue, lip and floor of mouth close to the midline can metastasise to nodes on both sides of the neck, while the posterior triangle (Level V in Figure 15.1) may be involved in aggressive tongue and posterior oral tumours. The more lymph nodes involved, the presence of metastases in lower cervical nodes and the extension of tumour beyond the node capsule (extracapsular spread) all herald a worse prognosis.

Distant spread

Distant spread tends to be more frequent in the later stages of the disease and may not be clinically apparent, although metastatic deposits have been found in the lungs, liver and bones in approximately 50% of post-mortem examinations carried out in patients dying with oral cancer.

Principles of management

The management of patients with oral cancer presents considerable challenges and it is mandatory that an experienced and specialised multidisciplinary head and neck oncology team is involved in all stages of assessment, treatment and follow-up (Box 15.2). The overall aim of treatment is to eliminate the primary tumour and any neck node metastases, while minimising patient morbidity. The basic principles applied to the clinical management of oral cancer are listed in Box 15.3.

Box 15.2   Multidisciplinary head and neck oncology team

Medical and dental staff
- Consultant head and neck surgeons (from maxillofacial, ENT and plastic surgery specialties)
- Consultant clinical oncologist (radiotherapy and chemotherapy expertise)
- Consultant in restorative dentistry
- Consultant in oral/head and neck pathology
- Access to consultants in radiology and diagnostic imaging
- Access to specialists in palliative medicine

Specialist nursing services
- Clinical nurse specialisation in head and neck surgery
- Macmillan palliative care specialists

Paramedical support services
- Speech therapists
- Dietitians
- Physiotherapists
- Maxillofacial laboratory and prosthetic services
- Access to psychological care services

Box 15.3   Principles of oral cancer management

1 Thorough evaluation of the patient and their disease
2 Tumour diagnosis, classification and disease staging
3 Comprehensive treatment planning
4 Co-ordination of therapeutic modalities (e.g. combination of surgery and radiotherapy)
5 Post-treatment oral reconstruction and rehabilitation
6 Psychological and social support

Evaluation of disease

Accurate assessment of the extent of disease is important and includes a detailed clinical history, general medical review and physical examination, a biopsy of the primary tumour to confirm the diagnosis and histology, possibly an examination under anaesthesia (EUA) to facilitate inspection, palpation and measurement of larger, painful and posteriorly sited lesions, and an evaluation of cervical lymph node involvement. Endoscopic examination of the rest of the upper aerodigestive tract may be carried out to identify other primary (synchronous) tumours. Table 15.6 details the important further investigations carried out during the assessment phase.

Classification and staging

Evaluation allows classification of cancers according to the size of the primary tumour (T), the involvement of associated regional lymph nodes (N) and the presence of distant metastases (M). Using the TNM system, it is then possible

Table 15.6   Investigations used in oral cancer assessment

Classification	Types	Specific aims
Histopathological examination	Incisional tissue biopsy	To confirm clinical diagnosis Classify tumour differentiation
	Fine needle aspiration (FNA) cytology	To confirm presence of metastatic carcinoma in enlarged lymph nodes
Diagnostic imaging	Plain radiography	
	• Orthopantomogram	To establish jaw bone or tooth involvement
	• Occipitomental view	To assess maxillary sinus or orbital involvement
	• Chest X-ray	Screening for bronchial cancer or metastatic metastatic lung disease
	CT scanning	Particularly useful in imaging bony involvement and antral and pterygoid regions
	MR scanning	Ideally suited for soft tissue tumours and cervical node assessment
Laboratory investigations	Haematology	To identify underlying anaemias or clotting disorders
	Blood chemistry	To identify renal or liver disease (e.g. cirrhosis metastases)

Table 15.7   Classification and staging of oral cancers

TNM classification	Clinical assessment of the anatomical extent of disease
Tumour	$T_1 < 2\,cm$
	$T_2 < 2$–$4\,cm$
	$T_3 > 4\,cm$
	T_4 Infiltrating deep structures
Nodes	N_1 Mobile palpable nodes $<3\,cm$ on same side
	N_2 Contra or bilateral mobile nodes 3–$6\,cm$
	N_3 Fixed node(s) $>6\,cm$
Metastases	M_1 Distant metastases present
Resultant clinical staging	Standard communicable description of individual patients' disease
Stage I	T_1 No Mo
Stage II	T_2 No Mo
Stage III	T_3 No Mo
	or
	$T_1/T_2/T_3 N_1$ Mo
Stage IV	T_4
	Any T N_2/N_3 Mo
	Any T/Any N/M_1

to stage individual patients' disease. This allows meaningful treatment planning and assessment of prognosis and helps advise patients and relatives, as well as providing a meaningful reference for data analysis between different treatment centres (Table 15.7).

Treatment planning

The fundamental decision of whether curative or palliative treatment is appropriate follows discussion within the multidisciplinary team and between patients and their relatives. While the aim of curative treatment is clearly the elimination of disease with minimum morbidity, palliative care aims to improve and prolong the symptom-free phase of the patient's life with the recognition that the disease is unlikely to be completely eradicated.

The choice is then whether to use surgery or radiotherapy as the primary treatment. If surgery is chosen, radiotherapy may be used in an adjuvant manner postoperatively. If radiotherapy is used as primary treatment, surgery is reserved for salvage therapy to deal with any residual disease. However, following radiotherapy tissues have a reduced blood supply and exhibit marked fibrosis leading to delayed healing and the risk of wound breakdown and fistula formation. The general health, age, life expectancy and wishes of the patient must be taken into consideration during treatment planning. While surgery may necessitate the loss of important functional units such as the lips, tongue or mandible, radiotherapy may produce immediate morbidity (stomatitis and xerostomia) or longer-term problems such as osteoradionecrosis.

Surgery

Surgical access

Good surgical access is fundamental to the effective exposure and complete removal of oral tumours. The approach adopted should be easy to repair and produce minimal scarring and deformity. While an intraoral technique may be sufficient for small anteriorly sited tumours, splitting of the lip, division of the mandible (mandibulotomy) and resultant mandibular swing fully displays the posterior tongue, retromolar and soft palate regions, and facilitates tumour excision in three dimensions under direct vision. Facial cheek flaps and maxillary osteotomies allow similar access to the posterior palate and retromaxillary regions.

Resection of the primary tumour

The principal objective of surgical treatment is to excise the entire primary tumour with a margin (ideally about 1 cm) of adjacent normal tissue in anticipation of microscopic spread, and to remove potential channels of metastasis such as nerves, vessels and lymphatics.

Lower lip cancers may be treated by wedge excision alone or combined with a lip shave procedure (removal of the entire vermilion) where there is extensive ultraviolet damage. Anterior tongue tumours may require partial, hemi- or subtotal glossectomy, depending on the size and position. While small buccal mucosal cancers can be excised intraorally, more advanced lesions may require excision of buccinator muscle and overlying skin.

Tumours of the floor of mouth, retromolar region and lower alveolus usually involve the underlying mandible and require mandibular resection. As bony invasion usually occurs from the superior aspect, a marginal resection may be possible, preserving the mandibular lower border. The inferior dental nerve canal, extending from lingula to mental foramen, should be included in mandibular body resections owing to the likelihood of perineural spread.

Mucosal excision, alveolar resection, palatal fenestration or maxillectomy may be required for tumours arising from the palatal mucosa and maxillary alveolus, depending on their size and position.

> **Box 15.4**   Neck dissection operations
>
> Comprehensive   (a) Radical (no structures preserved)
> (nodes excised from   (b) Modified radical (preservation of sternomastoid muscle,
>   Levels I to V)   internal jugular vein and accessory nerve)
> Selective   e.g. Supra omohyoid (nodes excised from Levels I to III/IV
>   only)

Management of the neck

Dissection of cervical lymph nodes containing metastatic disease is essential for the effective management of oral cancer, and is indicated whenever clinical examination or imaging techniques confirm enlarged, draining lymph nodes. Fine needle aspiration (FNA) may be carried out to confirm cytologically the presence of carcinoma deposits within enlarged nodes (see Chapter 16).

Neck dissection operations may be classified according to the various levels at which nodes are removed and the key anatomical structures that are either excised or preserved (Box 15.4). In oral cancer management, Levels I to III or IV are the most often dissected, with postoperative radiotherapy advised if multiple nodes prove positive or there is extracapsular tumour spread.

Neck dissection may be contraindicated, however, in extensive disease where involved lymph nodes may be fixed by tumour extension into vital structures such as the carotid artery or skull base. A complete surgical excision is either not possible or may produce significant morbidity or even mortality.

Reconstruction

Following ablative tumour surgery, reconstruction is essential to prevent facial deformity, maintain bone continuity and facilitate masticatory, swallowing and speech functions. Reduction of psychological morbidity and an acceptable quality of life outcome are equally important aims. Extensive removal of orofacial soft tissues and underlying mandibular or maxillary bone is often necessary for effective tumour resection and a range of reconstructive techniques are available (Box 15.5).

The use of free tissue transfer and microvascular surgery, in which free flaps (often comprising skin, muscle and bone) are transferred from distant sites and their dependent arteries and veins connected to vessels in the neck, enables reconstruction of complex defects with vascularised tissue at the time of tumour excision. The radial forearm osseofasciocutaneous flap, a groin flap based on the deep circumflex iliac artery (DCIA) or the fibula flap may be used to reconstruct the mandible (Figure 15.2).

Maxillary defects result in direct communications between oral and nasal cavities or the paranasal sinuses, with the inevitable production of nasal speech

---

Box 15.5　Reconstructive techniques

1 Primary closure (soft tissue defects)

2 'Simple' free grafts
　Skin　　　　　　　　Split thickness
　　　　　　　　　　　Full thickness
　Bone　　　　　　　　Cortical
　　　　　　　　　　　Cancellous

3 Local flap repair
　Intraoral tissue　　　Tongue flap
　　　　　　　　　　　Buccal fat pad
　Facial skin　　　　　e.g. nasolabial flap
　Muscle　　　　　　　e.g. temporalis flap
4 Regional pedicled flaps　e.g. pectoralis major muscle and skin flap

5 Free flaps (microvascular tissue transfer)
　Radial forearm flap
　Fibula flap
　Groin and iliac crest flap

6 Alloplastic techniques
　Titanium reconstruction plates, mesh trays and implants
　Acrylic dentofacial prostheses and obturators

---

and swallowing difficulties. The principal aim is thus to re-establish palatal continuity either with flap reconstruction or a prosthetic appliance and obturator, which fills the defect. Initially, such appliances may be secured with intraosseous screws to adjacent palatal bone holding skin grafts in position to reline mucosal defects. Later, they are replaced with specially designed removable appliances.

Radiotherapy

Radiotherapy is the treatment of tumours with ionising radiation and is potentially curative in oral cancer treatment (Table 15.8). X-ray, gamma ray and less commonly particulate radiation is delivered as external beams from outside the patient (teletherapy) or radioactive materials such as iridium wires can be implanted within or in close proximity to the tumour (brachytherapy).

External beams of supervoltage radiation converge on the tumour, so the latter receives a very much higher dose than the surrounding tissues. The total therapeutic dose of external beam therapy, usually 60 Grays (Gy), is fractionated into a number of smaller doses over 4 to 6 weeks. This increases the differential effect on tumour cells, which are less able to repair themselves compared with normal tissue. Brachytherapy treatment requires an intense radiation dose within the tumour and immediate vicinity, usually delivering a total of 65 to 70 Gy over 8 days.

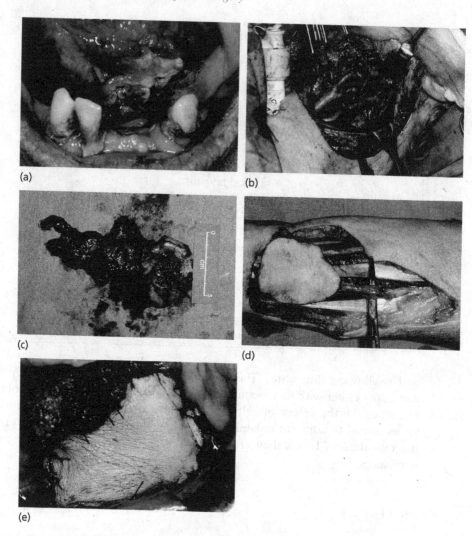

Figure 15.2   Stages in the surgical management of a floor of mouth cancer. (a) Typical clinical appearance of an exophytic and infiltrative floor of mouth squamous cell carcinoma; (b) functional neck dissection in progress demonstrating the internal jugular vein (V) and the common carotid arterial system (A). The sternomastoid muscle is retracted posteriorly and the fatty tissue containing the lymph nodes is being dissected anteriorly (N); (c) 'in continuity' resection specimen includes the mandibular gingiva, floor of mouth and anterior tongue, together with the draining cervical lymph nodes (N); (d) free fasciocutaneous forearm flap and vascular pedicle (radial artery plus venae comitantes) being raised; (e) forearm flap transferred to oral defect and secured in place with multiple interrupted sutures.

Table 15.8   The role of radiotherapy in oral cancer treatment

Indications for radiotherapy	Contraindications to radiotherapy
Patient unfit for major surgery	Previous local irradiation
Tumour inaccessible or technically unresectable by surgery	Large tumours, with bony invasion and cervical lymph node metastases
Surgery likely to produce severe deformity or functional morbidity	Unreliable patient attendance for outpatient therapy
Patient unwilling to undergo surgery	

Radiation may be given palliatively to incurable patients with a short life expectancy to relieve disease symptoms such as pain, bleeding or swelling. A cure is not attempted and the risk of acute reaction lessened by using a smaller dose, for example 20 Gy over 5 days.

Modern radiotherapy techniques utilise computerised methods and new forms of radiation to enhance therapeutic effect while trying to minimise irradiation of adjacent normal tissue.

Biological effects of radiation

Intracellular free radicals are formed leading to DNA damage and ultimately cell death when mitosis is attempted. Mitotic death occurs within a few days in rapidly proliferating tumours such as squamous cell carcinoma. The effectiveness of radiotherapy is increased in radiosensitive tumours, in the presence of increased oxygenation and in smaller tumours. In a successful treatment the tumour regresses and is replaced by scar tissue. Mitotic death of normal cells produces the side effects of radiotherapy.

Rapidly proliferating tissues such as oral mucosa and skin affected after 14 to 21 days (acute reactions) lead to mucositis, loss of taste, and erythema and alopecia respectively. These acute effects usually heal completely as the normal tissues proliferate and recover. Late reactions, which are irreversible, occur due to devascularisation of irradiated tissues as a result of mitotic death of slowly replicating vascular endothelial cells.

Xerostomia

Irradiation of salivary gland tissue produces an acute permanent loss of secretory cells. Salivary flow reduces during the first few days of radiotherapy, but within 6 weeks has stopped completely. The resulting dryness of the mouth can be distressing to patients, adds to their oral discomfort and impairs taste, chewing and swallowing.

Xerostomia carries an increased risk of rapidly destructive dental caries (radiation caries) and advanced periodontal disease. Artificial saliva preparations may be helpful, while oral administration of pilocarpine may help increase flow in patients with some residual salivary gland function.

Osteoradionecrosis

Bone irradiation lethally damages both osteoblasts and osteoclasts so that when stimulated to divide, as a result of a traumatic stimulus such as a dental extraction or localised infection, mitotic death occurs, precipitating necrosis. There is also diminished vascularity of the periosteum due to late effects on endothelial lining cells, particularly involving the dense and less vascular mandibular bone.

Clinically, the radionecrotic process usually starts as an ulceration on the alveolar mucosa with brownish dead bone exposed at the base. Pathological fracture may occur in the weakened bone, but the process may not be painful until secondary infection ensues, when severe discomfort, trismus, foetor oris and general malaise predominate. Radiographically, the earliest changes are a 'moth-eaten' appearance of the bone, followed by sequestration.

Treatment is predominantly conservative with long-term antibiotic therapy and careful removal of sequestra when necessary. In intractable cases, extensive surgical resection and reconstruction with compound muscle and bone flaps may be necessary. Hyperbaric oxygen and ultrasound therapy have also been recommended.

Dental care for oncology patients

Assessment of the general dental state by a specialist in restorative dentistry is mandatory for all head and neck cancer patients, especially for those likely to undergo radiotherapy. Extractions are advised for carious, non-vital, periodontally involved teeth or retained roots and their removal is performed carefully preradiotherapy to ensure rapid healing.

Subsequent to radiotherapy, meticulous oral hygiene is essential, especially during treatment when the mouth is inflamed and sore. Dilute chlorhexidine mouthwashes, topical fluoride applications, saliva substitutes and active restorative care may all be needed to preserve the remaining dentition. Should a tooth have to be extracted it is essential that an atraumatic surgical technique is used, together with antibiotic cover until healing is complete.

Chemotherapy

Chemotherapy has provided a major advance in the management of certain malignancies. As the primary form of treatment for lymphomas and leukaemias, for example, chemotherapeutic agents have markedly improved the long-term

Table 15.9   Chemotherapeutic drugs

Classification	Mode of action	Drugs used in cancer treatment
Alkylating agents	DNA damage by adding alkyl group	Busulphan
Platinum agents	DNA damage by adding platinum	Cisplatin
Antibiotics	Variable	Bleomycin
Antimetabolites	Impair synthesis and assembly of purine and pyrimidine DNA bases	Methotrexate 5-Fluorouracil
Mitotic inhibitors	Disrupt microtubules essential for cell division	Vincristine
Taxanes	Arrest cells at metaphase	Docetaxel
Antibodies	Interrupt growth stimulation	Rituximab

Table 15.10   Chemotherapy treatment regimens

Type	Administration	Aim
Induction	Prior to surgery or radiotherapy	To reduce tumour size and kill tumour cells
Sandwich	Between surgery and radiotherapy	To reduce risk of metastases
Adjuvant	After surgery or radiotherapy	To improve disease-free survival
Concurrent	In conjunction with radiotherapy	To sensitise tumour cells and increase destructive effects of radiotherapy
Palliative	After all other treatments	Shrink persistent tumour masses Pain relief

survival rates of patients. In general, however, chemotherapy is less effective in treating solid tumours in adults and is rarely of curative value in oral cancer treatment, but may have a role in trying to prevent secondary tumours developing from metastatic deposits.

Chemotherapy targets actively dividing cells to eliminate tumours while allowing normal cells to recover and repair. Drugs are thus usually administered in high doses intermittently and often in combination to aid synergy and overcome potential resistance. Many types of drug are now available (Table 15.9), and a number of different therapeutic regimes may be applied (Table 15.10).

The major side effects of chemotherapy are nausea and vomiting, bone marrow suppression, alopecia and oral mucositis. To reduce the severity of mucositis, a high standard of oral hygiene and careful attention to preventive and restorative dental care is essential.

Newer techniques combine cisplatin with irradiation as chemoradiation for locally advanced disease or as induction chemotherapy, with combined taxane, cisplatin and fluorouracil prior to palliative treatment for recurrent or metastatic disease. Future regimens may involve the use of monoclonal antibodies, immunotherapy, gene therapy and other targeted biological therapies in combination with traditional chemotherapeutic agents or irradiation.

Recent advances and current problems in oral cancer management

Unfortunately, overall survival rates for oral cancer have changed little over the past 20 years, although accurate disease staging and effective treatment planning (combination therapy involving both surgery and radiotherapy) have produced more effective loco-regional disease control. A greater number of patients now die, however, from distant metastases or from the emergence of second or even third primary tumours.

Quality of life is now recognised as an important determinant of therapeutic effectiveness and oral rehabilitation has a major role in promoting life quality and patient self-esteem.

Future developments in oral cancer therapy will require effective public health measures to target high-risk population groups and wider introduction of active preventive therapies. Accurate, reproducible and predictive clinico-pathological assessments of individual precancer and cancerous lesions are required, and further research is both necessary and ongoing into the potential therapeutic role of newer genetic and immunological therapies.

Further reading

Brown AE, Langdon JD (1995) Management of oral cancer. *Annals of the Royal College of Surgery Engand* **77**: 404–8.

Cawson RA, Langdon JD, Eveson JW (1996) *Surgical Pathology of the Mouth and Jaws.* Wright, Oxford.

Dimitroulis G, Avery BS (1998) *Oral Cancer. A Synopsis of Pathology and Management.* Butterworth Heinemann, Oxford.

Langdon JD, Henk JM (1995) *Malignant Tumours of the Mouth, Jaws and Salivary Glands.* Edward Arnold, London.

Lodi G, Porter S (2008) Management of potentially malignant disorders: evidence and critique. *Journal of Oral Pathology and Medicine* **37**: 63–9.

Napier SS, Speight PM (2008) Natural history of potentially malignant oral lesions and conditions: an overview of the literature. *Journal of Oral Pathology and Medicine* **37**: 1–10.

Silverman S (1998) *Oral Cancer*, 4th edn. American Cancer Society. BC Decker Inc, Hamilton, Canada.

Chapter 16
Surgical Treatment of Salivary Gland Disease

- Presenting complaints
- The minor salivary glands
- The major salivary glands
- Specific conditions

The salivary glands comprise the paired major parotid and submandibular glands located on the side of the face, together with bilateral sublingual glands in the floor of the mouth and the numerous minor salivary glands distributed intraorally (Figure 16.1). Disorders of salivary glands treated by surgery include cysts, salivary calculi, infections and tumours.

Presenting complaints

Salivary gland disease may present as acute inflammatory gland swellings, such as a viral or bacterial sialadenitis, recurrent swellings associated with mealtimes due to duct obstruction or stricture secondary to calculi, persistent diffuse whole gland enlargement as seen in Sjogren's syndrome or sialosis (a non-inflammatory, non-neoplastic enlargement seen in diabetes, alcoholism or anoxeria), or as nodular, intraglandular swellings suggestive of tumour or cyst formation (Box 16.1).

If a patient reports the appearance of a mass, the size and growth rate should be recorded, together with how long it has been present and the presence or absence of other symptoms. Rapidly growing, painful masses with symptoms such as facial nerve palsy, trismus and bony destruction are suggestive of malignant tumour progression, while a symptomless, slow-growing swelling is more likely to be benign. In addition, any change in consistency of the saliva or taste sensation should be noted and it is important to ascertain if there is involvement of other systems such as the eyes, liver, lungs or joints.

Principles of Oral and Maxillofacial Surgery, 6th Edition. Edited by U. J. Moore
© 2011 Blackwell Publishing Ltd

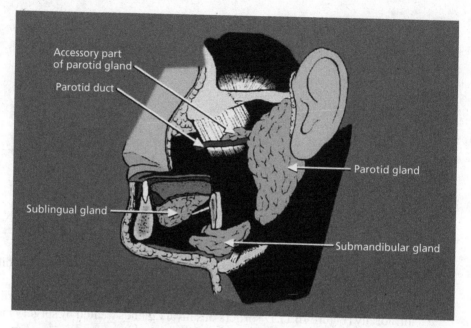

Figure 16.1 Diagram illustrating anatomical location of the major salivary glands.

Box 16.1	Classification of salivary gland disorders
Congenital	Aplasia
	Hypoplasia
Inflammatory	Sialadenitis – viral or bacterial infection
	Autoimmune – Sjögren's syndrome
	Idiopathic – necrotising sialometaplasia
	Sarcoidosis
Traumatic	Mucocele, ranula
	Salivary fistulae
	Post-irradiation sialadenitis
Obstructive	Sialolithiasis
	Atresia or ductal stenosis
Tumours	Benign – pleomorphic adenoma
	Malignant – mucoepidermoid carcinoma, acinic cell carcinoma, adenocarcinoma, adenoid cystic carcinoma
Idiopathic	Sialosis

The minor salivary glands

Cysts

Diagnosis and presentation

Common sites include the lips, cheeks, floor of the mouth and palate. The cause is usually trauma, especially cheek or lip biting which may lead to stenosis or rupture of the duct and accumulation of saliva. They are common in children and young adolescents. The types include the mucous extravasation cyst and mucous retention cyst. In the former, mucus ruptures through the duct and pools in the adjacent connective tissue; there is no epithelial lining and the saliva is contained by flattened connective tissue. In the latter, mucus is still contained by the epithelium lining the duct, which swells to form an epithelial-lined cyst (Figure 16.2).

Signs and symptoms

These cysts usually present as painless, smooth, bluish swellings containing fluid. At intervals they burst, discharging their contents, but if untreated they heal and form again. In the floor of the mouth, a cyst may arise from the sublingual gland and grow to a considerable size and is called a ranula (Figure 16.3).

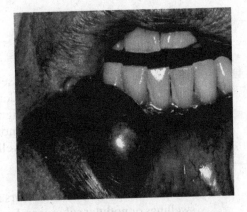

Figure 16.2 Salivary mucocele of lower lip.

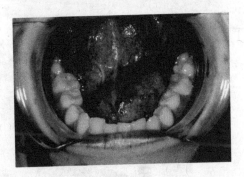

Figure 16.3 Ranula (mucocele) in the floor of mouth.

Treatment of cysts

Mucocele

Treatment involves delicate enucleation. An incision is made by drawing a scalpel blade lightly over the swelling and through the mucosa for a short distance beyond the lesion on each side. Alternatively an elliptical incision can be made to reduce the chance of rupture. The cyst is gently freed by blunt dissection and the gland concerned is also removed to prevent recurrence. Due to the fragile lining the lesion may burst during surgery. Other glands seen in the wound, which may already be traumatised, should be removed lest their ducts become blocked by scar tissue and give rise to new cysts. Primary closure is achieved by using superficial mucosal sutures.

Ranula

The ranula is more difficult to treat and care must be taken during floor of mouth surgery to avoid damage to the submandibular duct and lingual nerve. It is usual to have to excise the sublingual gland as part of this procedure and surgery is best carried out under general anaesthesia. More rarely, a ranula may extend through the mylohyoid muscle (a 'plunging ranula') into the upper neck requiring both intraoral and cervical approaches to facilitate complete removal.

Tumours

(See Chapter 15)

The commonest tumours to arise from minor glands include the benign, but locally invasive, pleomorphic adenoma and the malignant adenoid cystic and mucoepidermoid carcinomas (Figure 16.4). It is worth remembering that malignant tumours arise more commonly in minor salivary glands than in major glands, so intraoral glandular swellings should be regarded with suspicion.

Diagnosis

The pleomorphic adenoma occurs most frequently, with many arising as palatal swellings or nodular submucosal swellings within the upper lip or buccal mucosa.

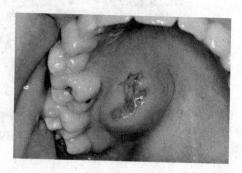

Figure 16.4 Pleomorphic salivary adenoma in the palate. An incisional biopsy has been performed.

It presents as a painless swelling of rubbery consistency, which may be fixed to either the overlying mucosa or the deeper structures. In the palate it is usually found to one side of the midline near the junction of hard and soft palate and may reach a large size.

The adenoid cystic and mucoepidermoid carcinomas may clinically resemble a pleomorphic adenoma but usually display more rapid growth, pain and ulceration of the surface mucosa.

Treatment

The pleomorphic adenoma is treated by excision with a margin of normal tissue because tumour outgrowths may be found within or outside the tumour capsule. Large defects may require a skin or mucosal graft, or rotational flaps or an oversown pack. Adenoid cystic carcinomas may spread far along the perineural lymphatics so that wide resection and reconstruction is necessary. Unfortunately, metastatic blood-borne spread may occur, leading to pulmonary tumour deposits. Mucoepidermoid carcinomas may be of low- or high-grade malignancy but again require wide excision. Radiotherapy is not often used because of the relatively slow growth rate and resultant radioresistance of salivary gland cancers.

The major salivary glands

Disorders of the major salivary glands requiring surgery include obstructions to salivary flow, infections and neoplasms. The surgical procedures available to treat these disorders are listed in Box 16.2.

Investigation of major salivary glands

Presentation and diagnosis

The clinician should record the presence of pain, swelling, altered salivary flow and a bad taste. The periodicity and duration of the swelling is often of great assistance in making a diagnosis. Clinical examination and gland palpation helps to determine the presence and nature of glandular swelling, tenderness and the presence of fixation, ulceration or local nerve involvement.

Box 16.2   Surgery of the major salivary glands

- Removal/Destruction of calculi
- Duct dilatation or repositioning
- Excision of sublingual gland
- Excision of submandibular gland
- Parotidectomy: superficial, total

Intraoral examination allows a subjective assessment of whether an increase or decrease in salivary flow is present. However, this is difficult to confirm except by physiological measurements, which are not always easy to perform.

Probing the ducts can be carried out with care to dilate strictures. A stepwise increase in the size of the probes is used. Salivary flow rates can be recorded for the submandibular and parotid glands following initial milking of the ducts and glands.

Obstructive sialadenitis or tumour formation may also arise in the accessory lobe of the parotid gland, giving rise to a firm nodular swelling within the cheek in the parotid duct region.

Plain radiography

Plain radiographs often reveal the presence of radiopaque calculi. The submandibular gland can be examined using dental panoramic tomography or lateral oblique projections of the mandible with occlusal views to show the duct. Parotid gland calculi may be visualised on soft tissue postero-anterior views of the mandible with the central ray directed parallel to the ramus of the mandible (Figure 16.5). Dental panoramic tomography shows both parotid and submandibular gland regions, but definitive diagnosis usually requires more specialised investigation.

Ultrasound

Non-invasive head and neck ultrasound techniques have improved dramatically in recent years and are now routinely performed to identify calculi, confirm glandular swelling and identify abnormal gland structure, distinguishing obstructive damage from tumour formation.

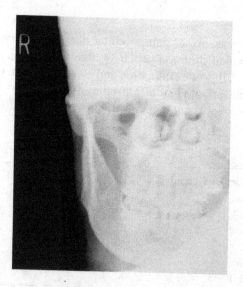

Figure 16.5 Soft tissue postero-anterior radiograph of mandible showing calculus in right parotid gland.

CT scanning/MR imaging

Modern imaging techniques such as computed tomography (CT) scanning and magnetic resonance imaging (MRI) are readily available in hospital radiology departments and are routinely performed in assessing tumour masses in salivary glands. This is particularly relevant in identifying the relationship of parotid lesions to the facial nerve, delineating benign tumour capsules from irregular malignant tumour margins and the presence of any associated cervical lymphadenopathy (Figure 16.6).

Sialography

This is an invasive radiological investigation that involves passing a fine cannula into a duct orifice followed by injection of radiopaque contrast medium to outline the ductal architecture. Its main advantage is the ability to illustrate filling defects, duct stenosis or dilatation proximal to localised obstruction (Figure 16.7). Sialography may also be therapeutic by flushing out minor calculi,

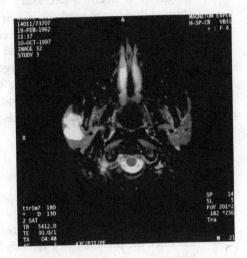

Figure 16.6   MR scan showing 'dumb-bell'-shaped right parotid tumour (pleomorphic adenoma).

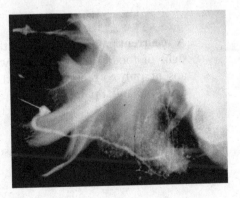

Figure 16.7   Sialogram of submandibular salivary gland and duct.

grit or mucous plugs during the investigation. Emptying of the contrast media from the gland also allows assessment of gland function which is helpful in assessing long-,term prognosis. The procedure must not be used, however, where there is acute infection in the gland.

Scintiscanning

This investigation has the advantage of examining all major salivary glands together. An intravenous injection of technetium is performed and the isotope is concentrated by the salivary glands. The head of the scanner picks up the radiation emissions producing a picture of the glands. Differential lack of isotope uptake helps identify specific gland disease.

Biopsy

Minor salivary gland excision biopsies may be performed if Sjogren's syndrome or other connective tissue disorders are suspected and histopathological diagnosis is deemed necessary. Major gland biopsies are not routinely performed due to the ready access in clinic of fine needle aspiration (FNA), which provides diagnostic cytology specimens without the risk of tumour seeding or salivary fistulae. Using an aseptic technique, a wide-bore needle, 18–20 gauge, is inserted into the gland. The target lesion is fixed between the index finger and thumb and the needle aimed in the direction of the shortest distance to the lesion. The lesion is aspirated and the cellular contents deposited onto a glass slide and fixed immediately. This can then be examined histologically in the normal way.

Obstructions to salivary flow

Aetiology

Obstruction may be due to stenosis of the duct papilla, sialadenitis, stricture of the duct, the presence of a salivary calculi or pressure on the duct from a nearby lesion.

Presentation

A recurrent painful swelling of the gland may be associated with meals or the sight of food. The swelling slowly goes down when the salivary stimulus is absent, only to recur at the next meal. Calculi can often be directly palpated using bimanual palpation.

Special investigations

These include radiography, ultrasound, sialography and judicious probing using lacrimal dilators.

Treatment of obstructions

Papillary stenosis

This more often affects the parotid papilla following trauma from dentures or the cusps of adjacent teeth. The submandibular duct may be affected where a salivary calculus causes chronic ulceration near the orifice. Treatment is by slitting the duct from its orifice for a short distance along its length and carefully suturing the margins to the surrounding mucosa.

A stricture remote from the papilla is not uncommon, though the cause if unrelated to trauma is not always clear. The stricture may be dilated using a series of dilators along the duct, but if this fails the stoppage is bypassed by surgery to bring the duct into the mouth proximal to the obstruction. Parotid strictures may require part of the duct to be reconstructed using a mucosal graft.

Sialolithiasis

Siaoliths, calculi or stones are more common in the submandibular duct, almost three times more frequent than in the parotid.

Submandibular calculi

The common sites include the anterior two-thirds of the duct, the posterior third at the distal border of the mylohyoid muscle and within the gland itself. They are frequently seen as a yellow palpable swelling, tender when inflamed or infected, which can be felt on bimanual palpation intra- and extraorally. Their presence should be confirmed by radiography, usually a lower occlusal radiograph (Figure 16.8).

When an acute infection is present first-line treatment requires antibiotic therapy even if the stone can be removed immediately. Stones in the anterior two-thirds of the duct may be removed under local anaesthesia through an incision made parallel to the duct in the floor of the mouth. First the stone

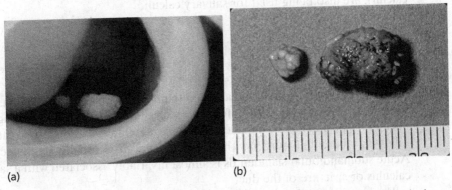

(a)   (b)

Figure 16.8   (a) Radiograph of salivary calculus in submandibular duct; (b) calculus after removal.

is accurately localised by palpation. A suture is then passed deep to the duct and posterior to the stone and tied fairly tight to prevent the sialolith moving back towards the gland. The assistant should push up the floor of the mouth from below to improve access. Blunt dissection is performed to identify the calculus. The duct is incised and the stone removed. A false opening is required where the incision was made. Small incisions are usually left open, but large ones may be partially closed and where necessary a drain is used to create a new orifice. Stimulation of saliva flow is important to keep the new opening patent.

Stones in the posterior part of the duct are more difficult to remove. Careful dissection must be performed to avoid damage to the lingual nerve, which crosses the duct in this region. Stones in the submandibular gland which cause symptoms are best treated by excising the gland. Complications of gland removal may include scarring, facial nerve palsy or lingual paraesthesia.

Parotid calculi

Parotid calculi may occur anywhere in the duct or gland. They are often poorly calcified and not easily seen on plain radiographs. Calculi in the duct can be removed through an intraoral approach, but the course of the duct through the buccinator muscle makes the operation difficult. Stones lodged in the gland usually produce minor symptoms and are best left untreated; others may have to be removed by excision of the part of the parotid gland in which they lie.

Non-invasive techniques

Newer, minimally invasive endoscopic and basket retrieval techniques are being introduced to aid calculus retrieval from within ducts, although these are often only available at specialist centres. Ultrasound and shockwave therapies, successful in the destruction of calculi at other sites in the body (such as renal calculi), are also being used for salivary calculi.

Infection

Acute sialadenitis

The parotid is more commonly affected than the submandibular gland and the sublingual is rarely affected. Infection reaches the parotid gland through the duct. Predisposing factors include xerostomia, debilitation or disturbed function following abdominal surgery. The causal organism is usually staphylococcus. Acute submandibular sialadenitis is almost invariably associated with a salivary calculus or stricture of the duct.

The gland is swollen, tender or painful and the patient is febrile. In the submandibular gland pus may be seen discharging from the duct. The floor of the mouth on the affected side is red and swollen. The parotid gland rarely discharges pus through the duct, though the papilla is often inflamed and viral sialadenitis (e.g. mumps) should be excluded.

Patients with severe gland infections should be admitted to hospital. Initially, vigorous antibiotic therapy is instituted and, where indicated, incision and drainage is performed. A salivary fistula is one of the complications. An incision a little way from the site of entry into the gland should avoid this. Oral hygiene should be carefully supervised. Where there is no obvious cause, a prolonged course of an antibacterial drug may be prescribed.

Chronic sialadenitis

Chronic sialadenitis commonly follows an acute attack and may result from prolonged obstruction to salivary flow. In the parotid gland it may be accompanied by sialectasis seen on sialography as dilatations of the ducts.

Treatment involves removal of any suspected underlying cause. Dilation of strictures to encourage salivary flow can be performed using lacrimal dilators. Careful use of antibiotic therapy may be required. If unsuccessful, excision of the submandibular gland is advised. Excision of the parotid gland is deferred whenever possible because of the danger to the facial nerve.

Tumours

Neoplasia usually presents as a non-tender swelling within the gland. The parotid gland is most often the site of tumours, the commonest of which is the pleomorphic adenoma, occurring 10 times more often than in the submandibular gland. Benign lesions are treated by local excision. Wide excision of a pleomorphic adenoma should include tumour outgrowths outside the capsule, which reduces the likelihood of recurrence. Malignant lesions require more extensive resection, with facial nerve preservation wherever possible. If directly involved with tumour, however, the facial nerve may have to be sacrificed and nerve grafting or facial reanimation surgery carried out.

Presentation and diagnosis

Benign tumours such as the pleomorphic adenoma present as slowly enlarging, persistent, painless swellings. They are not fixed to the skin or underlying structures and are usually mobile, rubbery, hard nodules arising within the gland. Imaging techniques such as CT or MR scanning delineate the extent and position of the tumour, while sialography shows a filling defect with obliteration of normal duct structure.

Malignant tumours in contrast usually enlarge quickly, with additional sinister symptoms such as pain, numbness, ulceration and trismus. Growth involving the facial nerve leads to facial weakness. Fine needle aspiration may be carried out to obtain a cytological diagnosis of malignancy, but open 'diagnostic biopsy' may be contraindicated as it can lead to tumour seeding and spread of the disease.

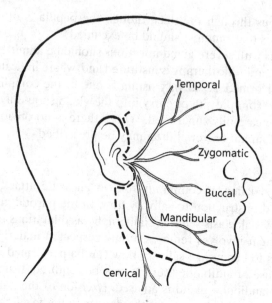

Figure 16.9 Surgical approaches to major salivary glands. The approach to the parotid is an extended preauricular incision. The submandibular incision should be placed 2.5 cm below the lower border to avoid branches of the facial nerve.

Treatment of tumours

The treatment of choice for lesions in the superficial lobe of the parotid is to excise the tumour with a wide margin of normal tissue (superficial parotidectomy), or in the submandibular gland to excise the whole gland.

Excision of the submandibular gland

A skin crease incision about 5 cm long is made in the neck about 2.5 cm below the lower border of the mandible to avoid the mandibular branch of the facial nerve (Figure 16.9). The underlying fascia and platysma are divided. The facial vessels are detected and ligated. Careful dissection is used to separate the gland from the connective tissue. In long-standing chronic conditions dissection may be difficult due to fibrosis. The facial artery has to be ligated again on the posterior aspect of the gland. Superiorly the lingual nerve, which may be embedded in the capsule, is carefully dissected from the duct. The duct is ligated as near the mouth as possible and cut. Calculi present within the gland or duct should be removed with the specimen to prevent further infection. A vacuum drain is inserted before closure to reduce postoperative swelling (see Chapter 7).

Surgery of the parotid gland (superficial parotidectomy)

The approach to the parotid gland is made through a sigmoid, preauricular incision extending from the temporal region to below the lobe of the ear, around the angle of the mandible and into a skin crease in the neck 2.5 cm below the

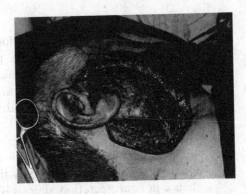

Figure 16.10   Operative photograph showing skin flap reflection during superficial parotidectomy.

lower border of mandible (Figure 16.9). A facial skin flap is taken forward to expose the gland (Figure 16.10). The facial nerve that runs in the substance of the gland must be identified and dissected from the gland, every effort being made to avoid production of facial weakness or paralysis. Dissection of parotid tissue from the facial nerve effectively excises both superficial gland and tumour, without compromising or rupturing the tumour capsule. With deeper sited or malignant tumours, a total parotidectomy may be required and on occasion facial nerve branches may have to be sacrificed to ensure tumour clearance. The auriculotemporal nerve may be damaged during parotid surgery, leading to a condition called Frey's syndrome, a profuse and embarrassing facial sweating that the patient suffers when salivating.

Specific conditions

Mumps

An acute, contagious viral parotitis usually caused by a paramyxovirus leading to salivary gland swelling, which commonly affects children under 15 years of age. The parotid is most often involved bilaterally, although unilateral mumps is described. Treatment is supportive, involving bedrest, analgesics and the encouragement of increased fluid intake.

Necrotising sialometaplasia

This unusual condition presents at the junction of the hard and soft palate and clinically and histologically can be mistaken for a malignancy. It is commonly unilateral and presents as an extensive, deep, crater-like ragged ulcer, which is usually painless. The condition is usually self-limiting over a period of 4 to 8 weeks. Antiseptic and local anaesthetic mouthwashes can be used if required.

Radiation sialadenitis

A common complication of head and neck radiotherapy, this irreversible acinar atrophy and fibrosis leads to severe xerostomia, radiation caries and chronic oral mucosal infection.

Sarcoidosis

This is a systemic chronic granulomatous disorder that most commonly affects young adults and may affect the parotid gland in approximately 6% of cases. There is persistent, diffuse painless gland enlargement and xerostomia. The combination of uveitis, parotitis and facial palsy in sarcoidosis is known as uveoparotid fever or Heerfordt syndrome.

Sialosis

A condition characterised by a non-inflammtory, non-neoplastic, recurrent, bilateral swelling of particularly the parotid glands. Probably due to a disturbance in neurosecretion, sialosis is associated with diabetes, alcoholism, eating disorders and a variety of drugs.

Sjögren's syndrome

This is a chronic autoimmune disease in which lymphocytic infiltration and acinar destruction of lacrimal and salivary glands leads to dry eyes and xerostomia. Bilateral parotid gland enlargement may occur and there is a risk long term of lymphoma development in affected glands. There is usually an associated autoimmune connective tissue disorder such as rheumatoid arthritis. Diagnosis is both from clinical presentation and identification of specific autoantibodies.

Further reading

Cawson RA, Langdon JD, Eveson JW (1996) *Surgical Pathology of the Mouth and Jaws.* Wright, Oxford.

Soames JV, Southam JC (2005) *Oral Pathology*, 4th edn. Oxford University Press, Oxford.

Chapter 17
Temporomandibular Disorders (TMDs) and Chronic Orofacial Pain

> - Broad overview of chronic orofacial pain conditions other than TMDs
> - Temporomandibular disorders (TMDs)
> - Trismus
> - Pathological states related to the temporomandibular joint

Surgery of the temporomandibular joint (TMJ) is indicated in only a tiny percentage of those presenting with symptoms from this structure. The TMJ and its supporting structures are however involved in a disproportionate number of referrals for management to oral surgery.

This chapter aims to give the reader a broad overview and understanding of the more commonly presenting chronic orofacial pain conditions with a specific focus on, Temporomandibular disorders (TMDs) which probably account for the largest proportion of the chronic pain referrals to oral surgery.

The chapter will firstly briefly outline the three other commonly presenting chronic orofacial pain conditions in order to allow the reader to distinguish between these and TMDs.

Broad overview of chronic orofacial pain conditions other than TMDs

Trigeminal neuralgia

This is defined by the International Association of Pain as 'a sudden, usually unilateral, severe, brief, stabbing, recurrent pain in the distribution of one or more branches of the fifth cranial nerve'. Triggers often include cold air or tactile stimulation of the area affected, for instance shaving or applying make-up. There is a female preponderance in the fifth and sixth decades of life and it most commonly occurs in maxillary or mandibular division of the trigeminal nerve.

Principles of Oral and Maxillofacial Surgery, 6th Edition. Edited by U. J. Moore
© 2011 Blackwell Publishing Ltd

Aetiology

Vascular compression of the trigeminal nerve root can sometimes be identified, while some cases are secondary to pathology such as multiple sclerosis (MS) or intracranial tumours. Cases attributable to vascular compression or with no identifiable pathology are classified as 'classical' trigeminal neuralgia, and those with identifiable pathology other than vascular compression are classified as 'secondary' trigeminal neuralgia.

Investigations

A thorough clinical history and examination including cranial nerve testing (see Chapter 1) is necessary before considering magnetic resonance imaging (MRI) to exclude intracranial causes:

- a space occupying lesion
- MS in patients presenting before 40 years of age
- a vascular loop compressing the trigeminal nerve root at the pons.

Management

Medical management

In the absence of any causative factors on an MRI, the drug of choice remains carbamezapine. Before starting carbamezapine the following tests should be taken: full blood count, urea and electrolytes, and liver function. These will help identify any pre-existing abnormalities and provide a baseline from which to measure any side effects of therapy. Haematinics should be repeated at intervals until therapy is discontinued.

Carbamezapine is started at 100 mg twice daily and increased in 100 mg increments gradually over a number of days until control is achieved. A maximum of 1200 mg/day can be given in divided doses. Alternatives prescribed in specialist centres include oxcarbazepine, gabapentin and phenytoin.

Surgical management

Neurosurgical management involves microvascular decompression, separating the trigeminal root from any vascular loop compressing it. Alternative surgical management includes gamma knife therapy and peripheral nerve procedures.

Burning mouth syndrome (BMS)

BMS is defined by the American Academy of Orofacial pain as 'a common dysaesthesia described as a burning sensation in the oral mucosa'.

Presentation

The tongue is commonly affected, but any part of the oral mucosa may be involved. Two subtypes have been delineated:

1 primary BMS – where no predisposing or exacerbating pathology, or deficiency can be found.
2 secondary BMS – where pathology or deficiency can be identified as exacerbating or causing the complaint. This subtype has a female preponderance in the fourth to fifth decades of life.

Primary BMS

The aetiology of this subtype is unknown, but recently a pathophysiological cascade theory has been proposed.

Secondary BMS

Factors identified that can exacerbate or cause the complaint include: candidosis; vitamin B_{12}, folate or ferritin deficiency; diabetic neuropathy; inadequate tongue space in complete dentures; drug reactions, e.g. ACE inhibitors; xerostomia.

Investigation

A thorough clinical history and examination including cranial nerve testing should give a good basis for diagnosis. Any of the factors related to secondary BMS need to be excluded, through careful history and examination, drug history, haematinics, random glucose and microbiological swabs.

Treatment

If factors related to secondary BMS are present, an appropriate referral should be arranged and the symptoms reviewed following this. If symptoms persist or there is no organic factor identified initially, consideration should be given to referring the patient to a specialist for cognitive behavioural therapy or pharmacotherapy.

A recent systematic review of pharmacotherapy has suggested that topical benzodiazepines may be of merit but that the use of systemic tricyclic antidepressants is not well supported by evidence.

Persistent idiopathic orofacial pain (atypical facial pain, atypical odontalgia)

This is defined by the International Headache Society as a 'persistent facial pain that does not have the characteristics of the cranial neuralgias and is not attributed to another disorder'.

Presentation

Patients present with poorly localised deep pain that does not follow anatomically defined patterns. The pain normally persists for the majority of the day and lacks consistency in its aggravating or relieving factors, while thorough investigation reveals no overt abnormality. Patients may have had multiple dental treatments to try and remove the pain. There is a female preponderance in the third to fourth decades.

Aetiology

The cause is unknown.

Investigation

A thorough clinical history and examination including cranial nerve testing to exclude any underlying pathology should be undertaken. An odontogenic cause should be excluded through careful examination, testing and, if indicated, radiographs of the dentition.

Management

If atypical pain is suspected the patient should be referred for specialist opinion and management. Irreversible or invasive procedures should not be undertaken on teeth to try and relieve the pain if the clinical picture, vitality testing or radiographic examination would not support the procedure. Specialist management will involve cognitive behavioural therapy with or without systemic pharmacotherapy, which may involve polypharmacy.

Temporomandibular disorders (TMDs)

Definition

'A *collective* term embracing a number of clinical problems that involve the masticatory musculature, the temporomandibular joint and associated structures, or both' (American Academy of Orofacial Pain).

For the clinician treating TMDs it is paramount to have an appreciation that TMDs are a group of chronic illnesses, which largely follow a benign course and mostly respond favourably to conservative therapy.

TMDs have been previously known by a number of other terms: Costen's syndrome, pain dysfunction syndrome, facial arthromyalgia, temporomandibular joint dysfunction. These terms are mentioned as some clinicians still persist in using them, although at the time of writing the accepted terminology for the group of conditions is TMDs.

Aetiology

The aetiology of TMDs is still undetermined, although five main factors have been suggested:

- parafunctional activities
- occlusal factors
- deep pain input
- trauma
- emotional stress (Okeson, 2003).

Invasive treatment of any of these factors in isolation is unlikely to produce success and conservative reversible therapy remains, therefore, the mainstay in treatment of TMDs.

Presentation, diagnosis and investigation

Patients can present with a variety of signs and symptoms including:

- clicking or crepitus in the temporomandibular joint (TMJ)
- pain or tenderness in the muscles of mastication or TMJ
- reduced mouth opening
- earache (related to pain in the TMJ)
- headache (related to pain in the temporalis muscles).

There is a larger proportion (20–45%) of the general population with signs and symptoms of TMDs than those that present for treatment (2–4%) and of those presenting the female:male ratio is 7:1. The age range of presentation is from the second to fourth decades. Those presenting in higher age ranges should be viewed with a greater degree of suspicion as TMDs are less likely to present late in life and there maybe another causative pathology that is mimicking the symptoms.

Established research diagnostic criteria (RDC) for TMDs take a dual axis approach to diagnosis (axis I – physical; axis II – psychosocial). The RDC/TMD physical diagnosis of TMDs falls into three main groups:

- group I – myofascial pain
- group II – disc displacements
- group III – other common joint disorders.

A modified, quicker, version of the RDC/TMD, the clinical examination protocol for TMD (CEP-TMD) has emerged. The CEP-TMD results in a RDC/TMD physical diagnoses (Box 17.1) and the examination form and process can be viewed online (see Further reading).

Diagnosis of TMDs is mainly based on clinical examination using protocols such as CEP-TMD or RDC/TMD, and plain radiographs are now rarely indicated except when signs and symptoms are suggestive of a more serious/sinister pathology, or when monitoring the progression/response to treatment of systemic pathologies such as rheumatoid arthritis. CT or cone beam CT would again be indicated by findings suggestive of a more sinister/serious pathology. Magnetic resonance imaging is accepted as the gold standard for examining articular disc derangements.

Management

Management can be divided into conservative (reversible) therapy and irreversible therapy. With the paucity of reliable evidence to support or refute treatments, especially irreversible, the consensus has become to institute conservative

Box 17.1   Diagnostic criteria for the CEP-TMD

Group	Criteria
Muscle disorders	
Myofascial pain Key: Painful muscles	1. Reported pain in masticatory muscles[1] 2. Pain on palpation in at least three sites[2], one of them at least in the same side of the reported pain
Myofascial pain with limited opening Key: Painful muscles + limited movement	1. Myofascial pain 2. Pain-free unassisted[3] opening < 40 mm 3. Passive[4] stretch ≥ 5 mm (from pain-free unassisted opening to 'painful' assisted opening)
Disc displacements	

Disc displacement with reduction
Key: Reproducible clicking
	1. No pain in the joint neither reported nor on palpation
	2. Reproducible[5] click on any excursion[6] with either opening or closing click
	3. With click on opening and closing (unless excursive click confirmed):
	  • click on opening occurs at ≥5 mm interincisal distance than on closing
	  • clicks eliminated by protrusive opening

Disc displacement without reduction with limited opening Key: Limited opening with no clicking	1. History of locking or catching that interfered with eating 2. Absence of TMJ clicking meeting DDR criteria 3. Unassisted 'painful' opening ≤35 mm 4. Passive stretch <5 mm (from 'painful' unassisted opening to 'painful' assisted opening) 5. Contralateral excursion <7 mm or uncorrected ipsilateral deviation on opening
Disc displacement without reduction without limited opening Key: History of previously limited opening – imaging needed to confirm DD	1. History of locking or catching that interfered with eating 2. The presence of TMJ sounds excluding DDR clicking 3. Unassisted 'painful' opening >35 mm 4. Passive stretch ≥5 mm (from 'painful' unassisted opening to 'painful' assisted opening) 5. Contralateral excursion ≥7 mm 6. Optional imaging (arthrography or MRI) to confirm DD
Other common joint problems	
Arthralgia Key: Painful TMJ/no crepitus	1. Pain on TMJ palpation either laterally or intra-auricular 2. Self-reported joint pain with or without jaw movement 3. Absence of crepitus and possibility of clicking

Box 17.1 (Continued)

Group	Criteria
Osteoarthritis Key: Painful TMJ + crepitus	1. Pain as for arthralgia (reported and on palpation) 2. Crepitus on any movement or tomogram evidence of joint changes[7]
Osteoarthrosis Key: Non-painful TMJ + crepitus	1. Crepitus on any movement or tomogram evidence of joint changes[7] 2. No reported joint pain, neither on palpation nor on any movement

[1] In the jaw, temples, face, preauricular area or inside the ear, at rest or function.
[2] There are 20 sites (10 on each side): posterior, middle and anterior temporalis; origin, body and insertion of masseter; posterior mandibular region; submandibular region; lateral pterygoid; tendon of temporalis.
[3] Interincisal opening plus overbite or interincisal opening minus anterior open bite.
[4] Passive stretch: the examiner's index and thumb are used to moderately force the mouth to open wider than unassisted opening. Patients are instructed to raise a hand to signal when the stretch becomes too uncomfortable.
[5] All clicks must be reproduced two out of three consecutive trials.
[6] Contra- or ipsilateral or protrusive.
[7] Erosion of cortical delineation, sclerosis of parts or all the condyle and articular eminence, flattening of joint surfaces, osteophyte formation.
There is an online resource showing the examination process for CEP-TMD at: www.ncl.ac.uk/dental/AppliedOcclusion/ (last accessed 25 May 2010).

(reversible) therapy as the initial management for all patients with TMDs due mainly to its high success rate in the majority of patients.

Conservative reversible therapy

All management should be prefaced by a careful and thorough explanation of, and reassurance over, the diagnosis of TMDs and the disorder's benign nature.

Conservative management can include any of the following either in isolation or in combination, dependent on the nature of the patients' complaint.

- Biobehavioural treatment. For example: stress management; relaxation strategies; habit modification – stop nail biting, pen top chewing, chewing gum excessively.
- Physiotherapy – self-physiotherapy through simple exercises and professional physiotherapy. The latter may involve manual therapy, acupuncture, local application of moist heat or ice, more advanced exercises or postural training.
- Simple pharmacotherapy – the use of non-steroidal anti-inflammatory drugs in patients with no contraindications may help in the early stages of TMDs.
- Advanced pharmacotherapy – in specialist clinics consideration will be given to the use of tricyclic antidepressants and other systemic pharmacotherapy for myofascial pain complaints.

- Simple splint therapy – the use of a lower soft 'suck down' splint at night time can be as effective as any other advanced type of splint and probably should be considered the first-line appliance to be made. It should be noted, however, that a lower soft splint can exacerbate a minority of individuals' complaint, but that this normally resolves with cessation of the use of the splint.
- Advanced splint therapy – this can include the anterior repositioning splint and the stabilisation splint. Full coverage appliances are favoured to reduce the risk of occlusal changes.
- Simple occlusal modification – this is limited to the removal of really gross interferences. A good example is TMDs clearly precipitated by the insertion of a new crown, denture or bridge within the recent past. It is likely in this case that the prosthesis is interfering and should be adjusted accordingly.

Irreversible therapy

Irreversible therapy is *very* rarely indicated due to the high success rate of conservative reversible therapy. There are two main types of irreversible therapy.

- Occlusal therapy – the equilibration of occlusal contacts so they are evenly distributed around the arch.
- TMJ surgery – there are several procedures historically associated with arthritic or disc displacement TMDs' subdiagnoses.

The indications for irreversible therapy are difficult to define, especially in the case of occlusal therapy. The indications for TMJ surgery have been suggested as absolute and relative.

Absolute indications include:

- some types of trauma
- organic pathology of TMJ
- developmental abnormalities of TMJ
- ankylosis.

Relative indications for TMJ surgery are harder to define and the failure of conservative reversible therapy should not automatically be assumed to be an indication for surgery.

The least invasive surgical procedures are arthroscopy and arthocentesis. Both these procedures involve the introduction of either instruments (-scopy) or needles (-centesis) into the *upper* joint space. The most frequent conditions these procedures might be used for are disc displacements or arthritic complaints of the TMJ. Both arthocentesis and arthroscopy can be used to perform lysis and lavage of the joint space. Arthroscopy's added value is that it can be used to perform some limited disc surgery.

Arthroplasty procedures (open TMJ surgery) such as disc repositioning or plication, discectomy, condylar shaves, etc., for TMDs are now rare but would involve similar surgical approaches to the temporomandibular joint as described later in this chapter.

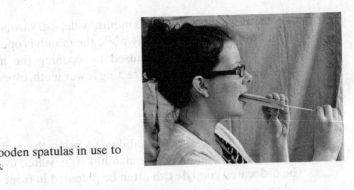

Figure 17.1 Wooden spatulas in use to improve trismus.

Trismus

This is defined as an inability to open the mouth normally. Trismus, together with pain and clicking, is one of the commonest symptoms associated with the temporomandibular joint (TMJ). As trismus is a **symptom**, *its cause should always be carefully sought, diagnosed and treated*.

Persistent trismus may occur due to tumours, intra-articular fibrosis or bony ankylosis following trauma, infection or certain diseases such as rheumatoid arthritis. It may also be secondary to extra-articular fibrosis or scarring.

Intra-articular bony or fibrous ankylosis must be treated by surgery, either by removal of the condyle (condylectomy) or by cutting through the neck of the condyle (condylotomy). In gross cases of bony ankylosis consideration may need to be given to a costachondral graft to reconstruct the condyle or a total joint replacement.

Trismus due to rheumatoid arthritis, ankylosing spondylitis or to extra-articular scarring may benefit from treatment with mechanical exercisers. Wooden spatulae in increasing numbers may be inserted between the teeth each day (Figure 17.1).

In more severe conditions the jaws are prised apart with Mason's gags used bilaterally under a general anaesthetic. Impressions are taken and an exerciser can be fitted, e.g. Therabite. Once a satisfactory opening (2.5–3.5 cm measured between the incisor teeth) has been obtained, this can be maintained by either the exerciser or by using wooden spatulae for about 10 minutes each day for 6 months.

Pathological states related to the temporomandibular joint

Dislocation of the TMJ

Dislocation of the condyle occurs usually in a forward direction over the articular eminence, and is often bilateral. The predisposing cause is laxness of the capsule and associated ligaments of the joint, which allow for excessive movement when opening the mouth wide, e.g. yawning. A blow can also dislocate normal joints, particularly while the mouth is open. Under a general anaesthetic dislocation can be caused by opening the mouth with a gag, or by downward pressure when extracting lower teeth, especially if the support to the jaw is inadequate.

Diagnosis

The patient complains of inability to bring the teeth together. In unilateral dislocation the midline of the mandible is deviated towards the unaffected side. The dislocated condyle can often be palpated in front of the articular eminence and radiographs will confirm this position.

Treatment

If reduction is attempted immediately it can usually be achieved without difficulty. However, if some time has elapsed muscle spasm may make reduction difficult and the use of an intravenous benzodiazepine or a general anaesthetic may be indicated. The operator places their thumbs (protected from the teeth by binding with gauze or by the use of tongue spatulas underneath them) over the external oblique line, retromolar fossa or molar teeth of the mandible on each side. The remaining fingers are cupped under the chin. While the thumbs press down very slowly, the fingers lift up the chin to slip the condyle head back over the eminentia. Often one side will reduce more easily, which facilitates the reduction of the second side.

The patient should be encouraged to relax their masticatory musculature during the attempted relocation of the condyle(s), because their natural reaction to the pressure applied by the clinician will be to contract their masticatory musculature, making the relocation more difficult. Asking the patient to consciously attempt to yawn inhibits the contraction of the jaw-closing musculature that may be preventing relocation. Once the condyles are relocated a crepe barrel bandage can be placed temporarily for 24 hours to help reduce the chance of immediate re-dislocation.

Chronic recurrent dislocation

Where the capsule is very slack the condyle may dislocate several times a day. Many affected patients can reduce their mandibles at will, but others require it to be done for them.

Surgery can be used for these chronic cases using one of two approaches to the problem.

- Reducing the range of movement of the condyle. This includes: down-fracture of zygomatic arch (Le-Clerc procedure); grafts to the articular eminetia; injection of sclerosing agents, e.g. autologous blood in to the joint space.
- Allowing the condyle to freely dislocate and relocate by performing eminectomies.

Arthritis of TMJ

There are multiple arthritic complaints that can potentially affect the TMJ. In the following section the two most commonly presenting arthritides affecting the TMJ will be covered: osteoarthritis (degenerative) and rheumatoid arthritis (inflammatory).

Osteoarthritis of TMJ

Osteoarthritis is part of the TMDs subgroup but is covered here for continuity and clarity.

Osteoarthritis is a degenerative condition of the articulating surfaces of the joint causing fibrillation of the cartilage (vertical splitting of the cartilage) covering the condylar head, exposure of subchondral bone and possible osteophyte lipping of the condylar head. One of the hypothesised causes of osteoarthritis in the TMJ is overloading of the joint, possibly through parafunctional activity, e.g. bruxism. Once loading of the joint is decreased the affected joint starts to adapt but the bony contour remains altered. This adaptive state is known as osteoarthrosis and clinically is distinguished from osteoarthritis through the fact that it lacks the pain associated with osteoarthritis.

Radiographic epidemiological studies have shown osteoarthritic degenerative lesions affecting the TMJ to be widespread among normal populations. However, patients only tend to present for treatment when they experience pain, possibly from a transient inflammatory episode.

Management of osteoarthritis is directed towards relieving symptoms and prevention of further degeneration. Conservative reversible therapy is the mainstay of management and consideration maybe given to dietary supplements such as glucosamine (not for those allergic to shellfish).

When the pathological changes are extremely advanced, more invasive procedures may be indicated. Those invasive procedures may include: arthrocentesis/scopy; a condylar shave (condylotomy) to reshape condylar head/remove the diseased condylar bone.

Rheumatoid arthritis of TMJ

Rheumatoid arthritis is not part of the TMDs subgroup. It is a chronic inflammatory disease affecting joints all around the body. It occurs in about 3% of the population, with a female preponderance.

Rheumatoid arthritis causes a synovitis to occur within the affected joint with consequent proliferation of the synovial tissues. The proliferation causes vascular hyperplastic folds of synovial tissues (pannus) to cover the joint surface leading to erosion of the bony and articular structures.

A large proportion of patients suffering from rheumatoid arthritis can have involvement of the TMJs but may not complain of symptoms. Symptoms can include trismus, pain and crepitus,. In severe cases occlusal changes can occur as the arthritis causes erosion of the condylar head. The occlusal change most commonly seen is an anterior open bite, although this level of severe disease in the TMJs is uncommon.

Management of rheumatoid arthritis affecting the TMJ is always in liaison with a rheumatologist. In mild or moderate cases management will centre on conservative reversible therapy previously outlined for TMDs but may also involve arthroscopy/centesis with or without steroid injection.

Surgical options for more advanced or severe cases include synovectomy (removal of pannus) and total joint replacement by use of costachondral graft or through alloplastic joints. Arrested disease that has caused occlusal changes may be a candidate for orthognathic surgery, especially in younger age groups.

Tumours of the temporomandibular joint complex

Primary tumours arising from the TMJ complex are rare. Tumours can be benign or malignant and can arise from any part of the TMJ complex and therefore can be: bony, cartilaginous, vascular, neurological, connective tissue or muscular in origin. Secondary metastases to the TMJ complex can occur from breast, liver, kidney, prostate and thyroid.

Despite the rarity of tumours of the TMJ complex the clinician must not let them escape their diagnostic attention. Complicating the situation are tumours occurring outside the TMJ complex that cause symptoms mimicking TMDs, e.g. nasopharyngeal carcinoma. The clinician must, therefore, have a high index of suspicion for neoplasia in any patient presenting with symptoms of TMDs plus any of the following symptoms:

- facial paresis or other cranial nerve involvement
- paraesthesia in the trigeminal dermatomes; swelling overlying TMJ or in ipsilateral lymph nodes
- changes in occlusion or facial symmetry
- persistent unilateral nasal obstruction with or without purulent discharge
- unilateral objective auditory changes
- rhinorrhea
- epistaxis
- anosmia or reduced sense of smell.

Surgical access to the joint

Open joint surgery access

The joint cavity is limited above by the zygomatic arch and posteriorly by the external auditory meatus. Surgery is made difficult by the facial nerve, which passes through the parotid gland (in which it is quite deeply buried) about 2 cm below the zygomatic arch, and by the internal maxillary artery deep to the joint. The approach is by a preauricular incision made in front of the tragus and above the attachment of the lobe of the ear up to the zygomatic arch and then

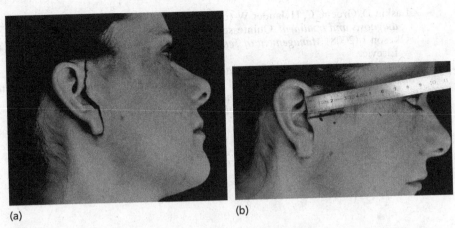

(a)   (b)

Figure 17.2   (a) One of the approaches possible to the TMJ – the preauricular approach. Note incision is designed to avoid facial nerve; (b) optimal entry points for arthrocentesis relative to the tragal-canthal line.

obliquely up and forward for 2 cm, or by a postauricular incision behind the ear which is then drawn forward to expose the joint (Figure 17.2a). The superior part of the parotid gland is drawn down, and the zygomatic arch cleared of the masseter. All stretching of the tissues to gain access is avoided as this may cause a facial nerve weakness.

Arthroscopic and arthocentesis access

The upper joint space is the target for arthoscopy and arthrocentesis. Previous to incising or inserting needles it is mandatory to palpate the joint during its full range of movements to ensure the patient being operated on does not vary from normal anatomical values.

Arthroscopic ports can be placed through small stab incisions (Figure 17.2b) along a line drawn from the middle point of the tragus to the ipsilateral lateral canthus. Variations on the positions shown in Figure 17.2b have been suggested.

Arthocentesis can be carried out by inserting needles through the same two arthoscopic sites, or slightly modified positions.

Further reading

De Leeuw R (ed.) (2008) *Orofacial Pain: guidelines for assessment, diagnosis, and management*, 4th edn. Quintessence Publishing, London.

Dimitroulis G (2005) The role of surgery in the management of disorders of the temporomandibular joint: a critical review of the literature. Part 2. *International Journal of Oral Maxillofacial Surgery* **34**: 231–7.

Gray RJ, Davies SJ, Quayle AA (1994) A clinical approach to temporomandibular disorders. 1. Classification and functional anatomy. *British Dental Journal* **176**: 429–35.

Laskin D, Greene C, Hylander W (eds) (2006) (*TMDs. An evidence-based approach to diagnosis and treatment*. Quintessence Publishing, London.

Okeson J (2008) *Management of Temporomandibular Disorders and Occlusion*. Mosby, Elsevier.

Sharav Y, Benoliel R (eds) *Orofacial Pain and Headache*. Mosby, Elsevier.

Woda A, Dao T, Gremeau-Richard C (2009) Steroid dysregulation and stomatodynia (burning mouth syndrome). *Journal of Orofacial Pain* **23**: 202–10.

Zakrzewska J (ed.) (2009) *Orofacial Pain*. Oxford University Press, Oxford.

Chapter 18
Facial Deformity

- Symmetric facial deformity
- The cleft patient
- Orthognathic surgery
- Asymmetric facial deformity

Facial deformity may be the result of a variety of different causes including congenital disease such as cleft lip and palate, developmental abnormality, trauma and infection. Deformity may also occur either as the direct result of a neoplastic disease or by its treatment, either with surgery or radiotherapy.

Very occasionally deformity may occur with other acquired conditions that may affect facial growth such as juvenile rheumatoid arthritis (Still's disease), or it may occur after growth has ceased as with Paget's disease or other disturbances of bone metabolism such as fibrous dysplasia.

It is also important to remember that the face is comprised of both hard and soft tissue elements, and that deformity may derive from either element, but very often one will impact on the other.

There is an obvious variation in facial form that gives us our individuality and ethnicity. Individuals who fall outside this acceptable range of variation may suffer from being labelled as either unattractive or ugly. This may cause the individual difficulties in social and sexual relationships and may deny certain employment opportunities. More severe facial deformity may cause social exclusion and can be associated with psychological problems.

This chapter aims to deal with the commoner types of facial deformity resulting from jaw growth disharmony, which often presents as malocclusion. The term 'dentofacial' deformity may be used to describe this problem. These problems usually result in symmetric facial deformity and are treated jointly by the maxillofacial surgeon and orthodontist.

The commoner conditions resulting from a disease process are also addressed, such as cleft deformity. Asymmetric facial deformity may result from conditions such as hemifacial microsomia and condylar hyperplasia. Again collaboration between surgeon and orthodontist is required.

Principles of Oral and Maxillofacial Surgery, 6th Edition. Edited by U. J. Moore
© 2011 Blackwell Publishing Ltd

Assessment of facial deformity

History

The patient may identify problems as:

- functional – difficulties associated with the bite, inability to chew or achieve incisor contact
- aesthetic – problems of their appearance as perceived by them, although some patients may be embarrassed to discuss this.

Patients are often referred by orthodontists who are unable to treat the underlying skeletal jaw disproportion by orthodontic means alone.

Examination

The patient is first examined by evaluation of the facial form, both from the profile and full face. It is helpful to divide the face into thirds (see Chapter 14). A full intraoral examination should include the state of the dentition as well as assessment of the occlusion. Poor dental health and hygiene are usually a contraindication to orthognathic surgery.

Radiographs

This includes a full radiographic assessment of the dentition, including impacted and buried teeth, associated pathology including caries and periodontal problems. The lateral cephalostat provides invaluable information for both the surgeon and orthodontist to aid in diagnosis and treatment planning.

Study models

Study models should always be available at the joint consultation; anatomically articulated models are used in the surgical planning.

Photographic records

Photographic records are extremely helpful in treatment planning as well as providing a clinical record. They should include both the face in profile and viewed from the front. Intraorally the occlusion should be shown from both sides and the front, and all photographs should be standardised and of good quality.

Special investigations

In some patients further information may be required, both as part of the diagnosis and in planning treatment. Patients with asymmetric deformity may require special scans; these are discussed below in the relevant section.

Diagnosis

Symmetric facial deformity may be diagnosed and classified according to the facial types shown below. This classification is useful in prescribing the correct form of surgical correction to maximise successful and stable outcomes.

Symmetric facial deformity

Classification

The following is a useful classification of symmetric dentofacial deformity.

- Type A. Class III malocclusion due to either a large mandible or small maxilla (or both). The vertical height of the face is not increased. Treatment may involve moving the mandible posteriorly or the maxilla anteriorly (or both) (Figure 18.1).
- Type B. Class III malocclusion with an anterior open bite. This is due to either a large mandible or a small maxilla (or both). The vertical height of the face is increased. Treatment will always involve superior repositioning of the maxilla to reduce the increased vertical face height, together with posterior repositioning of the mandible (Figure 18.2).
- Type C. Class II malocclusion with a deep overbite. This is due to a small mandible. The lower vertical face height is decreased. Treatment involves a mandibular advancement (Figure 18.3).
- Type D. Class II malocclusion with an anterior open bite. This is caused by an increased vertical growth of the maxilla in a downward direction. The mandible is of a normal size but has been rotated downwards and backwards by clockwise rotation due to the excess downward growth of the maxilla. Treatment involves superior repositioning of the maxilla, following which the mandible autorotates anticlockwise to become normally positioned in relation to the face, and comes into a normal class I occlusion (Figure 18.4).
- Type E. Class II with an anterior open bite. This is similar to Type D; however, the mandible is small and the surgical correction requires a mandibular advancement together with superior repositioning of the maxilla (Figure 18.5).

Treatment planning

At a joint surgical and orthodontic appointment, the orthodontic treatment plan and provisional surgical correction are agreed between the patient and clinicians, and the anticipated outcome discussed. The orthodontic aspects are discussed below.

Final surgical plan

The final surgical plan is formulated following completion of the initial orthodontic phase of treatment. A new cephalostat showing the position of the teeth following this orthodontic treatment is used to accurately plan the surgical procedure. This involves tracing the maxilla and mandible together with the dentition. A number of landmarks and references points are included to allow reproducible measurements.

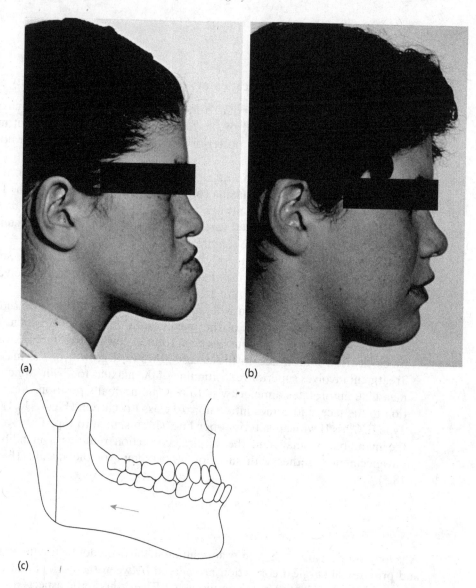

(a)

(b)

(c)

Figure 18.1 Type A. Class III malocclusion. The mandible has been surgically repositioned posteriorly and the maxilla advanced. (a) Preoperative appearance; (b) postoperative appearance; (c) operative scheme.

Presurgical orthodontics

Orthodontic treatment is invariably required prior to undertaking surgery. This normally requires fixed appliances. The orthodontist carries out decompensation of the dentition, together with alignment and co-ordination of the dental arches to allow a satisfactory postoperative occlusion to be obtained. Decompensation involves moving teeth back to their normal alignment and

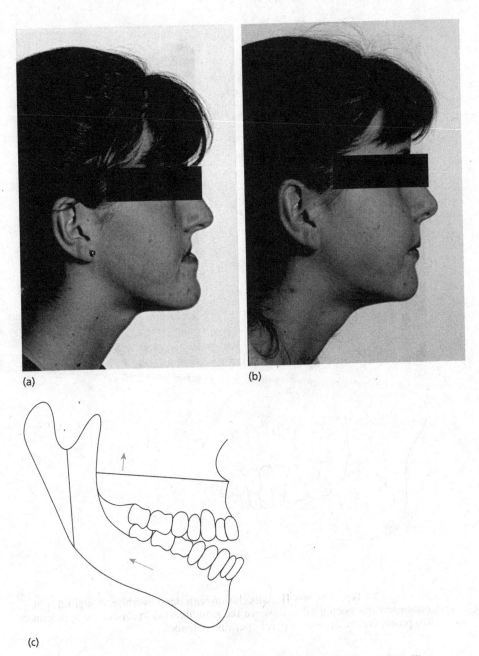

(a)

(b)

(c)

Figure 18.2 Type B. Class III malocclusion with anterior open bite. Bimaxillary procedures have been used to superiorly reposition the maxilla and move the mandible posteriorly. (a) Preoperative appearance; (b) postoperative appearance; (c) operative scheme.

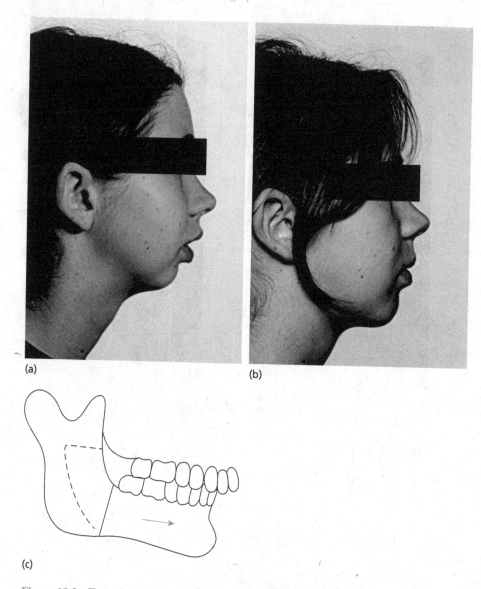

(a)   (b)

(c)

Figure 18.3 Type C. Class II malocclusion with deep overbite. A sagittal split osteotomy has been used to advance the mandible. (a) Preoperative appearance; (b) postoperative appearance; (c) operative scheme.

angulations to the skeletal bases, often revealing the true skeletal problem (Figure 18.6).

In type C cases it is recommended that flattening of the lower occlusal plane is not carried out presurgically. This allows the surgeon to produce a more satisfactory facial profile by lengthening the lower face. The immediate postsurgical occlusion achieved usually consists of 'heel and toe' contacts due to the

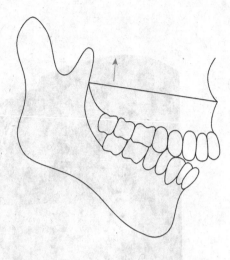

Figure 18.4 Type D. Class II malocclusion with anterior open bite. The maxilla has been superiorly repositioned. Operative scheme.

uncorrected curvature of the lower occlusal plane. Postsurgically the orthodontist is able to extrude teeth into a satisfactory, stable and final occlusion.

Postsurgical orthodontics

This involves fine-tuning of tooth positions in most cases. In type C cases the patient should be aware that a considerable amount of orthodontic treatment is required to establish the final occlusal relationship.

The cleft patient

Midface hypoplasia is commonly associated with cleft lip and palate patients. This is due largely to fibrosis from the primary repair disrupting normal maxillary growth. Thus maxillary advancement osteotomies are often required to establish a more normal facial profile and occlusion.

Alveolar bone grafting

Alveolar bone grafting is often carried out to re-establish continuity of the alveolus and allows eruption of the canine tooth.

Orthodontic considerations

Fixed appliance orthodontic therapy is required and will involve expansion of the contracted maxillary arch.

Special surgical considerations

Fibrosis following the primary surgery may impact on the surgeon's ability to advance the maxilla into a satisfactory position. It is also important to take into account the patient's speech, as nasal speech due to velopharyngeal

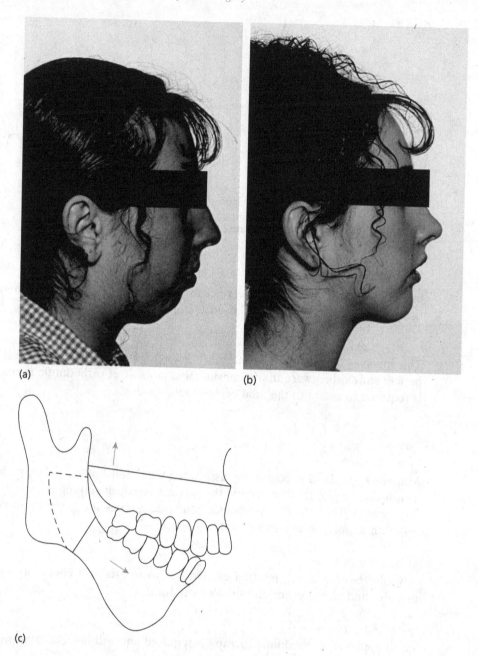

Figure 18.5. Type E. Class II malocclusion with anterior open bite and hypoplastic mandible. A bimaxillary procedure has been performed to superiorly reposition maxilla and advance the mandible. (a) Preoperative appearance; (b) postoperative appearance; (c) operative scheme.

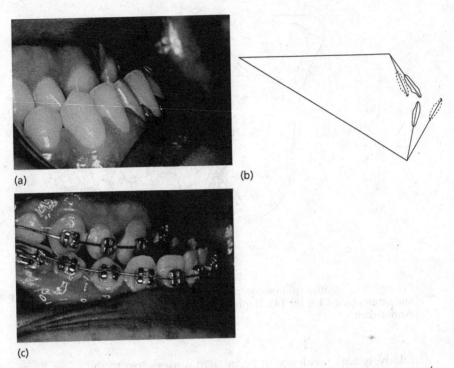

(a)

(b)

(c)

Figure 18.6 Presurgical orthodontics. (a) Prior to treatment; (b) apparent worsening of the malocclusion; (c) decompensation to achieve ideal angulation of the teeth.

incompetence may be exacerbated by maxillary advancement. Oronasal fistulae are often present and maxillary surgery may either produce or enlarge fistulae.

Orthognathic surgery

Orthognathic surgery is surgery to correct facial deformity and the associated malocclusion (ortho = to straighten, gnath = jaws). The surgery involves carrying out bone cuts (osteotomies). Patients are managed jointly by the maxillofacial surgeon and orthodontist and close liaison and joint consultation are essential for optimum outcome of treatment.

Mandibular procedures

Sagittal split osteotomy

A sagittal split osteotomy is used to reposition the mandible anteriorly or posteriorly. The procedure is carried out via an intraoral incision and can be internally fixated with screws or plates. The disadvantage of the procedure is the

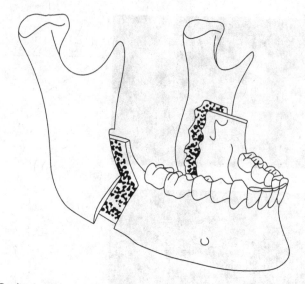

Figure 18.7   Sagittal split osteotomy. The bone cuts can be rigidly fixed using plates and screws (see Chapter 14). Reproduced by kind permission of VU Press, Amsterdam.

relatively high incidence of permanent sensory loss to the lower lip as a result of injury to the inferior alveolar nerve (Figure 18.7).

Vertical subsigmoid osteotomy

Vertical subsigmoid osteotomy is usually performed via an intraoral incision, although previously an extraoral incision was employed. It is only used for posterior repositioning of the mandible, and for minor mandibular asymmetries. It carries a low risk of injury to the mandibular neurovascular bundle. The major disadvantage of the procedure is that internal fixation cannot be applied when the procedure is carried out intraorally and thus intermaxillary fixation is required (Figure 18.8).

Genioplasty

Genioplasty has no effect on the occlusion but is used to adjust the facial appearance by reduction or augmentation of the chin depth and prominence. It can be used to achieve chin symmetry and is performed via an incision in the lower labial sulcus.

Maxillary procedures

Le Fort I osteotomy

The position of the maxilla can be altered in all dimensions except posteriorly. It is performed via an intraoral incision and disarticulation of the maxilla from the facial skeleton is achieved by a series of bone cuts.

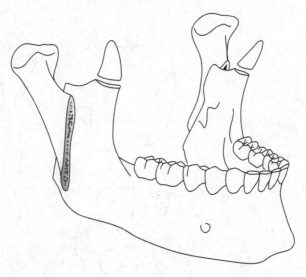

Figure 18.8   Vertical subsigmoid osteotomy. It is difficult to rigidly fix the bone cuts when performed intraorally. IMF must be employed (see Chapter 14). Reproduced by kind permission of VU Press, Amsterdam.

High Le Fort I osteotomy

The height of the bony incision can be raised to give more prominence to the mid part of the face following anterior movements (Figure 18.9).

Maxillomalar advancement

Maxillomalar advancement is used to improve deficient prominence in the region of the cheekbones.

Le Fort II and Le Fort III osteotomy

These follow the fracture lines following facial trauma described by Le Fort (see Chapter 14). They are performed less commonly and are used mainly to treat craniofacial abnormalities such as Treacher-Collins syndrome.

Segmental surgery is rarely required and indeed is a reflection of poor liaison between orthodontist and surgeon. Such surgery is often associated with poor outcome both in terms of the final facial appearance and iatrogenic periodontal problems or dental damage.

Intermaxillary fixation

Internal fixation can be used to avoid the need for intermaxillary fixation (IMF) in most cases, apart from those patients undergoing an intraoral vertical subsigmoid osteotomy when bone healing takes place without the support of internal fixation. Intermaxillary fixation is effected by means of the fixed orthodontic appliances for a period of up to 6 weeks. For other osteotomies IMF may be

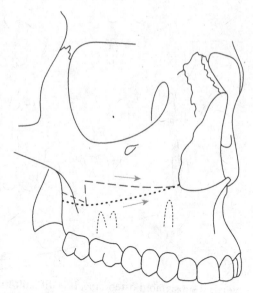

Figure 18.9   Le Fort I osteotomy. Once mobilised the maxilla can be moved anteriorly, upwards and downwards. Reproduced by kind permission of VU Press, Amsterdam.

applied with elastics in the first few postoperative days to guide the patient into their new occlusion.

Asymmetric facial deformity

Complete symmetry rarely (if ever) exists in nature and therefore asymmetric facial deformity may exist in a mild form in most individuals and may involve simply a lack of coincidence between the facial and dental midlines. Some individuals have a problem of sufficient magnitude to place them outside the range of normal variation, and often have an underlying pathology.

Individuals with asymmetric facial deformity often require special investigations to aid both diagnosis and eventual treatment planning, such as 3D imaging and the use of 3D models. If condylar hyperplasia is suspected then technetium isotope scans may be used to define if the condylar growth centre is still active prior to embarking on surgical correction.

Hemifacial microsomia

Hemifacial microsomia is a condition in which derivatives of the first branchial arch are incomplete or deficient. The ear is usually affected, together with shortening of the mandibular ramus and varying degrees of abnormality of the temporomandibular joint. Surgical correction is complex and involves collabo-

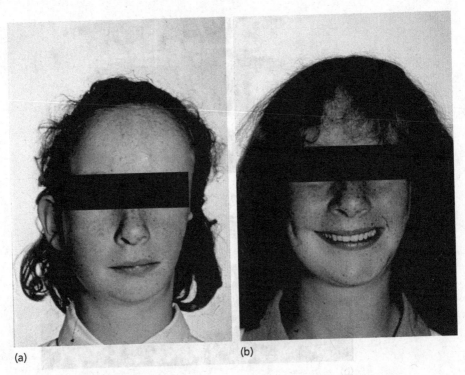

(a)   (b)

Figure 18.10   Hemifacial microsomia.

ration between the maxillofacial surgeon, orthodontist and facial prosthetist. Surgery will involve levelling of the occlusal cant due to the ramus shortening, and reconstructive surgery to restore facial symmetry (Figure 18.10).

Condylar hyperplasia

Condylar hyperplasia arises either when the condylar growth centre is reactivated after cessation of normal growth or when unequal activity during normal growth produces mandibular asymmetry. Correction may involve osteotomies of both the maxilla and mandible to correct occlusal cants and may also require presurgical orthodontics (Figure 18.11).

Distraction osteogenesis

See also Chapter 11.

Jaw width can be gained by applying forces with screw-based appliances between osteotomies in both jaws. Commonly this is applied in the midline of either jaw. Cuts are made in the bone in the midline to facilitate the process, which is controlled by the patient. Gradual opening of the screw over a period of weeks gives small increments of movement. The gains in jaw width and length coupled with orthodontics can avoid more major surgery.

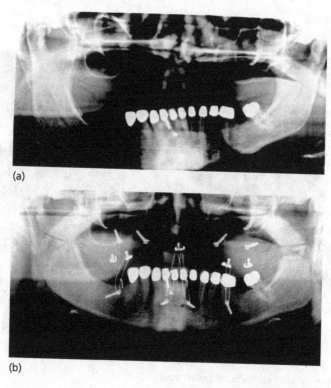

(a)

(b)

Figure 18.11   Condylar hyperplasia. (a) The occlusal cant can be clearly seen. The mandibular midline has shifted to the left; (b) a unilateral mandibular osteotomy has been performed on the right. The patient was edentulous in the upper jaw.

Further reading

Harris M, Hunt N (eds) (2008) *Fundamentals of Orthognathic Surgery*, 2nd edn. Imperial College Press, London.

Tuinzing DB, Greebe RB, Dorenbos J, van der Kwast WAM (1993) *Surgical Orthodontics – Diagnosis and Treatment*. VU University Press, Amsterdam.

Index

Principles of Oral and Maxillofacial Surgery, 6th Edition. Edited by U. J. Moore
© 2011 Blackwell Publishing Ltd

Printed in the United States
By Bookmasters